THE DRUGS
THAT CHANGED
OUR MINDS

THE DRUGS THAT CHANGED OUR MINDS

The History of Psychiatry in Ten Treatments

LAUREN SLATER

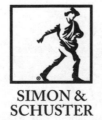

**SIMON &
SCHUSTER**

London · New York · Sydney · Toronto · New Delhi

A CBS COMPANY

First published in the United States by Little, Brown and Company, 2018
First published in Great Britain by Simon & Schuster UK Ltd, 2018
A CBS COMPANY

1 3 5 7 9 10 8 6 4 2

Simon & Schuster UK Ltd
1st Floor
222 Gray's Inn Road
London WC1X 8HB

www.simonandschuster.co.uk
www.simonandschuster.com.au
www.simonandschuster.co.in

Simon & Schuster Australia, Sydney
Simon & Schuster India, New Delhi

A CIP catalogue record for this book
is available from the British Library

Hardback ISBN: 978-1-4711-3688-7
Trade Paperback ISBN: 978-1-4711-3689-4
eBook ISBN: 978-1-4711-3691-7

Typeset in the UK by M Rules
Printed and bound by CPI Group (UK) Ltd, Croydon, CR0 4YY

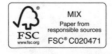

MIX
Paper from
responsible sources
FSC® C020471

Simon & Schuster UK Ltd are committed to sourcing paper
that is made from wood grown in sustainable forests and support
the Forest Stewardship Council, the leading international forest
certification organisation. Our books displaying the
FSC logo are printed on FSC certified paper.

For Lucas Henry Alexander
One and Only

Contents

Author's Note

Everything in this book is true. However, there are certain instances in which I have changed the names and identifying features of people I interviewed, at their request and to protect their privacy. There are other instances, however, in which names have not been changed. I allowed each subject to make that decision according to his or her comfort.

All autobiographical material emerged from my memory of events that sometimes happened as many as forty years ago or more. I composed my memories as they occurred to me and checked their accuracy by relying on family members who were with me at the time, when this was possible. I have made every effort to be accurate while also acknowledging that memories are friable, delicate webs held together by neuronal connections and chemicals we do not yet fully understand.

Introduction

I wrote this book because I have been taking psychotropic drugs for thirty-five years, with different drugs or drug combinations during different decades of my life. Some of these drugs have been miraculously effective for a time, while others have done nothing but leave me with side effects – increased sweating, a rapid heartbeat, a mouth so dry my teeth began to rot in their sockets. Of every doctor who has ever prescribed me a psychotropic drug I have asked the same questions: how does it work? And, more existentially, how do you know I need it?

What did I mean by that second question? I meant that while I had symptoms galore, I had no physical proof that anything was wrong with me at all. Several times during my adult years, for instance, I've wound up in the A&E department for a bad case of strep throat, and each time the doctor has instructed me to open my mouth and stick out my tongue while he peered into me with a torch and swirled a cotton bud around in the redness, after which he smeared my cells on a slide that would be tested to confirm the diagnosis and I would be prescribed the trusty cure, an antibiotic. Similarly, I keenly remember the morning of 26 September 1998, waking at dawn and popping my ovulation thermometer into my mouth, beep, beep, my temperature still high, a sign I might be pregnant. The night before, in the bathroom, I had lined up the kits, not one but three, all with their little wells and the plastic cup to collect my urine. I got out of bed carefully, so as not to wake my husband. The bathroom was dark, the sun just hitting the horizon and extending a single ray into the sky. I peed into the collection cup and then, using the dropper, deposited my urine into the wells and watched, transfixed, as the test wands changed colour, going from white to blue to red. A single line emerged, and then – was it? did I see it? – a second line began to form, faint but definite. The tests were telling me the most important piece of news I'd received so far in my life: I was gravid, with child, on the edge of my motherhood, a knowledge that filled me with fear and ecstasy. Because I'm compulsive by nature, I took a test every day for a week, watching the second line, the yes line, grow bolder and bolder, a sign that my HCG, a hormone secreted in early pregnancy, was rising.

There are no such dependable tests for determining depression. The truth is that while we have dozens and dozens of psychiatric drugs, while antidepressant use in England has doubled in just a decade, we still have no actual blood or urine or tissue test with which to determine the particular psychiatric illness a person suffers from. The body or brain of someone suffering from severe depression may very well be deeply different from the body or brain of someone who has what we call a normal mood, but if physical substrates of mental suffering do exist, psychiatry has so far been unsuccessful in definitively finding them. Therefore, when you take a psychiatric drug, you do so on faith. It is a great leap of faith, in fact, to take a drug when the doctor cannot actually find anything wrong with your body. Yes, you may be sleeping more or less than usual. Yes, you may be eating more or less. But these symptoms do not give rise to any particular chemical malfunction in your urine, your blood or your skin.

All I know for sure is that in my case, when I took my first psychiatric drug – imipramine for depression – at nineteen years of age, my body seemed to be healthy, even if my heart hurt. Now, thirty-five years and twelve drugs later, my kidneys are failing, I have diabetes, I am overweight and my memory is perforated. As the years close in on me, my lifetime now seems seriously foreshortened, not because of a psychiatric illness but because of the drugs I have taken to treat it – with diabetes and kidney trouble being just a couple of the well-documented side effects associated with the powerful antidepressant and antipsychotic olanzapine, a drug I've relied on like some do a walking frame, propping me up so I can sail through my days, going as fast as I can in the hope I will get everything done before I die. It would not be an overstatement to say that on the one hand, psychiatric drugs have healed me, while on the other, they have taken my life and my health and ruined me, drawing death near. Because of the diabetes, I get sores on my feet, festering sores that ulcerate and ooze. At fifty-four years old, my body is in the shape of an octogenarian with issues.

But I am not angry at psychiatry for limiting my life in the way it has, even as my decaying body scares me to my roots. Although the first psychotropic I took did me no good, the second one felt as if it had hurled me to heaven, where I lived a gilded life, rich and buttery, producing books and babies as fast as I could, because I knew the fluoxetine would wear off, and eventually it did. The next drug, the antidepressant venlafaxine, also eventually stopped working, and thus I became a consumer of polypsychopharmacy, sustained on a potentially lethal cocktail of drugs. My particular mix includes the risky olanzapine, another antipsychotic called aripiprazole, venlafaxine, the anti-anxiety medication clonaze-pam, the stimulant lisdexamfetamine, and probably one or two other tablets I'm forgetting because there are so many. Because of these drugs, I am able to think, to compose and to move pro-ductively through my life, although I do struggle with aphasia. What's a little memory loss, though, in exchange for a robust ability to cope?

My marriage of two decades recently dissolved, and yet I get up each day and find joy in being alive. That's what I call a robust ability to cope. That's what I call proof that these drugs work, maybe too well. Shouldn't I be shedding tears? I do, of course, but what I don't do is get sucked into the quicksand of despair. I feed my chickens. I ride my ponies. I make my gardens, which are right now blooming in the spring's first warmth, the salvia growing out of the ground in purple spires, the lupin sending up its coloured cones, the false indigo blooming its excess of blues.

Thanks to psychiatry's drugs, I have a mind that can appreciate the beauty around me, but then, thanks to psychiatry's drugs, I am dying faster than you are, my body crumbling as side effect after side effect sets in, messing up my metabolism, wreaking havoc with my glucose, polluting my urine. Thus in my world I live according to Descartes's central principle: my mind on the right, here and healthy, my body on the left, here and weak. Indeed his essential point, that there *is* a division between body and mind, proves to be terribly true in my case.

I wrote this book in part so I could examine some of the drugs I take, and others I never have. I wrote it in part hoping I would find, in my research, that there really are physical substrates to mental suffering. If psychiatrists could find them, it stood to reason there was a chance that drugs could be systematically made to correct the problem at its source, whereas now our psychiatric drugs are made too often in the dark, as serendipitous mistakes, with researchers trying a little of this and a little of that. The end result is that all of our drugs are in some sense dirty, casting their effects over the entire ball of the brain so that nothing is spared and the imbiber is left with the dreaded side effects. At the very least, finding the physical substrates to mental suffering would mean that one could be sure of a bona fide disease with a clear aetiology and course.

I wrote this book hoping I would encounter ample research on the long-term side effects of, say, the SSRIs, the selective serotonin reuptake inhibitors, which have been around for thirty years now, long enough for some good longitudinal studies to have been done. But I found very little. When it comes to examining these blockbuster tablets over the long haul, I met instead with an eerie silence, and almost no science at all. When it comes to studying side effects, virtually all we have are the original studies that Eli Lilly did to get Prozac (fluoxetine) approved in the first place, along with similar short-term studies by others in the years since, despite the fact that many patients, like me, have been sustained on a serotonin booster for decades. Why are so few really looking at the long-term effects? What is it we're afraid we'll find? I have grappled with this question and have tried to proffer some answers in this book.

I confess that I came to this book with a bias. I came as both a patient and a practitioner (I have a doctorate in psychology), and thus was hardly a blank slate when I began my research. My own experience has coloured what I chose to focus on and therefore what I've found. Luckily for me, however, my bias was not so severe as to blind me to some very sweet surprises. My assumption, when I started this book, was that drug discovery in psychiatry was dead, that through the ascension of 'Big Pharma' it had been reduced to a series of 'me too' concoctions geared towards profiting from variations on already approved medications, with nothing original in the pipeline. What I discovered, however, was a group of researchers remaking the field by reviving psychedelics and employing them in novel ways for those suffering from psychic pain. This is the far frontier of psychiatry right now, and I believe it promises rich rewards. A handful of practitioners are reaching back into the past and, in doing so, changing the future of a field that is desperate for innovation. While some psychedelics are old, even ancient drugs, they are in every instance being used in ways that are refreshingly unique and that offer relief to significant subsets of patients, many of whom would otherwise be out of options. MDMA, commonly known as ecstasy, shows potential in the treatment of social anxiety in autistic patients and for those suffering from post-traumatic stress disorder; psilocybin (the active agent in so-called magic mushrooms) can ease the anxiety that attends an end-stage cancer diagnosis and thereby remake the way we die.

The drugs I chose to write about in this book picked me more than I picked them. I was at no point aiming for something comprehensive but rather something riveting. I followed a linear timeline to some extent, but there is also a thematic thread that runs through these pages: these drugs tell the story of psychiatry's trajectory over the centuries, like lenses held up to the field of study. Through them we can see what there is to see, and observe a biology-based profession fall prey to psychoanalysis and then seize science again in a move that made the profession at once narrower and wider. Yes, biology is crucial to psychiatric medicine. After all, a single cell contains a whirling world. But the biology-based psychiatry of our day and age misses the need we all have to make myth out of the fabric and cuttings of our lives. Patients rarely seek psychoanalysis any more, in large part because talking therapies such as cognitive behavioural therapy (CBT) are preferred. This has made the field smaller than it once was, when Freudians and other theorists ruled the roost. I am not arguing for psychiatry to be led once more by the psychoanalysts, but the questions remain: where do patients go to be heard in a profession increasingly adopting the language and structure of science? Where do they go to sculpt, to create and revise the plot of their tangled lives?

I wrote this book because I love stories, especially ones that have not been fully told. While it was easy to get the details of how the earliest antipsychotics were discovered, for instance, I'd yet to read a really good account of the magic dye methylene blue and all it led to – the blue dreams it cast. As with each of my books, my goals were strictly narrative. I wanted to bring the seminal drugs of this century and the previous century forward as stories that could be told and retold, read and reread. The science is accurate, but in every instance I have endeavoured to embed it in the time-honoured tradition of telling tales, with a beginning, a middle and an end, with heroes and losers and plenty in between, struggling to make their way.

In a very real sense, my body holds a lot of the stories I've told here. It holds the history of psychopharmacology, with all the drugs I've taken having left their grooves in my flesh and in my brain, wherever they have worked or failed to work. Thus I wrote this book, in some inchoate sense, to discover my own body – its beginning, middle and end.

1

Chlorpromazine

Awake!

Breaking In

It is easy. I climb a crumbling low stone wall and push my hand through brambles to find an open window covered with torn strips of a metal screen, the trim rotten, the blistered white paint falling in jagged flakes as I part the remnants of the screen and, balancing carefully, thrust one leg through the old aperture. This very window was once barred, but now, lifetimes later, it yields with barely a nudge. It is as if this old building – heavy with history, loaded down with dreams and screams and maniacal memories – wants me to know all the horror it holds. As if it yields to me because I come as some sort of witness to days long gone, to a time when we treated the mentally ill in ways we might call mentally ill, plunging them into ice-cold baths, or nosing needles under their sunken skin to dose them with so much insulin that they hurtled into fathomless comas, lying on cots or in iron beds, their minds frozen until light finally made its way in and the patients re-emerged. If insulin didn't cure patients of their monsters and bi-headed beasts, we sometimes severed the fibres of their burning brains, leaving them docile as dolls.

Inside, this old asylum is mostly dark. Outside, it is a beautiful summer evening redolent of roses that grow along the low stone wall and pour across the upper fields overtaken with white-headed weeds and pink clover. Years and years ago, these same fields were closely mowed, as if by controlling the scalps of grass the staff could somehow also leash the brains of the madmen and women this institution contained. The grounds were quite lovely back then. The buzz-cut green and the exuberant roses and the stone walls lent a bucolic look that stood in stark contrast to the insides of the actual hospital building, where I stand in the late dusk of a June day, the sky outside the colour of periwinkle. The outside smells of damp summer, the inside of mothballs and something stale but impossible to name.

By crawling through the window I have officially trespassed on state property, and yet I feel I must see these haunted halls. As my eyes adjust to the dimness of this dead place I can make out doors, dozens of them lining a corridor littered with medicine trolleys. The impression is of a place humming and hurried one moment and abandoned the next, as if an announcement came down from above to jump ship and people left everything in mid-motion, the trolleys haphazardly strewn about, the prescriptions now faded and lying curled on the floor. I bend to right an overturned flask and then pick it up, holding it to the evening's last light, against which is visible a faint golden glow from the liquid it once contained. I set the flask aside, then make my way forward through the murk and bump into a stack of books, toppling it to release a flutter of wings and the shrieking of birds – tiny birds with yellow waistcoats who have built their nest amid the disintegrating tower of tomes.

Metal beds on wheels flank the long hall, with its aged linoleum floor warped and bulging, broken in spots. The walls, painted a seasick green, are shedding, and there are cupboards stacked with rolled-up towels, and rusty medicine cabinets. A while later, having ascended the stairs to the fourth-floor hall, I pass a canvas cot, and then, in a small room, a long bed over which are suspended the wires and suckers that were attached to shaved skulls for electro-convulsive treatment, current fed through the cranium that for some reason seemed to have some positive effect.

Crammed into a corner on the highest floor, the fifth, is a tiny square of space with a single caged bulb screwed into the buckling ceiling, the damp dirt floor beneath it clawed by who knows how many hands. This could well have been the 'quiet room', where patients were sent when their behaviour could no longer be con-trolled. Down below me, and beyond the fields that surround the structure, the city streets thrum. Through one of the dirt-speckled windows I can just make out a pair of women pushing pushchairs. A man walks by with a baguette tucked under his arm as vendors hawk their wares beneath bright umbrellas striped and swirled and spotted – a picture of perfection that serves only to deepen the gloom of this building soon to be razed, sent tumbling into a heap of broken brick by the crane's wrecking ball.

Founded in 1833, this state hospital was once a bustling insti-tution, forty miles west of Boston. In the 1920s, '30s and '40s, this hospital, like a host of other mental hospitals (called then insane asylums) scattered around the US and abroad, was a place to send the crazed and 'idiotic', a place equipped with what today seem like terribly primitive tools to handle the screaming, sweaty bodies of men and women hounded by hallucinations in an era long before managed care and medication. A hundred years ago, even eighty years ago, very few people were confident that chemicals could mend the mind, which as recently as the nineteenth century was believed to dwell not in the brain but somewhere in a spirit or soul immune to chemical intervention. Those afflicted with serious mental illnesses – schizophrenia, bipolar disorder, severe depres-sion and autism – often lived out their lives between the walls of hospitals just like this one, undergoing questionable cures that, while never intended to harm, rarely worked.

In 1991, more than 150 years after it first opened, this hospital at last closed its doors, meeting the same fate that had already befallen many other such mental hospitals in the decades following the deinstitutionalisation movement that gathered momentum in the 1960s, when US President Kennedy, whose sister Rosemary had been the victim of an early and failed prefrontal lobotomy, provided funding for community mental health centres, a move that was further encouraged by the passage of President Johnson's Medicaid and Medicare bills. In 1955, at their peak, American mental hospitals held 560,000 patients nationwide, double the number at the turn of the twentieth century. By 1988, three decades later, that figure had fallen to 120,000.

One of the phenomena that truly made this sea change viable – allowing patients to be treated in the least restrictive setting possible, whether that was in a community health centre or at home with their families – was the discovery, in the early 1950s, of a blockbuster drug called chlorpromazine. When branded and marketed as Thorazine in the United States and Largactil in Europe, this new drug stabilised untold thousands of schizophrenic, psychotic and otherwise mentally ill patients and eventually brought about a sustained exodus from mental hospitals in the United States and abroad.

Great and Desperate Cures

One way of grasping the meaning of chlorpromazine is to know the types of treatments that preceded it, treatments which the former University of Michigan psychologist Elliot Valenstein has called 'great and desperate cures'. There was, for instance, insulin coma therapy, first used by Austrian psychiatrist Manfred Sakel in 1927, in an attempt to treat opiate addicts in withdrawal with small doses of insulin. Some of these patients, however, slipped into hypoglycaemic comas, and when they awoke, following an emergency administration of glucose, their personalities seemed altered. Addicts who had been defensive, angry, difficult were now 'tranquil and more responsive'. This led Sakel to wonder whether deliberately inducing comas in schizophrenic patients might produce a similar recovery. He set about trying this and claimed miraculous results after inducing comas, sometimes as many as sixty times in a two-month period, in his schizophrenic patients. Perhaps unsurprisingly, patients emerging from these comas did appear more docile, but the treatment carried severe risk – including death and irreversible coma.

Convulsive therapies were also popular during the first half of the last century. Before electroconvulsive treatment (ECT) was developed, convulsions were brought on by injecting patients with drugs. Ladislas Meduna, a psychiatrist working in Budapest, noted that epileptics who also had schizophrenia appeared to have fewer seizures and that, conversely, schizophrenics who suffered from epilepsy would often have spontaneous remissions of their psychoses after a seizure. Meduna chose first camphor and then pentylenetetrazol, a white crystalline drug employed as a respiratory or circulatory stimulant, to induce seizures in schizophrenic patients. Afterwards, his first test subjects rose from their beds and asked, in perfectly lucid ways, when they could go home. 'I felt elated and I knew I had discovered a new treatment,' Meduna said. 'I felt happy beyond words.'

What was the operating theory behind pentylenetetrazol therapy? Some claimed that it gave the mentally ill a near-death experience that set them straight once the seizures were over. Instead of scaring schizophrenics to death, the thinking went, it scared them back to life. Patients coming out of pentylenetetrazol shock often called for their mothers, or begged the nurses to hold them, childlike behaviour which their doctors considered proof that the seizure had altered their personalities for the better. No longer raucous or caught up in the clutch of hallucinations, pentylenetetrazol patients were frequently friendly and cooperative, and this led doctors to believe that with enough treatments, the positive behaviour would become habitual.

Pentylenetetrazol therapy, however, had a host of thorny problems. When asylum doctors beyond Meduna tried it on their patients, the seizures the drug caused were horrific. The treatments filled their patients with dread, and they begged to be spared the injections, which caused their whole bodies to writhe and spasm in convulsions of such ferocity that they frequently suffered fractures: dislocated shoulders, broken femurs, clavicles, scapulae. One patient compared it to being 'roasted alive in a white-hot furnace'. And yet it was not uncommon for patients to have as many as forty pentylenetetrazol injections.

Other treatments, some of which caused patients degrees of discomfort we can only imagine, since seemingly they left behind no record of their experiences, involved the injection of animal blood and castor oil and massive doses of caffeine. For quite some time, sleep therapy became a popular intervention in the treatment of schizophrenia – a kinder although no less dangerous undertaking. Patients were fed a cocktail of tranquillising tonics and drugs meant to send them into slumbers that, in some cases, lasted as long as two or three weeks. The rationale: in states of deep rest the nervous system might find its precarious balance again. It's true that some schizophrenics were actually helped by sleep therapy, but there were a number of fatalities as well. Patients' lungs filled with fluid, pneumonias developed or vomit was aspirated – all in a time before penicillin.

In 1938, Italian psychiatrist Lucio Bini discovered that he could cause convulsions in mental patients using electricity instead of drugs. Bini tried his new therapy on catatonic patients, some of whom were helped by this charge to their systems, as they emerged from their catatonia and began conversing with those around them. Others, however, as they lay on the table, seized to no effect at all, the voltage so high they flopped like fish, again and again, as the body was charged and changed, in a mode of treatment that seems barbaric to the modern mentality. (Electroconvulsive therapy, which actually can be extremely effective in severe depression that has failed to respond to antidepressant medications, is still used today, the theory being that the electrical current 'resets' the brain. But the voltage is much lower, the treatment is typically used on only one hemisphere and patients are given muscle relaxants so they do not have violent seizures.) Other hospital-based therapies of the time included ice wraps, freezing baths or just plain old restraints, with the patient simply tied to a chair while his dreams and demons wafted.

Were the lengths to which these psychiatrists went to calm the mad mind heroic, or simply cruel? Canadian doctor Heinz Lehmann, for instance, noting that the psyches of his schizophrenic patients seemed much clearer when they were felled by high fevers, sought out ways of inducing in his patients the most extreme temperatures he could, going so far as to inject turpentine into the abdominal wall of one female patient in the hope that the infected abscess formed in the wake of such a procedure would cause a fever high enough to quell her hallucinations. Some have criticised Lehmann for what they consider cruelty, but it's more likely that this doctor, who would later become one of the first North American prescribers of chlorpromazine, had the best of intentions, so driven was he to find ways of suppressing psychosis.

The zenith – or, depending upon your outlook, the nadir – of these fervent efforts to cure, or at least subjugate, the mentally ill was the 1936 development, by Portuguese doctor Egas Moniz, of psychosurgery. At its best, psychosurgery was a vanguard technique that – though we are now loath to admit it – healed some patients, allowing many to be released back into the community. For instance, there is the case of the doctor, decimated by depression, who, after psychosurgery, re-established a medical surgery with nine other colleagues – and became a pilot to boot. There is also the case of a former virtuoso violinist, unable to play anything but her jangling, screeching nerves once her schizophrenia set in, so much so that she set the instrument aside for a dozen years. She too submitted to the destruction of her frontal lobes and found, afterwards, that she could make music again, such that music was still her livelihood almost twenty years later. At its worst, however, psychosurgery was an ice pick thrust carelessly through the orbit of the eye. Indeed, the very first transorbital lobotomy in the United States was performed by the notorious Walter Freeman on a housewife in Washington DC, using an ice pick from his own kitchen drawer.

What this string of experimental treatments reveals is that while we tend to think of the last century and the centuries before it as eras when there were few or no viable biological therapies available to mental patients, this is at best half true. Yes, there was a period when psychoanalysis and its psychodynamic offshoots did grip the American imagination, assuming pre-eminence over medication in the 1950s, '60s and even the '70s, but both in the United States and in Europe we have never been without biological treatments for those suffering from mental disease or distress. Equally significant, some of these biological treatments were actually effective, even if only briefly and for uncertain reasons. For the deeply disturbed there was insulin, camphor, electricity, enemas, ice and ice picks, and for the walking wounded, from antiquity on, there were all manner of tonics and brews, this in a period when whatever medication was available was easy to procure, before pharmacies controlled the flow of chemicals.

In the early twentieth century, for instance, opiates were widely used for all sorts of ills, even sold in syrup to calm colicky babies. Lithium baths prospered – vats of cool bubbling water said to soothe the troubled soul. Extract of conium, either on its own or coupled with iron, quinine or Fowler's solution, was used to treat depression, as was the plant extract nux vomica. Hyoscyamus, from the passion flower, was used to diminish sleeplessness or extreme excitement. There were tinctures of veratrine and belladonna and stimulants such as ammonia, lytta and all kinds of aromatics in small amber bottles you held just below the nostrils, sniffing in comforting draughts of lavender, rosemary or cinnamon. So prevalent were and are attempts at biological cures, and so available for such a great span of time, that non-physical therapies such as psychoanalysis and other 'talking cures' are in fact the real oddity, a brief blip in what has otherwise been a mostly somatic approach to the treatment of human suffering in all its manifestations.

But despite the steady and ongoing reliance on brews, tonics, leechings, electrical current, ice baths and lithium waters, on aromatics and extracts made from the garden's crushed stamens and leaves, on convulsions and comas and high-flying fevers, prior to the development of chlorpromazine no one had ever really conceived of a drug to help *heal* serious mental illness. The tonics and brews of yesteryear were for the most part intended merely to manage the most severe symptoms. And while barbiturates were synthesised as early as 1903 and brought to market in 1904, and opium even earlier, these were used mostly as sedatives, to send patients into states of slumber so that doctors could attempt deep-sleep therapy. No one was trying to develop a tablet that might somehow steady the brain, because the notion of such a thing lay outside the imagination, seemingly beyond conception.

The mind, back then, was mythic. It was a vast and uncharted territory, an Antarctica, unreachable, unfathomable, arising not from neurotransmission and chemical signalling but from, it was believed, electrical impulses impossible to decode, or, still more abstract, from one's singular and God-given spirit. Very little was known about neurotransmitters, the chemical messengers that convey nerve impulses across a synapse, because while the neuro-transmitter acetylcholine had been discovered in 1921, it was the only one researchers knew of, and it would be decades before they began to understand how or why it worked. Serotonin, noradren-aline, endorphins and complex chemical cascades – these all lay far in the future, yet to be uncovered in laboratory experiments.

Thus while the emphasis on biological cures was not at all new, before chlorpromazine and then a second antipsychotic, reser-pine, these biological treatments were largely contradictory, even paradoxical, given that measurable materials were being used to treat what many saw as the immeasurable soul. Had anyone in the nineteenth or even the early twentieth century suggested that schizophrenia arose from an 'imbalance' of chemicals in the brain, that person would have been seen as speaking nonsense, because schizophrenia arose, in the popular imagination, from the twisted soul and, in the medical imagination, from either a fixed and ill-fated inheritance, meaning a bad bloodline passed from person to person, or from humours – blood, bile, phlegm – gone wildly out of whack. When we finally did discover antipsychotics in the 1950s, we discovered much more than drugs. We discovered, along with capsules containing crushed and potent powders, the 1.3-kilogram (3-lb) mass of matter between our ears which, we now believe, serves as the seat of our humanity. For many people, this was a brand-new belief.

Brilliant Colours

Chlorpromazine was a long time coming. In fact it took almost a century to finally become what it was, a chemical called chlorpromazine hydrochloride made by chlorinating the antihistamine promazine in a laboratory at Rhône-Poulenc, a French pharmaceutical company which, from the 1930s to the 1950s, specialised in antihistamines. But although Rhône-Poulenc and the pharmacists working under its roof can be credited with creating, in 1950, the drug that came to be known as chlorpromazine (sold as Thorazine in the United States), its existence really began in the mid-nineteenth century, when organic chemists discovered that by distilling coal tars they could make brilliant colours, which they sold as dyes.

One of these dyes, named methylene blue, turned out to contain medicinal properties (and, in fact, is still today included on the World Health Organization's list of essential medicines, being used as an affordable antimalarial drug and also showing promise for the treatment of Alzheimer's). In 1886, in the process of researching a cure for malaria, against which the dye did prove to be effective, German scientist and eventual Nobel laureate Paul Ehrlich discovered that this strange and potent blue liquid would selectively stain the nerve cells of the frogs he dissected, and thus seemed to have an affinity for nerves, the motorways and byways of everything we feel and are. Ehrlich, observing how the blue dye sank into and saturated only the frogs' nerve cells, leaving the rest of the dissected animal untouched, thought to treat neuralgia with methylene blue; it didn't work, but more than a decade later, in 1899, an Italian doctor named Pietro Bodoni, aware of Ehrlich's research, used it to treat manic excitation in psychotic patients with good, even grand success, calming their fevered fears and rat-a-tat agitations. This makes sense in hindsight, because of all the dyes discovered in the heyday of organic chemistry, it was methylene blue that would eventually be transformed – distilled and finally synthesised – into chlorpromazine fifty years after Bodoni first tried the dye on the deeply distressed of Genoa.

Despite the success methylene blue had in calming manic excitation in psychotic patients, the dye never quite had a chance to come into widespread use, thanks to the introduction of barbiturates, in 1904, just five years after Bodoni's initial treatments in Genoa. Barbiturates were faster acting and cast a wider net, their highly sedative effects able to calm virtually any kind of patient with any kind of mental illness diagnosis, and to do so more effectively than methylene blue, which was not a sedative. Methylene blue, in addition, could not be used in deep-sleep therapy, while the barbiturates could.

It is common, or even fashionable, for people to think that prior to chlorpromazine and the drugs that followed, psychiatrists were operating in the Dark Ages, using these 'great and desperate cures' in ways often painted as almost, if not outright, barbaric. The real story, however, is much more nuanced. Without doubt the large asylums of the past could be gruesome places, but the doctors and their proffered treatments must be seen as separate from the settings in which they practised. In addition to the successes of psychosurgery, with patients such as the doctor-cum-pilot and the violinist, there are similar stories about patients who underwent insulin coma therapies, electroconvulsive therapies and sleep therapy, and achieved happy outcomes.

Our predecessors, then, were not practising in the Dark Ages any more than we are practising in an Enlightenment. There has always been consistent confusion, a range of questionable cures, and then the occasional goal. This is the case today as much as it was back then. Methylene blue was a kind of goal that disappeared from psychiatric use not because it was ineffective or barbaric but because, according to British psychopharmacologist David Healy, 'patents had been obtained on newer agents and no drug company would market an old drug even if it worked.' In the case of methylene blue, then, 'there were competing therapies or interest groups likely to make more money out of other therapies than they would from methylene blue.' In the 1970s, methylene blue re-emerged as a means of treating manic depression, for which it was highly effective, but ultimately corporate profit-seeking interests rather than therapeutic outcomes won the day.

What matters here is how we view the past. We tend to construct the story of psychiatry as a tale of ever-upwards progress – cure upon cure, each one better than before – with a triumphant emergence from the Dark Ages once chlorpromazine was synthesised. This, however, is not actually true, as is so aptly demonstrated by methylene blue, a perfectly good psychiatric drug developed a half century before chlorpromazine but relegated, temporarily, to the rubbish bin of time because of a shift in allegiance to the barbiturates, which were celebrated in their day but which in fact can be highly addictive. A close examination of the past reveals reasonable, and in some cases excellent, treatments, while a close examination of the present reveals the same. Progress has been made, but many treatments of today are no more effective than those of prior centuries. In actuality, there were no Dark Ages, nor was there a sudden coming into the light. Rather there has been a steady search for cures that has gained ground as technology has improved. But even with this technology, psychopharmacologists, if they are honest, will admit that they are still operating largely in shadow, unable to see the aetiology of the illnesses they are trying to treat, operating on hypotheses that are, in many cases, no more sound than those which existed before our time.

Where methylene blue is concerned, thankfully the dye never went away completely. The phenothiazine nucleus, a three-ring molecule that sits at the centre of what was then a newly discovered blue dye, became the platform from which new drugs were developed well into the twentieth century, especially in France. That nucleus, it turned out, had antihistaminic effects, an area of focus for the drug company Rhône-Poulenc. It produced drowsiness and eradicated seasonal allergies, the drippy nose and weepy eyes irritated by pollen-packed air in the spring and summer. Rhône-Poulenc used the phenothiazine nucleus to create drugs we still take today, like Benadryl, as well as drugs that have fallen out of favour, like promethazine, a powerful antihistamine synthesised in 1947 and the direct precursor to chlorpromazine.

Henri Laborit

The French military doctor Henri Laborit, soon to be chlorpromazine's earliest champion, was born in Hanoi, in 1914, and first served as a medic in Indochina. He was unusual in all sorts of ways. Laborit was passionate about science, but he was also deeply interdisciplinary, producing in his lifetime not only reams of scientific articles but also novels and plays and poems. He preferred his private research to federally funded projects, desiring the freedom to pursue the questions that most captivated him. A loner by nature, he cast his professional allegiance with no particular person or place and was thus uniquely positioned, as a free-spirited individual open to experimentation, to recognise the potential of chlorpromazine, a drug that, he believed, could be useful to a variety of medical disciplines.

During the Second World War, Laborit had served aboard the destroyer *Sirocco*, which was torpedoed by German S-boats in the battle of Dunkirk, suffering several explosions and promptly beginning to sink, tilting first with one side submerged before finally going under the choppy frozen sea, where several hundred sailors lost their lives. Laborit spoke little of this incident during his lifetime, little of the fact that the ship had taken him with it before he resurfaced and began to swim from the doomed vessel, spending hours in an icy ocean, his chin thrust just above the frosty froth, before he reached shore. Years later, during his tenure at the Val-de-Grâce military hospital in Paris, Laborit began to study what he termed 'artificial hibernation', inducing in his surgical patients a kind of hypothermia in the hopes of slowing the body's response to the insult of the incision, the flood of histamines, the heaving of the heart. He would pack his patients in ice and cool their bodies, so that all the physical reactions to surgery went into a kind of suspended animation while he sawed and sutured. One wonders if Laborit's hypothermic experience in the ocean inspired in him this idea to encase his patients in ice and bring their body temperatures so low that every system slowed to a creep, thereby stemming the stress response to his scalpel.

But before he ever tried artificial hibernation on patients, Laborit had been especially fond of the antihistamine promethazine during his surgery days in Tunisia, where he was stationed immediately after the war, at the naval hospital in Sidi Abdallah. The area was heavily mined with leftover explosives from the war, and many young soldiers suffered casualties in their efforts to clear them, often arriving at the hospital in a state of shock. Laborit operated on patients with missing limbs or with their chests blown open, the human heart visible, that vermilion pump. In these surgeries he began using promethazine, because he had observed that it instilled in his patients a 'euphoric quietude' – a unique kind of calm, or even indifference, that allowed him to slide his scalpel into skin and limbs with no cries of protest or pain. The antihistamine served as a 'potentiator' that permitted Laborit to use smaller doses of other dream-making drugs, like morphine and barbiturates, both of which, when given in large amounts, compromised the body's metabolic systems even as they were decreasing pain. He was so taken with promethazine as an anaesthetic potentiator that, after arriving at Val-de-Grâce in 1951, he asked his colleagues to come watch him operate on some of his 'tense and anxious Mediterranean types', all of whom succumbed to promethazine's blow, lying glassy-eyed and listless as Laborit carved and cut.

It is hard for the modern mind to grasp the hurdles our predecessors faced not even a hundred years ago. These days, a large percentage of surgeries are done laparoscopically, with minimal anaesthetic and with the patient sitting up and sliding off the table on to two stable feet once the procedure is complete. While every surgical patient still signs a consent form which says, in small print, that you might well expire from the endeavour, outpatient surgery today is almost as safe as driving your car to the corner shop. But in the 1930s, '40s and '50s, when Laborit was practising and morphine and barbiturates were the drugs of choice, many patients died not from their illnesses but from the stress, or shock, of surgery itself, a phenomenon called surgical shock, described by Philadelphia surgeon Virgil H. Moon in 1942:

> The patient is profoundly depressed. Metabolic functional activities are low. The skin is pale and moist with cold perspiration. The eyes are sunken, the features drawn and anxious in expression … The flesh has a lifeless doughy feel and the superficial veins are collapsed and bloodless. There is a constant thirst but efforts to relieve it are ineffectual because of constant vomiting. The respirations are shallow and are interspersed with deep

sighs. The pulse is rapid and weak ... The patient is restless ... and may become delirious. Death is preceded by stupor or coma.

It was this constellation of symptoms that so seized Laborit's mind, that worried him and urged him on to find innovative ways to avoid surgical shock and the resultant deaths. Artificial hibernation – packing his patients in ice – was one method, and using promethazine as a potentiator another. But while each of these helped sometimes, Laborit wanted something better, quicker, cleaner, something that would once and for all eradicate the deadly condition that V. H. Moon had so aptly described, the pale and doughy flesh, the stuporous coma and deep delirium that always preceded the end.

Discovery

Rhône-Poulenc knew of Laborit's use of their antihistamine pro-methazine and Laborit knew of Rhône-Poulenc's ongoing interest in developing novel antihistamines with effects on the central nervous system. The great pharmaceutical house was especially interested in Laborit's observation that promethazine, with or without cooling, seemed to dissociate the mind from pain. With that information in hand, the company set about trying to create a still more powerful antihistamine that would build on and exceed promethazine's strength, an antihistamine that would so stabilise the body and so limit the stress response to the scalpel that surgical shock would, once and for all, become a thing of the past.

Thus it was that chemist Paul Charpentier, in 1950, began to further explore promethazine and its phenothiazine nucleus. The company's main goal was to develop a drug capable of potentiat-ing other narcotics. Rhône-Poulenc had no intention of creating a psychiatric drug, not because they thought a psychiatric drug might fare poorly in the marketplace, but because, as previously mentioned, the very idea of a drug to treat madness was marginal at best. What Rhône-Poulenc wanted, and what Laborit wanted, was something *stronger* than promethazine, a drug that would sever the mind from feelings of pain while allowing the patient to retain some modicum of consciousness and the surgeon to avoid the dangers and shortcomings of morphine and barbiturates.

Charpentier, along with his colleague Simone Courvoisier, began to toy with methylene blue's phenothiazine nucleus during the autumn and winter of 1950. The two chemists chlorinated promazine, an antihistamine related to promethazine, thereby producing 'a completely different molecule', and creating, as a result, a more potent drug called chlorpromazine, a novel compound which in its US incarnation was eventually christened Thorazine, though it's known as chlorpromazine in the UK.

Charpentier and Courvoisier were familiar with Pavlov's work with dogs that had been conditioned to salivate when they heard the ringing of a bell. Pavlov's dogs had learned that when the bell rang, they would get food; in time all it took to moisten their mouths was the tinny sound of the clapper. Pavlov demonstrated, through these experiments, that animals, including humans, could be trained to form strong associations and that these associations were, in many instances, the fundamental building blocks of learning and memory. With this in mind, Courvoisier set out to test chlorpromazine on rats trained to climb a rope in order to escape an electrical shock that was administered along with the sound of a buzzer. The scientist electrified the floors of the rats' cages and hung a rope from the ceiling to the floor with a non-electrified platform, partway up, where the rats could rest in safety. Courvoisier then set about training the rats to climb the rope in order to escape the shock, something they all quickly learned to do.

Once her rodent subjects were trained, Courvoisier dosed them with the newly developed chlorpromazine, at that time simply called 4560RP (the RP standing for Rhône-Poulenc). The buzzers sounded. And something strange happened. Under the influence of 4560RP the rats did not climb the rope in order to flee the electrical surge. Instead they simply squatted in their cages, their tiny feet absorbing the jangling current, their eyes open and alert but oddly impassive. This new compound, unlike the antihistamines that had preceded it, was able to undo the associative learning that is the bedrock of classical conditioning. With a seemingly simple swipe, it was gone. Had the compound put the rats to sleep, their responses might have made more sense; the animals could have been so heavily sedated that they ceased to feel the surge of current in their bodies. But this was not the case. Every rat was awake, alert, but indifferent to the shocks and uninterested in the rope as a means of escape. This suggested to the chemists that 4560RP – descended from methylene blue – was more powerful than promethazine, so powerful it was able to alter deeply ingrained habits, responses, reactions and reflexes.

Throughout the winter of 1950, Courvoisier and Charpentier tested chlorpromazine on rats, rabbits and dogs. They discovered that the new drug could outperform promethazine in several areas. Its strong anti-emetic properties meant that it could eradicate nausea and the vomiting that often accompanied it. It was also anticholinergic, meaning it could suppress muscle spasms, while the drug's obvious hypnotic and sedative effects were an advance beyond promethazine, in that they caused still more indifference in the patient.

Of all the research Courvoisier and Charpentier did with chlorpromazine, Rhône-Poulenc was most interested in the drug's capacity to eradicate the conditioned reflex response. Although the lab rats' muscular strength and agility were clearly unimpaired, under the influence of chlorpromazine they showed no interest in climbing the rope to escape the shocks coming from the electric grid of their floor. This suggested to the pharmaceutical company that this new drug was more than a simple sedative, and that it was acting on the central nervous system in profound ways.

Accordingly, in the spring of 1951, Rhône-Poulenc distributed eighteen ampules of their novel compound for clinical testing, which meant something very different in those days from what it does in ours. Doctors 'tested' a new drug in one of two ways: either by taking it first themselves and recording in a notebook their own responses, or by handing it to a small sample of patients and observing the effects. Researchers had only recently begun to conduct randomised double-blind, placebo-controlled trials, which have become the gold standard of drug testing in our day. (A double-blind trial is one in which neither the patient nor the researcher knows who is taking the actual medication and who is taking the placebo, and is meant to guard against biases on each side.) Pierre Koetschet of Rhône-Poulenc admitted: 'We had no clear idea of what "chlorpromazine" would do in man. We had the strong impression that it was an interesting non-toxic product that would be useful.' Rhône-Poulenc released the drug with the idea that it would act as an anaesthetic potentiator, not as a psychiatric drug. According to David Healy, 'The idea of an antipsychotic was all but inconceivable at that time.'

Because Laborit and Rhône-Poulenc already had a close working relationship, and because of his enthusiasm for promethazine, Laborit was one of the first doctors to receive chlorpromazine. He received five samples and was quick to try them out on patients as part of what he called his 'lytic cocktail', an anaesthetic made up of different drugs that produced drowsiness and indifference. Now, with his five samples, Laborit substituted the new antihistamine, chlorpromazine, for promethazine. He also went so far as to recommend that chlorpromazine be included in soldiers' battlefield kits, as a kind of first aid that could be self-administered in case of injury, to help manage stress responses and the flood of histamines into the body. Adhering to this recommendation, the US military did include chlorpromazine in the medical kits of its soldiers during the Korean War. So marked was the apathy caused by chlorpromazine that the soldiers who took it lay languidly on the battlefield, indifferent to their wounds and unworried about their situation, in some cases foregoing opportunities for rescue, to the point where some may have died as a consequence. Chlorpromazine as a battlefield staple was quickly discontinued.

Clearly this new drug altered one's mental as well as physical state. Laborit's clinical notes reveal from early on his awareness that chlorpromazine might have psychiatric relevance. There was potential, he believed, for 'possible use of the product in psychiatry, its potentiating action permitting, among other things, a sleep treatment with barbiturates that has an improved margin of safety'.

Laborit went further than suggesting the use of chlorpromazine in psychiatry in his published papers. He also discussed it forcefully, if informally, over lunch in the canteen at Val-de-Grâce, urging his psychiatric colleagues to try this new compound, saying that if they did, they might not need to resort to the straitjacket, the ice pick and the isolation. His colleagues, however, with hypnotics and barbiturates already at their disposal, showed little interest in experimenting on their raving charges. Their indifference did not dissuade Laborit. There is no record that he ever administered chlorpromazine to himself, but his next subject, rather than a patient, was a 28-year-old psychiatrist friend named Cornelia Quarti, who agreed to test the drug on herself. At 11 am on 9 November 1951, at the Villejuif psychiatric hospital, and with Laborit and three of her associates watching, Quarti submitted to an intravenous injection of chlorpromazine, after which she lurched to the lavatory and returned nearly fainting.

Laborit, along with colleague Léon Chertok, propped up their now dosed subject in bed with pillows and watched her closely. Despite her descent, Quarti was still game and she communicated to Laborit all the subjective states she was experiencing under the influence of chlorpromazine. About a week later, on the basis of Laborit's tape recording of their session, Quarti wrote out how the drug had affected her:

No subjective change was felt until 12.00, when I began to have the impression that I was weaker, that I was dying. It was very painful and agonising ...

At 1.00, an intense affective change appeared ... the painful feeling of imminent death disappeared to make room for a euphoric relaxation. I had felt all along that I was going to die, but this new state left me indifferent. I began to talk more volubly, although my voice was still very weak, very faint. I tried to joke; I felt incapable of being angry about anything; irresistibly optimistic, and full of love for the whole world. Although very much in touch with my surroundings, I was more and more overcome by an extreme feeling of detachment from myself and from the others. My perceptions were normal, but their tone had changed; everything was filtered, muted ...

The weakness and difficulty in speaking persisted for several days before gradually disappearing. The affective changes lasted for about a week, but became more complex than the simple dysfunction felt during and immediately after the experiment. Contrary to my customary manner, I felt very jovial, with a facility for puns ... a complete detachment or neglect, and a certain lessening of self-control. The mood was of perfect euphoria, unaffected by all the little traumas of daily life.

More convinced than ever about the relevance of this new drug for psychiatry, Laborit continued to make his case at the hospital canteen until finally, on 19 January 1952, Colonel Joseph Hamon, the hospital's director of neuropsychiatry, and two of his associates gave the drug to 24-year-old Jacques Lh., afflicted with severe manic agitation, a 'revolving door' kind of patient who had been institutionalised at Val-de-Grâce several times in the past and had received, all told, fifteen electroconvulsive treatments and four treatments with the sedative thiopental for mania between 9 September and 10 October 1949, and then again, from 6 February to 6 April 1951, nine electroconvulsive treatments and fifteen insulin comas. Given that he was considered a hopeless case, per-haps the doctors at Val-de-Grâce thought they had little to lose in shooting him up with this largely mysterious compound. Jacques Lh. took his chlorpromazine intramuscularly, along with a strong dose of a drug called pethidine, a sedative, as he lay supine on his pillows. The needle sank into his skin. He lay very still, without moving. The doctors watched, wondering. They spoke to him and he responded. Then he stuck out his tongue and fell straight into a deep sleep.

For the next twelve days Jacques Lh. received the same cocktail, chlorpromazine and pethidine, every day, after which he slept. Hours later, as the sedative wore off, he would awaken and step out of bed and into a period of unusual calm that at first lasted no more than a few minutes before he returned to his typically psychotic behaviour, but that gradually, as the days went by, began to stretch out for longer and longer allotments of time. Eventually he ceased tearing his sheets and trying to burn his blankets. He no longer put flowerpots on his head. He lost interest in giving disjointed, impassioned speeches about the loss of liberty on the planet Pluto. The violence he was prone to packed up and went away. After twenty days, this supposedly hopeless case, having now received in total 855 milligrams of chlorpromazine, was judged by the Val-de-Grâce staff to be 'adaptable à une vie normale' ('fit for a normal life'), and he was discharged and never heard from again. No one knows the long-term fate of Jacques Lh. No one knows if he returned home, or if he even had a home to return to. No one knows what happened to his dreams and his demons, although since he was not maintained on the drug, it is hard to believe that they didn't return. We know only that he was not seen at Val-de-Grâce again.

In the early 1950s, with chlorpromazine just making its first rounds, none of the doctors, scientists, psychiatrists or researchers involved knew a thing about psychopharmacology. In fact, the word barely existed in the normal lexicon. Jacques Lh.'s doctors saw his illness go away, and they had no reason to think anything but that the drug had cured him, just as penicillin cures the patient of strep and, once cured, the patient can cease the medication. Jacques Lh. himself probably thought he was cured, and while there is no record of his response to the clarity that came with his particular drug cocktail, we can imagine he must have experienced it as a real relief, because psychosis is a dreadful state in which a person is hounded by hallucinations, the head crammed full of squeals and screams, the body wracked by daytime dreams of steep stairs and burning bonfires and pitiless gods who demand idiosyncratic sacrifices at altars no one can see. Jacques Lh. trudged out into the world with his head mercifully emptied of the cruel chaos that constitutes a psychotic illness, having been briefly blessed with a state of 'normal' calm that must have made his symptoms, when they returned, as they were bound to, that much sharper, fiercer, hotter, harder – the sanguine self a dim memory if even that.

Sainte-Anne

Less than a mile from the Val-de-Grâce military hospital, where Laborit laboured in search of the safest anaesthetics, stood another imposing institution, right in the heart of Paris, surrounded by city streets to which vendors flocked on market days to sell their wares – buckets of bright flowers, fish, their silver scales aglitter in the sun, laid out on beds of ice, oranges stacked in pretty pyramids, and healthy rotund watermelons, their thick rinds striped with the palest seams of green. This institution was called Hôpital Sainte-Anne, one of Paris's only mental hospitals, housing in the early 1950s over five thousand patients who crowded its dimly lit halls, who crouched in corners or paced the corridors talking to invisible rivals. These five thousand patients were divided into wards – locked and open, male and female – all of which were presided over by one thousand nurses and other staff members, and then, supervising the nurses, the junior psychiatrists, and supervising the junior psychiatrists the senior psychiatrists, and, sitting at the helm, a deeply intelligent and fiercely hierarchical patrician named Jean Delay, considered one of the most brilliant doctors of his generation.

Delay's father had been a respected surgeon in the south of France who wanted his son to follow in his footsteps, which Delay did, passing all of his examinations with perfect or near-perfect scores, despite realising, at some point in his medical education, that surgery did not interest him half as much as the human head. Diverting from the path his father had laid out for him, Delay veered into neurology while also studying psychiatry at the Sorbonne, with a thesis on memory and its pathology. Unlike Laborit, who abhorred hierarchy and who would, after sharing the Lasker Prize in 1957 for his role in the discovery of chlorpromazine, set up his own private lab in which he could pursue his own interests unencumbered by the daily demands of life on the medical fast track, Delay thrived on the rat race, keen to prove his considerable merits and, in the process, to earn his seat at the tip of the top. Thus, when he was appointed full professor and head of the department of psychiatry at the University of Paris, which was housed within the Sainte-Anne complex, Delay easily and keenly took this coveted position, overseeing the jam-packed wards from a benevolent distance, always with his assistants, Pierre Deniker and Pierre Pichot, by his side.

Perhaps in part because of Delay's wide and learned mind (he read deeply in diverse subjects and had a love of literature), Sainte-Anne, despite its wretched patients and mediocre resources, attracted many talented psychiatrists and researchers. For a time Jacques Lacan came there to give weekly seminars, which drew audiences much larger than Delay's, a fact that bothered Delay so much he eventually sent Lacan across town, to opine elsewhere. He was that sort of man, grandiose but benevolent, full of himself and hitched to his hierarchy but prone to jealousy, and yet so smart, so superbly educated, that it was hard to quibble with his position.

Yet despite Delay's stature, the breadth and depth of his mind and his education, Sainte-Anne in the early 1950s was like any other insane asylum of its time. Patients were treated in the typical manner, with enemas given in the hope of detoxifying their colons and emptying their innards of illness, electroconvulsive shock therapy performed minus the muscle relaxants, so that the patients' entire bodies were wracked with current, and lobotomies practised, going in through the eye sockets, with an ice pick, or in through the skull, into which two holes were drilled before inserting the knife blade or spatula, a quick *swish swish* and it was done. Baths were drawn in attempts to soothe manic agitation, with water rumbling into ancient claw-foot tubs and the tiled rooms dense with steam, the moist mirrors dripping and distorting in a Dalí-esque way. One female patient in Sainte-Anne suffered second-degree burns because she was tied into her bath and the cold water pipe ceased working, scalding her, the nurses ignoring her screams as they were so used to such sounds.

People walking to and fro on the busy city streets below Sainte-Anne regularly heard the wails and slams and tilted laughter of the madmen and women behind those brick walls. Not even a man as learned as Delay could do much to help his charges, and this may be why he kept a careful distance between himself and the patients, seeing only the most difficult cases and only on occasion. His aristocratic bearing was entirely at odds with the reality of the hospital he had to run. He ran it by delegating, by sealing himself inside his well-appointed office, where he received the crème de la crème of the psychiatric, scientific and artistic community. He was close friends with André Gide and received visits from the poet Henri Michaux, who regularly used psychedelic mushrooms to stimulate his muse.

Delay and his main assistant, Pierre Deniker, who oversaw the male locked wards, knew nothing about chlorpromazine, even after Rhône-Poulenc released samples of it into the medical community. They did not know about patient Jacques Lh.; they had not read Laborit's published paper in which he ended by suggesting that the compound might have a place in psychiatry. They did not know about Cornelia Quarti or about psychiatrists Jean Sigwald and Daniel Bouttier, who had successfully used the drug – alone, rather than as part of a blend – on Madame Gob, a fifty-seven-year-old psychotic patient at the Hôpital Paul Brousse, also in Paris, in December 1951. Sigwald and Bouttier were the first ever to use chlorpromazine on a patient for psychiatric purposes (as opposed to Laborit's surgical, anaesthetic use), but they did not publish their results until 1953, while Colonel Hamon and his colleagues released their results on Jacques Lh. in March 1952, making them the first psychiatrists to publish an account of chlorpromazine's psychiatric use, with barbiturates.

Delay and Deniker first learned about chlorpromazine at the end of 1951, when Deniker's brother-in-law, an anaesthetist – who had himself heard of Laborit's use of chlorpromazine with artificial hibernation and had tried the drug on his own patients – suggested to Deniker that he might be interested in it for its tranquillising properties. Thus, on 2 February 1952, at Deniker's request, Rhône-Poulenc sent to Sainte-Anne some samples of chlorpromazine. Deniker, who had tried all sorts of somatic treatments on his patients, with no luck, was likely not expecting much. He chose a group of six male patients, in whom he would induce a kind of artificial hibernation while simultaneously administering the drug, much like Laborit. At this point chlorpromazine had been in circulation for several months and a number of psychiatrists had tried it, many with good, if not outstanding, results, but none of the psychiatrists, except Sigwald and Bouttier, had tried chlorpromazine alone. All of them had used it in conjunction with other drugs. Deniker set out to use chlorpromazine all by itself, although he did request, and receive, slabs and buckets of ice from the hospital pharmacy. The patients were packed in these cold cubes and then shot up in an arm or a buttock while Deniker sat by their side and nurses rushed to and fro, replacing melted ice with more and more ice until at last the pharmacy could not keep up with the demand and the frozen component was abandoned and the drug administered entirely alone.

Here is what happened. Although science and magic are exactly the opposite of each other, the latter accomplished through impenetrable mystery or miracle, the former undergirded by replicable results that prove to have relevance and validity in the material world, chlorpromazine's effects on the minds of the mad, while clearly rooted in the science of pharmacology, nevertheless had a distinctly magical feel. This was made all the more so because in 1952, little was known about the biochemistry of the brain; no one knew about serotonin, dopamine, noradrenaline or the synaptic cleft. So when chlorpromazine worked – and work it did, extraordinarily well – it seemed less like a drug had been given and more like a wand had been waved, all the junk and rumble and static and screams stuffed inside the wracked minds of the insane just emptying out, leaving in their wake the tender but beautiful fabric of cogent thought, of untainted language, of intact memory, longing and love. Nameless patients suddenly had names. They had histories and hopes their illness had smothered but not snuffed, and now the hope was here again. They had humour and abilities of which their doctors had had no idea.

There was, for instance, the case of Phillippe Burg. Burg had been enveloped in a deep psychotic state for years, utterly unreachable. He hadn't walked, or even talked. Nothing had helped him, and every treatment had been tried. Once given chlorpromazine, however, and over a series of weeks, Burg began to emerge from his madness. The torpor that had trapped him diminished and then disappeared. The man began to move about, to stretch, to place one foot in front of the other, carefully, cautiously, as if to test that the floor beneath his feet was real. It was. He walked, for the first time in more years than anyone could count. And then, after he began to walk, he started, also, to talk. He said his name – *Phillippe Burg* – and then he asked his doctors what their names were, and suddenly a real relationship began where before there had been only handling. Burg progressed so rapidly on chlorpromazine that eventually the hospital staff allowed him to attend an outing with his mother. The pair went to dinner at Hemingway's favourite haunt, the Closerie des Lilas.

Other patients, too, in other hospitals around France, began to emerge from their murk as news of chlorpromazine spread. Catatonic patients tended to respond almost immediately, whereas others needed days or weeks to stabilise. Either way, the responses were often incredible. One newly awakened patient in an asylum near Lyon had a severe sickness that had kept him cloudy for years. But now, on chlorpromazine, he told his doctor, Jean Perrin, that he knew who he was and where he was. He reported that he was a barber from Lyon and that now, well, he would like to go back to work. His psychiatrist responded with a challenge. 'Give me a shave,' the doctor suggested intrepidly to the barber, whose skills must have been at the very least rusty, dulled from years of disuse and disease. Nurses produced a bowl of warm water, a stack of clean and folded towels, some soap and an unsheathed blade, which was placed in the barber's hand. The doctor sat in a seat while the recently revived patient smocked him with the towels and soaped up his chin and cheeks. Then, with sane and steady hands, the barber raked the razor over the iron filings of stubble until the psychiatrist's skin was perfectly smooth and satiny.

At the Bassens Hospital, in Rhône-Alpes, was another patient about whom nothing was known. Like the barber from Lyon, this patient also had been stuck in an interminable series of rigid postures, and, also like the barber, had been failed by all the treatments the doctors had tried. As with the barber, this patient responded to chlorpromazine in a single day. After receiving an intramuscular injection, he suddenly began greeting the nurses, calling each one by name, correctly, as if, over all these years, facts had indeed seeped beneath the snow of his psychosis, and the real world, the nominal world, had made its way into his scrambled mind even as his mouth was unable to articulate what he had absorbed. After he'd greeted the nurses, he had an odd request: some billiard balls, please. Billiard balls? Yes, billiard balls. With some misgivings the staff produced for the now walking and talking patient three bright billiard balls, which the patient began to juggle expertly, keeping up a steady tempo as the balls rose and fell into his cupped and careful palms, managing it all with elaborate and expert finesse. He had been a juggler in his former life, it turned out, before insanity had come to claim him, and now, like the barber, he wanted to return to his vocation.

On wards all across France, scenes like this played out as papers were published and word spread through the psychiatric grapevine. There was a drug! At last there was a drug! It really worked! Patients who'd been cast for years in catatonic postures were dusting themselves off and walking away into the world, whistling. Many French psychiatrists looked and listened with a deep and tired scepticism, because for years they'd been trying this and that and that and this, going so far as to drill holes into the sides of their patients' skulls and cut the connections, bringing the wires down. Other psychiatrists, however, especially the younger ones, were quicker to believe that this new drug might be a brew worth trying. In fact, in Sainte-Anne and other psychiatric institutions, the younger psychiatrists started to appear in the admissions centres, offering to bring the trickiest and most troubled patients back to their floors because, well, there was a drug!

Nurses crushed capsules of chlorpromazine into patients' food, or doctors injected it into their striated muscles, and everywhere across France patients responded by waking up and looking around, oftentimes with as much confusion as relief. The world was not as they recalled it. Some of these patients had been sunk in inaccessible psychoses for decades. Now they looked outside the barred windows of their wards and saw streets full of cars and no horse-drawn carriages anywhere – where had they gone? The cars whizzed by, their horns tooting, their colours all gloss and glow. The patients were allowed to go on outings and discovered that prices were so much higher than they remembered. It was a world of quickened time and tempo. It was a world where electric lights lit the streets at night, casting shadows on the floors of the patients' hospital rooms. It was a world that was in many ways as strange as their psychoses, as if they'd been kissed by a prince or a princess, or been the unwitting subject of some chemical abracadabra.

With so many patients awakening within the walls of their asylums, screams replaced with coherent speech, crazed laughter now hushed, one imagines that the streets around asylums quieted. Outside of Sainte-Anne's, for instance, there was a busy market that sold produce and fish and fresh eggs and cream. Jean Thuillier, the psychiatrist who had treated Phillippe Burg, would sometimes leave his office and wander the open-air market to shop for his family. 'During the spring and summer the windows of the hospital would be open on to the street and you could hear the wailing and the screaming of the patients,' he said. 'But the first year of the neuroleptics I remember one fish dealer who knew me well pulling me aside and asking me with wonder, "Doctor, what are you doing with the patients up there? We don't hear them any more." "I'm not killing them," I told him.' The fish dealer was not the only one to notice the sudden silence that had come over the wards. The glaziers, called in to replace the panes of glass that were so frequently smashed, also found themselves with far less work to do.

Rhône-Poulenc took note of the psychiatric success stories and began issuing what they called 'provisional notes' with each new batch of the drug. These notes suggested that the drug might have uses beyond being an anaesthetic potentiator and an anti-emetic, that, specifically, it might have uses in psychiatry as well. Laborit suggested that Rhône-Poulenc give the drug the name Largactil, meaning 'large action', a drug appropriate for many different needs and states, and thus chlorpromazine became known, in France (and the UK), as Largactil, chosen to express 'the extreme diversity of the drug's psychodynamic activities'. The company decided to market the drug not only to psychiatrists and surgeons but also to anaesthetists, obstetricians and gynaecologists.

Chlorpromazine in the United States

As all across France, and then Europe more generally, patients locked inside psychotic states were beginning to wake up and psychiatrists, who had often previously felt marginalised, were tasting their triumph, finally possessing a drug that made their fringe status in medicine more a thing of the past (or so they hoped), Rhône-Poulenc was thinking about how to maximise profits not just in Europe but worldwide. In 1952 the French pharmaceutical company approached Smith, Kline & French, a US pharmaceutical firm, about licensing chlorpromazine. The president of Smith, Kline & French responded to Rhône-Poulenc's inquiry by writing, 'The compound is exceedingly interesting at first glance and I wonder if you could arrange to send us, as soon as possible, 500 grams of the pure substance for our use in tests here.'

Rhône-Poulenc sent 200 grams of 'the pure substance' and SK&F set out to do its own testing. The atmosphere in the United States was very different from the atmosphere in Europe, vis-à-vis the treatment of mental patients. The French had always prized somatic treatments, whereas, in 1952, the United States was in the grip of psychoanalysis. Many psychiatric illnesses, even some of the most severe, were seen as stemming from repressed sexual desires or repressed rages turning and twisting the mind. SK&F knew this and thus decided to mine this new compound for its anti-emetic properties, having more solid clinical data supporting chlorpromazine's anti-emetic function and believing, probably correctly, that it would be far easier anyway to get a drug that controlled nausea and vomiting approved than it would be to get an antipsychotic approved, especially as none had ever existed before. They retained every intention, however, of pushing chlorpromazine's off-label uses in as many markets as possible, psychiatry prime among them. Their advertisements for chlorpromazine, as Thorazine, show that the company was soon hawking the 'anti-emetic' for every kind of ill imaginable, claiming it as a veritable panacea capable of treating everything from alcoholism to the pain associated with severe burns to the distortions and deliriums of dementia.

Although officials at SK&F worked hard to get their product into the hands of North American psychiatrists, the introduction of the drug was tainted almost from the start by resistance and controversy, 'especially from people who had emotional commitments to the psychological type treatments', said Henry Brill, who ran Pilgrim State Hospital in New York, then the world's largest mental hospital, home to almost fourteen thousand residents at its peak, in 1954. 'These were the practitioners who defended psychoanalysis and psychotherapies and psychodynamic procedures of one type or another – the talking type of treatment. They were very unhappy and weren't able to believe what was taking place.'

The resistance to this new therapy reveals the degree to which psychoanalysis had developed cult-like qualities, sealing itself off from outside interventions and insisting on a kind of religious adherence by both practitioners and patients. Psychoanalysis and its psychodynamic offshoots in fact *were* a kind of religion, in that they operated on faith and an articulated system of beliefs. To try anything different or new was tantamount to sin. The resistance to the new drug also betrays the degree to which even supposedly 'enlightened' people can have a built-in knee-jerk conservatism when it comes to the novel, although, to be fair, in this case the novel threatened the entire underpinnings of psychoanalytic practice. If a drug could cure schizophrenia, then entrenched theories about bad mothering and repressed sexual conflicts as the seed of the illness would have to be shed.

Even those North American doctors who were using biological

rather than psychoanalytical treatments were not using drugs. Heinz Lehmann, the same Montreal psychiatrist who had once gone so far as to inject turpentine into a patient's abdominal wall to bring on a fever, became one of the first to try the new drug on that side of the sea. 'No one in his right mind was working with drugs,' he admitted. 'You used shock or various psychotherapies.' Lehmann tried chlorpromazine on his patients not because Smith, Kline & French pushed him towards trial but because he had read the European reports one Sunday afternoon while taking a bath. He practised at the Verdun Protestant Hospital, living with his family on the grounds of the asylum, having emigrated from Germany in 1937, a Jew who would almost certainly have been exterminated by the Nazis were it not for a letter from a family friend inviting him to Quebec for a skiing holiday. He left Germany with his skis and enough luggage to last him for two weeks, intending never to return. Once in Canada, he was granted refugee status and a temporary medical licence.

Lehmann was an enormously dedicated clinician, dealing with a personal load of more than six hundred patients, trying any- thing and everything to jolt his charges back into reality, but with little success. After reading the reports coming out of France, he obtained samples of chlorpromazine from SK&F and tried the drug on a group of seventy patients, many of whom began to respond. 'Nowadays, of course, this would take years but in those days it didn't take very long,' Lehmann said. 'We just chose seventy and we did them all, practically simultaneously, within one or two months. Also I didn't have to ask permission from the Director of the Hospital. I didn't have to get permission from the FDA [the US Food and Drug Administration] or the government. There were no ethical committees at the time, no guidelines, laws or regimen- tations ... I don't remember – this was in 1953 – whether I even asked the patients.'

Like the psychiatrists in Lyon and Paris, Lehmann was aston- ished by what happened. Within just four or five weeks, many of his schizophrenic patients were symptom-free. 'I thought it was a fluke – something that would never happen again,' he said. 'In 1953 there just wasn't anything that ever produced something like this.' Indeed the patients' turnarounds were so dramatic and positive that Lehmann later called it 'unthinkable – hallucinations and delusions eliminated by a pill! I suppose if people had been told, "Well, they'll die two years later," they'd still have said it's worth it. It was so unthinkable and so new and so wonderful . . . Chronic schizophrenics who had been divorced because they had been psychotic for ten years, now all of a sudden they were symptom-free and their husbands or their wives were married again. It was a very strange time.'

By publishing his results, Lehmann, along with American psychiatrists who also tried chlorpromazine on their patients with successful results, was instrumental in getting the medical establishment in North America to accept that chlorpromazine was not simply another sedative that briefly covered up the real symptoms of schizophrenia. These doctors believed, in large part on the basis of the conditioned avoidance tests done with rats by Courvoisier and Charpentier, that chlorpromazine had specific antipsychotic properties and that it was acting in some distinct and unique fashion to rebalance a brain that had lost its bearings.

Entering Asylums

Despite its initial marketing as an anti-emetic in North America, chlorpromazine quickly made inroads into psychiatry, in part because of the published studies coming out of France and then the United States. With the initial resistance to the drug from psychotherapists and doctors in private practice, in many ways it was the state asylum systems, particularly large institutions like Pilgrim State, that brought chlorpromazine as an antipsychotic into circulation in this country, by proving that it had a profoundly positive effect on the schizophrenic mind. Before the introduction of chlorpromazine at Pilgrim, Henry Brill, the hospital's clinical director, described the wards as dark and desperate places where each psychiatrist had 165 patients under his or her care, making it virtually impossible to practise any form of psychodynamic therapy. Mary Holt, a doctor there, wrote that a few years prior to the arrival of chlorpromazine, the women in the two buildings she was in charge of were so 'wild' that she 'just couldn't keep them decent. They'd soil themselves, tear their clothes, smash the windows and gouge the plaster out of the walls. One of them would even rip radiators right off the wall.' What Brill and his colleagues wanted was a quick, clean somatic approach, something sweeping and easy to administer on a large scale that would not necessarily cure their charges but that would allow them some specks of humanity and decency.

Working in the basest conditions, with the sickest subjects, and with the impossible mandate of practising depth psychology or psychoanalysis on thousands of raving mental patients incapable of stringing a simple sentence together, psychiatrists at asylums like Pilgrim had little to lose and much to gain by trying chlorpromazine. And so, by the mid-1950s, that's exactly what they did. Brill, encouraged by the early literature he had read about the new compound, was tentative but hopeful. 'Once I had seen a small handful of cases that confirmed what had been said, I had no more real doubts,' he wrote. 'The most memorable experience I remember was walking into the dayroom and seeing this small group of patients dressed, quiet, cooperative and in surprisingly good contact – with their psychiatric symptoms wiped away. That was perhaps the most spectacular demonstration anyone can ask for.'

Pilgrim transformed. The park-like grounds became places for play and conversation among patients now able to socialise. Brill conceived of a medicine cabinet that would be hung above patients' beds and in which they could keep the private possessions that had previously been stripped from them upon entering the ward. Glasses, penknives, money – all this and more would be returned to the patients, who could now be trusted to tend to themselves. One psychologist described visiting Pilgrim in the late 1950s and witnessing a group of patients parading up and down the walkways, making music with tambourines and trombones, others laughing and clapping as the procession made its way down the lane. In short, the entire tenor of the hospital was profoundly altered, and previously useless activities, like occupational therapy, now provided patients with the chance to try tools that would have been much too dangerous for them prior to the drug. Patients worked with saws and drills, gaining skills and feeling for the first time in who knows how many years the particularly human pleasure of making things.

Martin Fleischman, an asylum psychiatrist in California, also saw his hospital transformed by chlorpromazine: 'Patients became quieter, wards became quieter and psychiatric aides became quieter. Lest everything be evaluated in terms of decibels, let it also be recalled that delusions and hallucinations decreased, and the understandability and predictability of patients increased. In short, patients became people and even more important, they became identified as people by the people who took care of them.'

Given these remarkable results, why, one wonders, in a country that has always prided itself on its biomedical breakthroughs, on its technological finesse and prowess, were so many psychiatrists in private practice set against this new drug? Why did it take so much time for these private practitioners to accept that there might be a chemical cure for their sickest patients? 'In those days, the idea of treating psychosis was considered ridiculous, because psychosis by definition was an incurable disease,' said Belgian scientist Paul Janssen. 'The idea that it could be cured with a pill was ridiculed as simply too childish an idea.'

Another possibility: in the United States, psychiatry in general and psychoanalysis in particular had a large number of Jewish practitioners, many of them émigrés from Nazi Germany, who had escaped concentration camps and come across the sea seeking asylum. These Jewish practitioners had seen firsthand the Nazi obsession with biomedical technology, the terrible experiments performed upon mental patients and Jews, all in the name of progress. It could be that for them, any type of chemical treatment smacked of Germany circa 1935–1945, while a talking treatment ensured a gentleness and humanity these Jewish psychiatrists sought above all for their patients. Whatever the reason, chlorpromazine was at first roundly rejected by those tightly tied to Freudian notions, and it made its way into psychiatric circles largely through the very back door, the underground door, if you will, which is to say the locked doors of the toughest mental institutions set high on hills and isolated from the public, places of such deep desolation that the doctors, even if sceptical, were willing to try new treatments that came their way.

As news of psychiatric success stories spread, however, it was no longer merely asylums but hospitals all across the United States that were asking Smith, Kline & French for samples of chlorpromazine and using the drug on vast swathes of patients who came to clarity under its influence. Wards were revolutionised. Patients walked and talked appropriately. Reports of atmospheres in asylums being completely altered came in from Alabama, Maryland, California, Arkansas, Arizona and Colorado, to name just a few states. In 1955, the year after chlorpromazine was approved by the FDA, SK&F took in $75 million. (At least one psychopharmacologist was so impressed with the profits and the power of the drug that he double-mortgaged his house to buy shares in the company.) As evidence of the drug's rapid adoption and broad application, within a year of its being marketed, 4 million prescriptions for chlorpromazine had been written. Within a decade, the drug had been taken worldwide by 50 million people, and SK&F's profits doubled three times in the fifteen years after the drug was introduced.

It is safe to say that every state asylum was profoundly changed by chlorpromazine. The use of other types of somatic therapies waned. Straitjackets gathered dust in locked cupboards. Quiet rooms were transformed into dayrooms where patients could mingle and mix. Psychosurgeries – previously used on thousands and thousands of patients, leaving a considerable portion of them with a blunting of personality, or a literal loss of voice – finally began to decrease, and this was another of chlorpromazine's great victories.

Then the inevitable happened. No longer wracked with symptoms, and in many instances clearly coherent and capable, patients became ready for ever-increasing amounts of independence. At Traverse City State Hospital in Michigan, for example, in 1955 far fewer patients needed to be spoon-fed – a drop from twenty-seven to two. The number of patients now fit to eat in the dining hall went up by 150 per cent, while soilers decreased markedly as well, down from twenty-five to five. All of this in a single hospital, although asylums across the country were reporting similar statistics. Eventually, patients became ready to be released back into the community, to be treated by psychiatrists in their own hometowns or at community mental health centres that sprang up everywhere to meet the needs of those flowing out of the huge and soon-to-be obsolete asylums. Within twenty years, the population of mental hospitals fell to less than a quarter of what it had been before chlorpromazine came on the scene.

While these discharges represented clinical triumphs, they did not come without problems. As in France, patients who had been locked in inaccessible psychotic states for years found themselves in a completely changed world and in some cases on their own. Family members did not always welcome the newly released patients back into the fold. Job skills were rusty or nonexistent.

Setbacks

Perhaps it was equally inevitable, then, that the seemingly unstoppable good news about chlorpromazine was not entirely unalloyed.

Baltimore psychiatrist Frank Ayd, who received the first official permit from the FDA to use chlorpromazine in the treatment of schizophrenia, discovered troublesome side effects. Within the first six weeks of using chlorpromazine, two of his patients got jaundice. The first had viral hepatitis, so Ayd could not be sure that the jaundice was from the chlorpromazine. The second, however, whom Ayd described as 'chronically agitated', though clearly jaundiced as a result of the chlorpromazine prescription, did not want to stop taking the drug. 'I do feel better,' she insisted, 'even though I'm yellow.' Ayd also reported that women on chlorpromazine began to lactate. He had the breast milk analysed, curious to see its components, and found that it was precisely the same as normal breast milk. Ayd was also one of the first to discover and report on the phenomenon of false pregnancy tests that occurred as a result of chlorpromazine use, evidence that the drug was interfering with normal hormonal processes in women in ways we don't understand.

But perhaps most troubling to Ayd was the discovery that, when given in hefty doses, the drug produced what is called a dystonic reaction, a rigidity in muscle movements and an awkwardness of gait, a shuffling sort of step – and sometimes still worse symptoms. In 1955 Ayd shot a film of a patient on a high dose of chlorpromazine who had become twisted up like a pretzel, his limbs entwined. Concerned, and perhaps confused, Ayd showed the film to pharmacologists at Smith, Kline & French, who in turn asked for input from neurologists, some of whom, still under the psychoanalytic sway in this country, dismissed the reaction as 'hysterical'. In those days, even Parkinson's disease, an affliction of dopamine deficiency which leads to loss of motor control and causes patients to spasm and stiffen, tended to be seen as a condition related to repressed anger immobilising the victim.

But the dystonic reactions that Ayd had observed could not be easily dismissed. As doctors experimented with doses, raising them in the hopes of making a good effect great, over time some patients displayed bizarre behaviours – tongue thrusting, lip smacking, restlessness, involuntary movement of their torso and limbs, a constellation of symptoms known as tardive dyskinesia. The condition could in some, but not all, cases be reversed with the administration of anticholinergic drugs, which are intended to counteract the release of the neurotransmitter acetylcholine at neuromuscular junctions and thereby prevent muscle contraction. Tardive dyskinesia eventually affects 32 per cent of patients taking neuroleptics after five years, 57 per cent after fifteen years and 68 per cent after twenty-five years. Given the severity of the side effects, one would think that the newfound enthusiasm for chlorpromazine might have been dampened, but it wasn't. The profits of SK&F continued to rise while newly released patients slowly felt their way into lives so quiet and calm they must have seemed almost as strange as their now defunct hallucinations once had.

Whence the Magic

Whatever its pros and cons, the invention and dissemination of chlorpromazine is ultimately as significant for what it did not do as for what it did. Yes, the drug reversed states of psychosis so severe they had trapped patients for years. Yes, by doing so, the drug helped to birth the deinstitutionalisation movement and the corresponding rise of the community mental health centre. And in the United States the drug finally put a dent in the deeply held American affinity for psychoanalysis, as even the clinicians most dedicated to 'the talking cure' had to concede that this capsule could clear the mind more effectively and efficiently than could any leather sofa and conversation. But the drug did not, at least initially, spur anyone to ask *how* or *why* it was working. No one had the slightest idea. It was simply enough for everyone that it *was* working. Clearly the capsule suggested that mental illness, at least in some respects, was a brain-based phenomenon, but beyond that, few had a clue.

Indeed it would be years before any viable theories arose. The double-helix model of DNA was just being discovered, but its role in schizophrenia is only partially understood even today. English researcher Gregory Bateson developed, in the mid-1950s, what he called 'the double-bind theory of schizophrenia', a theory that suggests the disease arises when parents send conflicting messages to their child. A child might become schizophrenic if, for instance, he or she was praised with words but also frequently punished with actions. (This theory has been largely discarded as researchers have uncovered other, more persuasive possible aetiologies that have to do with brain morphology, genetic predisposition and, perhaps most importantly, the neurotransmitter dopamine, which we will come to.)

Was it therefore irresponsible of doctors to be giving a drug about which they had no hypotheses, never mind theories, as to how and why it worked? It seems so, and yet think of the alternative – to withhold a drug that can restore a life because its mysteries have not been mapped. Chlorpromazine reveals to us the sheer power of empiricism. In many ways it helped to set the stage for the other, more targeted psychotropic drugs that followed, about which, in truth, we still know much less than we'd like to. So much of psychopharmacology happens in the dark, which, one might say, is its premier weakness, or its defining strength, if you appreciate its willingness to persevere in shadow, propelled by faith and whatever facts can be unearthed along the way.

Back in the 1920s, German researcher Otto Loewi, a professor of pharmacology at the University of Graz, had confirmed the function of the first neurotransmitter, no more, no less than a wet chemical, a part of the brain's primordial soup that dwells in tracts within our neural tissue. Today scientists know that there are over forty different kinds of neurotransmitters in our brains, but Loewi knew of only one, discovering that the brain chemical acetylcholine mediated the transmission of nerve signalling from one cell to the next, a discovery for which he would eventually be awarded the Nobel Prize. In response to this newly found knowledge, psychiatrists in the 1930s had repeatedly tried giving acetylcholine to their schizophrenic patients in the hopes of achieving a remission, with no success. But between the discovery of acetylcholine in the 1920s and the phenomenon of psychiatry's penicillin – chlorpromazine – in the 1950s, few other brain chemicals had been unearthed. In fact, back then, not all scientists even accepted that the brain operated via the chemical signalling of nerve cells; many suspected that any signalling going on was electrical rather than chemical in nature.

Thus chlorpromazine was released into the world with no notion of what it was doing and no real way of finding out. After all, lobotomies notwithstanding, you cannot very well carve open the skull of a patient and start poking around in his head in the hopes of tracing the medicine's path or impact. And while one *can* do some form of this to animals, by giving them the drug and then sacrificing them to study their brains, in the first half of the twentieth century, prior to the discovery of chlorpromazine, the field had no antipsychotics with which to make such a study. Beyond that, there is and was no way of creating an animal model of schizophrenia. It would take the discovery and introduction of a second antipsychotic, reserpine, to change this state of affairs.

An alkaloid from the Rauwolfia plant that had been used in India to treat fever, vomiting, snakebite, insomnia and insanity for thousands of years, reserpine was introduced in the United States at around the same time as chlorpromazine, but while chlorpromazine was used clinically, reserpine was used more experimentally. In 1955 Robert Bowman, a researcher at the National Institutes of Health, invented the spectrophotofluorometer, a machine that allowed scientists for the first time to detect other neurotransmitters in animal brains. Bowman's fellow researcher Bernard Brodie investigated serotonin (the same neurotransmitter that fluoxetine would eventually seek to manipulate), using the new machine to discern whether the reserpine administered to rabbits that had been sedated with the alkaloid correlated with the serotonin levels in their brains. Brodie found that administering reserpine to rabbits decreased the amount of serotonin in their neural tissues. This in turn appeared to cause the rabbits to become lethargic, apathetic in just the same way that depressed people display these behaviours.

The new technology was a significant moment in the fledging field of the neurosciences, and a solid step towards a more scientific psychiatry. With the invention of the spectrophotofluorometer – and the concomitant discovery that the administration of reserpine decreased serotonin in the brains of bunnies, making them seem slow and sad – researchers could now crack the capsule open, so to speak, and squeeze from chlorpromazine its chemical secrets and signatures in the hopes that, by understanding how it helped, they might discover something about the substrates of psychotic affliction.

The Search for the Physical Substrates

Given that in the early stages of chlorpromazine no one knew how it achieved its results, the drug did more than mend the minds of chronic schizophrenics; it also eventually pushed scientists to discover its hidden mechanisms and to try to reveal, in the process, the neural glitch that they had begun to believe schizophrenia must surely be. Chlorpromazine set off a biological revolution in psychiatry. It made the discipline medical by allowing for a new language and structure of thought to emerge. A discipline that had its origins in the humours of Hippocrates was now governed by words like *neurotransmission* and *chemical signalling* and the logic that underlay them.

The revolution that had started with the spectrophotofluorometer accelerated when, in 1957, Kathleen Montagu, a researcher at the Runwell Hospital, outside London, demonstrated the presence of dopamine in the human brain. Swedish neuropharmacologist (and eventual Nobel Prize winner) Arvid Carlsson followed up on Montagu's research by showing that dopamine, previously thought to have been just a precursor to noradrenaline, was a neurotransmitter in its own right. Curious to see what would happen to dopamine when mediated by chlorpromazine, scientists then gave the drug to mice and found that, under its influence, their dopamine levels decreased. These findings led to a spate of other dopamine experiments, and from these experiments emerged what is called the 'dopamine hypothesis of schizophrenia'. The hypothesis at its most basic suggests that the schizophrenic brain is awash in dopamine; that excess dopamine is responsible for the voices and the visions; and that drugs which block or otherwise occupy D_2 (dopamine) receptors in the brain are successful antipsychotics. The dopamine hypothesis was further supported by the fact that amphetamines, which increase dopamine production in the brain, make schizophrenia worse. The reason why chlorpromazine was working on psychotic patients, according to this hypothesis, was that it was lowering the level of dopamine in the schizophrenic brain.

At the same time that psychopharmacology – motivated by the clinical success of chlorpromazine – was discovering endogenous chemicals and receptor sites in the brain, neuropathologists, inspired by the notion that the field of psychiatry could be made medical again, began looking for an anatomic explanation for mental illness. Some psychiatrists believe that schizophrenics at birth have often endured far more obstetrical trauma than had those subjects untroubled by the disease. But neuropathologists studying schizophrenia found that the problem had most likely occurred earlier, in the womb – an error in the way the foetal brain is wired. The dilemma was twofold. There were areas of the brain in schizophrenics where the neurons were jumbled, and even when properly arranged, the neurons weren't uniformly sized, when compared to the brains of those unafflicted by schizophrenia.

Scientists believe it's highly improbable that these patterns could develop at any time other than during embryogenesis. By using PET scan and fMRI technology – neuroimaging procedures developed in the wake of the spectrophotofluorometer that are able to measure brain activity by detecting changes linked to blood flow – researchers were getting a look, for the first time, at the brains of schizophrenics versus those of controls. As a result, they were also able to demonstrate that schizophrenics have enlarged cerebral ventricles (the ventricles hold cerebral spinal fluid in the brain), and, more significant, that the degree of enlargement is proportional to the degree of impairment.

At the present time no one really knows what the relationship is between the dopamine hypothesis of schizophrenia, which posits that excess dopamine is at the root of the disease, and the observations of the disorganised neurons and the enlarged cerebral ventricles found in many (although not all) schizophrenic brains. Does excess dopamine somehow scramble the neurons or cause the enlargement of cerebral ventricles? Or are these phenomena merely two distinct symptoms of what is a multifaceted syndrome? Some people with the illness, for instance, become catatonic; others become paranoid. We know of several strains of schizophrenia, and there may be still subtler variations of the illness, perhaps dozens, in which case it may also be that just as healthy brains are vastly different, so are sick ones, which means that a unified theory of schizophrenia, while appealing, may be misleading.

The New Antipsychotics

All of this neurological research has been the guiding force behind efforts at refining our antipsychotics over the past sixty years. At the present time we have a wide array at our disposal, some of them similar in their pharmacological action to chlorpromazine, while others, the newest antipsychotics – aripiprazole, ziprasidone, olanzapine and quetiapine, for example – act on entirely different brain chemicals, such as serotonin and noradrenaline. The new antipsychotics are now a multibillion-dollar industry in the United States alone, and by 2011 they had surpassed statins – cholesterol-lowering agents such as atorvastatin and simvastatin – as the bestselling category of drugs in that country, a truly mind-boggling fact when one considers how rare psychosis is in the population. Schizophrenia in particular and psychosis in general affect no more than 1 per cent of the population, around 3 million people in the United States, but far more than 1 per cent of the population is imbibing some sort of antipsychotic drug. For instance, by 2011, the total number of annual prescriptions written for the group of drugs known as atypical antipsychotics (which includes aripiprazole and quetiapine) rose to 54 million from 28 million in 2001, almost doubling in the space of a decade, meaning that psychiatrists and psychopharmacologists are likely prescribing the new antipsychotics for off-label conditions not approved by the government. The astounding rise in the number of prescriptions for the newer antipsychotic drugs may be due to psychopharmacologists' belief that, when added to a depressive's diet, so to speak, an antipsychotic boosts the action of the antidepressant and more effectively irradiates the iron grip of despair than does an anti-depressant alone.

As for chlorpromazine, the loudly touted penicillin for psychiatry, the drug responsible for initiating pharmacological and neuropathological inquiries into the human head, it has fallen by the wayside, outshone by the newer offshoots that emerged in its wake, drugs that boast a supposedly safer side effect profile and a more efficacious antipsychotic action, which may not be at all true. Chlorpromazine's reputation was done in primarily by its link to tardive dyskinesia, combined with the rampant anti-psychiatry movement that started in the 1960s – initiated in part by books like Thomas Szasz's *Myth of Mental Illness* and in part by the rise of the civil rights movement and feminism, both of which employed a rhetoric later adapted by the anti-psychiatry movement to insist that mental patients were another oppressed minority, 'their psyches manipulated by therapists'. Thus the drug once hailed for saving the minds of many madmen and women the world over is rarely prescribed any more, so out of fashion has it fallen. Indeed, with some exceptions, the drug has been relegated to the veterinary world, where it goes by the name acepromazine and is given to circus elephants with pre-performance jitters and high-strung horses whose owners are hoping to bring home a blue ribbon.

For a drug that so effectively and completely, if temporarily, cleaned up the chaos of entrenched psychotic conditions to be relegated to the dustbin of the back ward, so to speak, seems odd, but it reveals how susceptible psychiatry is to fashion and fad, how hard a time psychiatry has holding on to the very science it seeks, too often falling prey to the new and the nifty. Psychiatrists, of course, will not admit that their preference for newer antipsychotic drugs has anything to do with trend, and will insist instead that it has everything to do with research and patient safety, but the fact is that the new antipsychotics on the market carry their own significant risks, some of them far more severe than the motor dysfunction that chlorpromazine, in excessive doses, can cause. It is well documented that some of the new antipsychotics can cause enormous weight gain, leading to metabolic disturbance, which in turn can develop into type 2 diabetes. 'When it comes to antipsychotics', said McLean Hospital's psychopharmacologist Alexander Vuckovic, who is also a Harvard professor, 'you have to pick your poisons. Which would you rather be in two years – a circus freak or a diabetic?'

Of course, if you are not afflicted with schizophrenia or another psychosis, you can cull a third choice from Vuckovic's comment and say 'neither', but if you happen to be a person in need of an antipsychotic in order to see straight, a person who is persecuted by voices or sees filmy beings flying before his eyes, a person who can rarely speak a sane sentence then 'neither' is not an option. Such a person is faced with unfortunate choices indeed. The very starkness of the choices suggests that, while psychiatry has come far, it still has a long way to go. The bare basic facts reveal a profession still stuttering, with at best a slippery grasp on the science behind its tablets and potions, a legion of medical men and women who can help you in one way but hurt you in another. The misgivings and doubts that many people feel about this inherent risk are in part what gave rise to the anti-psychiatry movement.

The Anti-Psychiatry Movement

In 1961, after a year spent working as an orderly in a mental institution, a Stanford student by the name of Ken Kesey began to write a book. What emerged from his experience is *One Flew Over the Cuckoo's Nest*, which eventually inducted millions of readers into the putative world of the ward. Kesey's cuckoo's nest featured traumatic shock treatments, forced medication, a nurse named Ratched who would have whipped her charges were it legal, such was her dislike. *One Flew Over the Cuckoo's Nest* portrayed the mental hospital as a dark and demeaning place where people were regularly stripped of their humanity and shocked again and again on a cold steel slab until they were empty-eyed and crippled, while orderlies without care or concern held down the doughy bodies of people imprisoned in pitiless wards for years, with no end in sight.

Kesey's fictional account, along with works by intellectuals like Thomas Szasz, Michel Foucault and Erving Goffman, to name a few, ignited the fledgling anti-psychiatry movement of the 1960s, which began to flourish in the United States and abroad. Suddenly mental illness was a myth designed to punish what was in fact just another variation of creativity, and the wards were really prisons, places whose purpose was to repress the wayward tendencies of those who lived on and mined the margins of society, gifted people whose voices and visions should be celebrated rather than treated or in any way tamped down. The drug that had freed, the drug that had redeemed the seemingly hopeless mentally ill, became the chemical straitjacket, and now the juggler, the barber and all the other patients brought back to reality by chlorpromazine did not have, and never had had, anything wrong with them in a strictly medical sense, because madness was just a social construct used to suppress and repress. The celebrated silence of the wards now became proof of oppression.

In 1969, prominent anti-psychiatrists such as Szasz and R. D. Laing visited Tokyo University, inspiring students there to revolt, which they did, occupying the department of psychiatry and tossing out Hiroshi Utena, a professor of psychiatry who had done biological work in the 1950s. For a full decade the department remained occupied by students, and all inquiry there screeched to a halt. All across Europe, similar scenarios played out. In France, fired by the ideology of the anti-psychiatrists, students stormed the venerable Sainte-Anne asylum and assaulted Delay's office. One imagines university kids upending his handsome desk, tossing his gilded pens out windows, emptying his drawers and shredding his papers. In an instant, it seemed, this giant of psychiatry and the huge institution he ran were ransacked and a whole new kind of madness now swirled around Delay, one for which he had neither clue nor cure.

HELP

But it seems wrong to end the story of chlorpromazine here. Without a doubt, schizophrenia is a dreadful illness, perhaps *the* most dreadful of all the psychiatric conditions, and so even if we don't have all the answers we need, we should be grateful for the story of chlorpromazine, the *fact* of chlorpromazine, which started a ball of knowledge rolling that has not stopped. Perhaps, then, this story should end where it started, with methylene blue, that brilliant transparent dye the colour of the Caribbean Sea, out of which sprang promethazine, which then gave way to chlorpromazine, which turned the world of psychiatry on its tender head.

It is fitting that psychiatry's first drug was born from blue, a kind of creation myth suggestive of sky and sea, salt and spray, primitive elements giving way to gelatinous capsules that doused the fantasias made by madness, leaving the heads of the mentally ill mercifully quiet and clean, empty and ready for new stories that might grow like shoots in the fresh soil that sanity allowed. When I was prowling through that old abandoned mental hospital, I tried to imagine what some of these new sane stories might be, and tried also to imagine what preceded that release – what it would be like to be completely claimed by dancing demons and taunting clowns in a cruel and never-ending circus where flamethrowers forced fire down your throat and no one could see it and save you. I tried to imagine the horror of schizophrenia, the perpetual feeling of persecution, the high keening clarity of paranoia, a clarity so compelling it shatters the mind, which is terrified, always.

I have had my fair share of psychiatric difficulties, and at times, in depressions too deep for words, I have seen my world drained of colour, the trees flat and stark, a strange black hat rolling across a midnight road. This is as close as I have ever come to madness, too close for comfort but not nearly close enough to really comprehend. Thus, meandering around that old asylum which was emptied during deinstitutionalisation, I look for clues. I touch the suckers that were once attached to scalps to deliver current straight through the cranium, causing the patient's brain to seize again, and then again. I riffle through dusty tomes in a library where stacks of books are home to beetles and other bugs. I watch a spider spin her lair in a patient's long-abandoned room, and remember the experiment in which spiders were dosed with hallucinogens and, under their influence, made ever more complex and wild webs, each one a work of silk and art, impermanent and impossible to replicate. I put my hand on the flat pillows on each of the dusty beds and try to conjure the hurting heads that each night rested here, with their squalls mixed up in the sweaty sheets, the blue dreams that might lie ahead as yet unknown.

In room number 332, on the second floor, the glass in the window is crazed with cracks, and the last light is leaving now, the sun visible only as an orange seam at the very edge of a summer-time sky. Below me on the street walk people in sandals and skirts, oblivious to the huge history this asylum holds. I lift up the pillow on the bed and beneath it find a scrap of paper so thin and soft my touch almost turns it to talc. Written on the paper, a single word: *HELP*. Is it the delusion of a patient who believed an alien was lifting him up towards a cruel and cryptic planet? Or a simple statement made once chlorpromazine finally cleared a confused mind, emptying its screams and shards? Impossible to know. *HELP*. A sign of illness or recovery? *HELP*. Something every one of us wants to have, in whatever fashion it arrives. I think about bringing the scrap back home with me, but it seems wrong to remove it from its intended place beneath the pillow, and so I put it back and cover it up, as it was, and will continue to be, until the wrecking ball brings this edifice down. In the place where this building now stands – what will come? I imagine a field of flowers, a pretty park, a deep pond in which fish float like lamps beneath the clear surface. A wishing pond that collects the pennies of those who close their eyes and toss.

If I had one wish to make, it might be for a perfect preparation, an ultimate drug that works according to the precise needs of its imbiber, eradicating depression, turning mania into happiness, schizophrenia into simple creativity. I'd wish for a blue concoction that could give birth to something like serenity for everyone who wants it – and who would not? I'd wish for a drug with no side effects except supreme mental health, a robust brain packed with well-proportioned neurons all speaking smoothly to one another and, under the influence of this ultimate recipe, a world brimming with good, with great intentions and a happily-ever-after kind of ending. But that is not what we have here. We have, instead, a single word – *HELP* – which signals something ambiguous at best. Was the juggler helped for his whole lifetime? Or did side effects make the medication impossible for him? What happened to the barber from Lyon? For how long was he helped before the strange and scary motor movements came to claim him? Would we ever have an antipsychotic that removes symptoms without causing crippling side effects? Chlorpromazine brought psychiatry very far, but in the end, not far enough, not nearly.

2

Lithium

A Salted Stone

An Ancient Element

Unlike other drugs, lithium is older than we are, born in the big blast that gave our universe its considerable kick start. An element found in meteors and stars and space, lithium appeared within twenty minutes of our universe's initial explosion. The element is so light that it atomises on contact with air, bursting into crimson flames. It was first discovered on Earth more than two centuries ago, in 1800, by Brazilian geologist José Bonifácio de Andrada e Silva, who was working in an iron ore mine on Utö, a rocky island off the coast of Sweden rich in minerals, including a new one that Andrada called petalite. If you were to travel to Utö today, chances are fair that you, too, might come across petalite – crenellated and raspy to the touch. Scientists in the nineteenth century who later studied petalite found that it contained not only silica, alumina, manganese and water – elements embedded in other rocks as well – but also a small amount of an odd salt no one had ever seen before. Curious, investigators passed an electric current through the salt, which melted with a red flash and a crackle. The salt came to be called *lithion*, after the Greek word for 'stone'.

The Uric Acid Diathesis

The lightest of all the metals, grand and timeless, an ingredient in sun and stars, meteors and comets, lithium came to be used for mere mankind. Though an unstable element itself, it has the ability, perhaps ironically, to confer on its users a kind of quiet calm. But in the nineteenth century, long before the drug was commonly applied for psychiatric purposes, lithium came to be prized for its ability to alkalinise excessively acidic urine. According to the doctors of yesteryear, uric acid was responsible for all manner of serious problems, not only gout, which in fact does arise from too much uric acid in the joints, but also bladder stones and renal stones, feelings of faintness, migraine headaches, instability of mood, low tone, lack of appetite, swathes of sadness, surpluses of delight, irritable excitement, epileptic fits, tumours and tics and flus and fevers of every sort. Many doctors further believed that lithium, this strange white salt, could eliminate uric acid, meaning that lithium was therefore seen as a salve for practically every illness.

But because the vast majority of diseases and disorders are not, in fact, caused by or even in any way related to high uric acid or to gout, it stands to reason that most patients treated with lithium in the nineteenth century and beyond did not get well. It is true that lithium salts make urine more alkaline, but that's irrelevant if one is suffering from, say, diabetes, a disorder rooted in insulin resistance, and one that would therefore not have responded to a change in urine metabolism in any way. And yet treatment with lithium salts for all kinds of physical and mental complaints continued well into the twentieth century, and did not disappear from texts like *The Merck Index* and *The Pharmacopoeia* until as late as 1940. In other words, a treatment that we now know to have had no effect on almost all patient complaints, a treatment that failed time and time again, nevertheless lived a long and healthy life. Why, when the diabetic remained diabetic even after lithium administration, or when the migraine sufferer still had hammers in his head, did these mounting failures not put an end to what seems, in our day and age, to be an overly simplistic if not outright foolish notion, the linking of complex and varied diseases to a simple stream of urine and the acid found within it?

There is one possible explanation for the long and vital life of what has come to be called the uric acid diathesis: the treatment – administration of lithium salts – made patients feel good. Even if their bodies were still suffering, the patients' minds were nevertheless soothed by what we now know is a potent psychoactive drug. Researchers, for instance, have measured the amount of naturally occurring lithium in tap water in twenty-seven counties in Texas and found a negative association between lithium levels in the water and suicide rates, meaning the higher the level of lithium in the water, the lower the suicide rate. Similar studies have been carried out elsewhere, such as in Japan, where researchers studied the tap water of eighteen districts of the Ōita Prefecture and noted that even very low levels of lithium in the water supply may be protective against suicide, and by extension against depression as well. Until 1948, the lemon–lime flavoured soft drink 7UP, popular in the United States, contained lithium citrate, a little boost contained in a drink. F. Neil Johnson, the author of a history of lithium therapy, published a letter he received from an unnamed correspondent whose mother, a depressive, was prescribed lithium for something unrelated, and who recalled its effect on her:

I was born in 1917 and soon afterwards my mother ... suffered a depressive illness for which she was admitted to [the hospital] ... When I was quite a young child she suffered from 'gravel' for which she was prescribed lithium citrate and this she took for almost all the rest of her life ... Aged 73 she began to be incontinent ... and at operation the urologist removed a pear-sized stone from her bladder ... Post-operatively she discontinued the lithium citrate as there seemed no need for it. Six months later ... she suddenly broke down with agitated depression from which she suffered for seven and a half years until her death.

The medicinal use of lithium was first discovered by Alexander Ure, a Scottish surgeon, who gave a talk in 1843 about how lithium, 'a substance of which no therapeutic action has been heretofore made', could dissolve bladder stones. Ure went on to show his audience an actual stone that had significantly shrunk after immersion in a lithium bath. Sir Alfred Garrod, at one point Queen Victoria's doctor, repeated Ure's experiment but this time on gout deposits rather than bladder stones. Garrod reasoned, correctly, that gout was caused by excess uric acid in the body, and it was he who went on to promulgate the theory that many other diseases could also stem from this excess, thereby conceiving of the uric acid diathesis.

Lithium Spas

Lithium was usually administered to patients in a carbonate solution until, in the mid-nineteenth century, spas and springs became popular. Various regions in England and continental Europe boasted natural mineral springs said to contain high concentrates of lithium, and doctors would 'prescribe' a dip in these springs to their ailing patients, who were usually well-to-do and willing to travel, sometimes hundreds of miles. Entrepreneurs took note. By the late nineteenth century, hydropathic establishments were proliferating. At the same time, companies selling potable lithium water in bottles made of clear green glass, with pop-off tin tops, flourished both in the United States and abroad as well-known doctors endorsed lithium, making public statements about the benefits one could derive from the spas and springs and drinks. The list of ailments that the waters could putatively cure included prostate enlargements, gonorrhoea, cystitis, portal vein congestion, jaundice, hepatic diabetes, obesity and atonic dyspepsia, to name just a few. So many famous doctors chimed in that a powerful consensus formed about how potent these waters really were, with medical journals publishing report after report of hydro successes.

But as the coffers of the spa resorts and the bottled-lithium makers rapidly filled, some scientists began to question just what these waters were made of. The first sceptical report, published in 1889, came from a chemist who announced that the lithium content of commercially available spring water was in fact much lower than the label advertised. Similar reports followed, including an 1896 claim that an analysis of three of the most widely consumed brands of lithium waters had found absolutely no lithium in two of them. It took a while, but by 1914 a lawsuit again Buffalo Lithia Water finally reached the Supreme Court of the District of Columbia, which rendered this unequivocal opinion: 'For a person to obtain a therapeutic dose of lithium by drinking Buffalo Lithia Water he would have to drink from one hundred and fifty thousand to two hundred and twenty-five thousand gallons of water per day ... Potomac River water contains five times as much lithium per gallon as the water in controversy.'

Unsurprisingly, the happy hydro industry went south, and by the early 1920s bottled lithium water was no longer widely available. With it, one might surmise, went the uric acid diathesis. Instead, although the credibility of the hydropathic establishment went to waste, the uric acid diathesis stayed as strong as ever. In place of bottled water, lithium tablets were brought to market, which allowed any sufferer to make his or her own liquid concoction and control the concentration at the same time.

Lithium for Depression

While, in the nineteenth century, lithium was used primarily to treat a variety of illnesses beyond the brain, some doctors of the time did note the drug's efficacy in reversing states of depression or despair, as had happened with the dye methylene blue. In 1888, British doctor Alexander Haig, following a series of experiments on both himself and others, suggested that high uric acid was correlated with certain sorts of depression, and that any drug that lowered uric acid levels, as lithium did, would be a beneficial psychiatric treatment. Two years later Carl Lange, a Danish internist familiar with Haig's work, published a description of what he called 'periodical depression', a psychological state that many of his patients seemed to suffer from. This sort of depression wafted like the wind; it came and then it went, but it always came back again. Lange was the first to use lithium prophylactically – and for a psychiatric condition. Around the same time, John Aulde, a Philadelphia doctor, also began to give it to his patients prior to their plunges and advised them to take it continually, in this way warding off 'the old trouble coming back'.

The prophylactic use of lithium in the treatment of depression would emerge again in the mid- to late twentieth century as a major and contentious issue, but at the time of the article in which Lange described his treatment protocol, no one took much notice, except perhaps his brother Fritz, who oversaw the Danish asylum at Middelfart. Fritz Lange followed his brother's lead by giving lithium to several hundred patients suffering from depression, in doses similar to what we would prescribe today. In 1894 Fritz published a book stating that the benefits of lithium treatment for depressives appeared just a few days after commencing the drug. Not as quickly as chlorpromazine would eventually act on psychotic patients, but swifter and more effective than any other medication then available.

The Collapse of the Uric Acid Diathesis

Given the prevalence of lithium and the iron grip of the theoretical rationale that underscored its use, how and why did the uric acid diathesis ever die out? Thomas Kuhn, writing about paradigm shifts in science in the twentieth century, describes how one set of beliefs gives way to another, seemingly more relevant set, and thus the scientific field progresses in fits and starts. But when it came to lithium and the uric acid diathesis, there was no single paradigm that displaced what was by all accounts a deep belief. Instead there was a series of pivotal discoveries – antibiotics, anaesthesia and the resultant advancement of surgery among them – that one might say eventually, and incrementally, stole the show.

The 1930s, for instance, saw the introduction of sulphonamides, a group of bacteria-inhibiting drugs, followed a decade later by the mass production of penicillin, which made its entry into medicine with a dramatic flourish. In 1942, in Boston, Massachusetts, a packed nightclub called the Cocoanut Grove caught fire, with people trapped in the flames and unable to escape. Nearly five hundred died, and hundreds more suffered burns over much of their bodies, their skin crisped and blackened. Ambulance after ambulance rushed the charred survivors to area hospitals. Inevitably, infection started to set in. Antibiotics were still in trial and thus not available, but Massachusetts General Hospital made a special plea to the pharmaceutical company Merck, located in New Jersey, to release some of the product to its doctors as soon as possible. Merck responded by sending 32 litres (7 gallons) of antibiotic ampules packed in ice, carried in a car flanked by policemen on motorcycles, the whole caravan making its way across one state and into another in a grand and solemn procession. Once the yet-to-be-tested antibiotic arrived at the hospital, the doctors broke open the ampules and delivered this new medicine to their burn victims, whose wounds by now were suppurating, festering with pus. Within hours these wounds began to clear up, and within days, when the bandages were unwrapped, newborn skin, as pink as the inner lip, was visible, the burns healing rather than rotting. The new drug, penicillin, a breakthrough miracle, was celebrated in print, on the radio and in conversations across the country.

But penicillin wasn't the one thing that eradicated the uric acid diathesis. The theory had been steadily fading for years, diminished by the arrival of antibiotics, along with the emergence of advanced anaesthetics, the development of steroids and diuretics, and anti-hypertensives and hypoglycaemic agents, many of which were mass-produced as chemical companies turned into pharmaceutical houses with corporate capitalistic agendas that shifted the emphasis away from the dinosaur days when urine ruled the roost.

Eventually the uric acid diathesis fell out of fashion, like cargo trousers and lace curtains. In an era that witnessed the first successful heart transplant, the notion that the whole of human pain could be explained by your urine had been rendered quaint. Into the vacuum created by this theory's exit rushed all manner of new inventions and discoveries, not only in medicine but also in astrophysics, in genetics, in biology. The world widened. The moon moved closer as NASA developed rocket fuel and dreamed of the travel that would one day come. We learned that stars have life cycles, that they begin as disorganised gasses and end as black holes, fathomless infinite pits of emptiness that are enough to make human depression look like a playdate in the park. Can it really be a surprise, then, that the diathesis slipped away, trampled by technology which was, every day, exceeding even itself in its range and reach?

The twentieth century left behind the diathesis and its sidekick, lithium, a little old salt from an old wives' tale that we once believed might help us, even heal us. Lithium slipped into the sea of old ideas, washed up on a beach littered with rocks and other discards. By the 1940s you couldn't get your hands on a lithium tablet if you tried. The drug was gone, long gone, except here and there, in preparations no one had ever heard of and certainly had never used.

Luckily for us, while the uric acid diathesis could and did die, taking lithium with it, the *substance* itself could never be completely extinguished. Of everything psychiatry has in its armamentarium, lithium is one of the only drugs that is not man-made. It is in and of Earth, or better yet the solar system, or better yet the universe, an element that pre-existed any human being and is therefore protected from propensities, from fashion. Gone was Buffalo Water, gone were the tablets from which one could concoct one's own soothing, but lithium is ineradicable. Thus when we returned to it – or when one specific, unusual and modest man returned to it, in 1946 – it was waiting there for him, in all its blinding white abundance.

A Beginning Down Under

The story starts again in suburban Australia when a young and keenly curious Australian doctor named John Cade was released from a Japanese POW camp at the end of the Second World War and sent back home to his family to begin a new life, a life he'd have to create in good faith, despite the atrocities he'd witnessed as a prisoner of war. It involves a gaggle of guinea pigs, a Melbourne mental hospital and a single hypothesis Cade had developed and nursed all through his wartime imprisonment.

Born in 1912 in a small country town in Victoria, Cade became a major in the 2nd/9th Field Ambulance, and was stationed in Singapore during the war. When the country fell to the Japanese, in February 1942, he was captured, shackled and blindfolded, with a bayonet pressed against his neck. Thereafter Cade was held as a prisoner of war for three and a half years, during which time he closely observed his fellow prisoners trying to cope with the brutality of their captors. The men at Changi camp were starved, a watery soup their only food, with vermin and filth everywhere.

It was during these three and a half years that Cade began to develop his hypothesis of mental illness and mental health, watching men as they broke beneath the stress of frequent beatings and starvation, their minds going waywards and opening to voices and visions, to extreme excitability in some cases or abject despair in others. Cade stayed sane throughout all the horrors by turning his imprisonment into a psychological and anthropological study that had at its heart a single question: what caused a mental breakdown, and why did some succumb while others remained steady? As he toiled in the camps, as he spooned watery soup into his mouth, as he lay on his pallet of crushed leaves and moss and listened to the moaning of many men, Cade developed this idea: mania, he believed, must be caused by an excess of some normal metabolite the body produced, while depression must be caused by a dearth of the same metabolite. Interned, he had no way of testing his notion, but as soon as he was freed, he returned 'mourning the wasted years and determined to pursue the ideas that had germinated in that interminable time'.

After his release, Cade was at last reunited with his wife and two young sons, the older of whom had been only three when his father left for Singapore. He resumed psychiatric work on New Year's Day in 1946, at the Bundoora Repatriation Mental Hospital, which had become Victoria's chief mental hospital for war veterans. Haunted by the lost years in lock-up and spurred, as always, by his curiosity, Cade went to work trying to discover what this crucial metabolite that he had theorised might be. Right from the get-go, then, his emphasis was on aetiology. He was a man who sought the source of human suffering, which set him apart from his colleagues in other countries, such as Delay and Deniker at Sainte-Anne, who did not really reflect on the pathophysiology of their patients' illnesses, and who, when presented with a drug to treat the delusions and hallucinations of schizophrenia, used it but appeared not to wonder *why* it worked, focusing instead on the purely empirical fact that it did. Cade, one might say, was a more ambitious scientist, seeking right from the start the biochemical substrates of mental pain, and willing to offer his own hypothesis based on nothing more than a hunch. He had his mental antennae tilted towards a world of molecular constellations, at the same time always observing the nuances of human gesture and language.

Cade's wife told a story from many years later of walking with him in the woods near Melbourne one time and happening upon some droppings still moist on the emerald leaves. Cade bent down to study them. After a moment, he straightened his spine, brushed off his knees and pronounced that an elephant had been there.

'John,' his wife said. 'Have you gone mad? We're in Australia.'

The couple continued to walk. After some time, the woods gave way to a clearing, in which stood a circus, complete with elephants. Astonished, Cade's wife turned to him and asked him how he had known. Cade explained that he remembered how the droppings looked from photographs he had taken of these massive mammals at the zoo.

Now, with his psychiatric work resumed, he was ready to turn his highly absorbent brain towards the problems and possibilities of madness – the madness of deep despair, when all the world is stripped of contour and colour, and the madness of mania, with its high-flying colours and tossing trees and swirling skirts and screams. Where, however, to start? This metabolite, whether in excess or dearth, could be anywhere in the body or in the brain, which is itself crammed with billions of neurons. 'Because I did not know what the substance might be,' wrote Cade, as he stood on the threshold of this moment, 'still less anything of the pharmacology for lower animals, the best plan seemed to be to spread the net as wide as possible and use the crudest form of biological test in a preliminary investigation.'

Cade and Guinea Pigs: The First Experiment

Cade and his wife by now had several children – three more were born after his return – and to the children the guinea pigs were pets. The family kept their guinea pigs caged in the back garden and they quickly became Cade's first experimental subjects. Influenced by his predecessors, Cade opted to start his search for the metabolite with urine. The protocol: manic, depressed and schizophrenic patients on the wards of the Repatriation Hospital were to abstain from fluids for twelve to fourteen hours (overnight) before the following morning's samples were collected, so long that the concentrated urine was swimming with sediment. Cade also took urine from controls, individuals not suffering from a mental illness.

Once he had adequate samples, which one of Cade's sons remembers his father storing in the family refrigerator, Cade set about injecting the urine – both the 'clean' urine and the urine from schizophrenic, manic and depressed patients – into the abdomens of his guinea pigs. What he found was that the urine 'from the manic patients proved to be far more toxic than from the other groups, although all the samples led to deaths among the animals.' As Cade acknowledged, though, 'all that had been demonstrated so far was that any concentrated urine in sufficient quantity would kill a guinea pig, but that the urine from a manic subject often killed much more readily.'

Thinking that the uric acid might be the element in the urine responsible for the deaths, Cade began to investigate the effects of uric acid on overall urea toxicity. Because uric acid is insoluble in water, Cade began adding lithium salts to his samples, in an effort to make the uric acid dissolve. He noted that the presence of lithium made the urea less toxic. That made him wonder how lithium used alone would affect the guinea pigs. He injected large doses of it into the abdomens of the animals.

Cade was surprised, even stunned, by what happened next:

After a latent period of about two hours, the animals, although fully conscious, became extremely lethargic and unresponsive to stimuli for one to two hours ... Those who have experimented with guinea pigs know to what extent a ready startle reaction is part of their make-up. It was thus even more startling to the experimenter to find that after the injection of a solution of lithium carbonate they could be turned on their backs and that, instead of their usual frantic righting reflex behaviour, they merely lay there and gazed placidly back at him.

Cade thought he was on to something here, and clearly he was. He had administered to usually timid, anxiety-prone animals a solution that eradicated these propensities and produced a quiet calm. For a psychiatrist at a large asylum jam-packed with raving patients, it must have been mere moments before Cade wondered what effect this lithium would have on his charges. Before conducting that experiment, however, Cade tried the lithium solution on himself. We don't know if he was scared or worried or confident, although surely he was curious. Surely he must have sat very still once he was done, waiting to feel whatever effects there might be. He must have been alert, and if the wind was in the trees, he must have heard it more keenly and wondered whether this was the drug or simply his heightened senses. Trying it several times over the course of a few weeks, Cade felt only mild ill effects: some transient nausea but nothing else. At that point, he surely must have smiled.

After all, this might be very good news for an asylum crammed full of maniacal people with bent and broken ideas: men who believed spies lived in the white walls and whispered to them day and night. Women who careened down the corridors wearing lipstick so poorly applied that it made their mouths look brutal, pulped. Patients who could not sleep and so stayed up, dreamless and full of despair. People in such severe pain that even modest movement seemed too much of an effort – all purpose, all point, having been drained from lives lost years ago. Worst of all, though, were the ones who believed they were brilliant, whose chatter never ceased, words surging from their mouths in a stream of nonsensical sounds, their eyes bright with ideas that formed so fast they toppled one over the other like a house of cards continually coming down, unable to be soothed, clenched in a continual saga of operatic proportions that exhausted everyone around them, especially the nurses.

Cade must have thought of them, and then thought of his guinea pigs resting easy on their backs, willing to be scratched, to be touched. Many hospital dispensaries had huge vats of lithium left over from the nineteenth century, so theoretically the drug would have been available to Cade. Even if the canister was furred with dust, as long as it was still sealed, the salt would be pure.

A Night Drive

I've never lived in a large asylum like the one over which Cade presided. The mental hospitals I've lived in have all been decidedly undramatic, single floors in general medical centres, the meal trolley wheeled off the lift three times per day, the forks and knives always plastic. As a thirteen-year-old girl, I used to watch Rosemary, a wisp of a woman, young and pretty, her eyes spilling a perpetual overflow of tears, until the liquid snaked slowly down her face, dangling at the edge of her chin and finally falling with a noise I swear I could hear, the quietest kind of crash. I used to listen to Gerry as he sprinted up and down the halls belting, 'Some people sit on their butts, got the dream, yeah, but not the guts.' While Rosemary was silent and still, Gerry was the opposite, a constant whir of motion and a continuous spew of sound, a carousel of Shakespeare and Ethel Merman and passages from huge tomes he'd drag into the dayroom to either stand on or read from. *The Count of Monte Cristo* was one of his favourites. Gerry had so much energy he hardly ever slept, not even after his nightly tablet, which was big and blue and which he'd only pretend to swallow, spitting it into his cupped palm once the night nurse turned her back, winking at me as he did so. 'Kiddo,' he called me. 'Poet.' He claimed he was a professor at Harvard, and who knows, maybe he once had been. But mania had got its teeth in him just as depression had seized hold of Rosemary, both of them pinioned in entirely opposite ways.

As for me, I was just a mixed-up adolescent who modelled herself after Sylvia Plath. In the beginning at least, mental illness for me was some form of drama, of dangerous play, the razor so sharp it sliced the skin on my arms with barely any pain, blood rushing up and welling in the wounds I made, every one of which fascinated me. I flirted with mental illness when I was a teenager, but by the time I turned twenty the flirtation was over and I was seriously sick. Fluoxetine rescued me for decades when I was in my twenties, thirties and forties, enabling me to write several books and marry a man who was gentle and give birth to two babies. But even with all my abundance and all that extra serotonin, the sickness came back and back, morphing each time like a cruel chameleon, manifesting sometimes as obsessive-compulsive disorder and other times as generalised anxiety disorder, which is a name far too banal and clinical to adequately describe the terror of that condition, a terror so true and fanged that it can loosen your bowels as you crouch in some corner and cry.

My last breakdown occurred seven years ago and involved, like lithium itself, stones. I became, at first, enamoured of stones; they were everywhere and each one was precious. No one knew this but me. I was living on a planet rife with precious heft, and I'd rush down the street collecting these gems, filling my pockets. Soon my study at home was piled high, and the heaps spilled into the hall and clattered down our steep stairs as my children and husband looked on in a kind of horror. I was gleeful, exuberant, because we were rich, we had stones, and it was just a matter of time before everyone else realised that when you held a simple rock you were clutching all of human history in your plain old palm, the rock millions, maybe billions of years old, its veins and pathways and sedimentary layers suggesting song and deep space and even the Big Bang itself. So excited was I by stones that I stopped sleeping and stayed up all night polishing my treasures with an electric grinder, and indeed I can say in sanity that there was something lovely about seeing a plain old stone with its grit gone, seeing its speckled or mottled hide, its blue hue or emerald artery. Yes, stones can be lovely, but in my manic state they were everything and I was on to something so special that sooner rather than later the whole world would go along with me.

The major problem with mania is the inevitable depression that comes in its wake, and the more manic you are, the more depressed you will get, as if there is some law, or even some kind of divine punishment, for going up so high, because you will then go down proportionally so low and for the same period of time. True, there are the *rare* cases of people who have only mania; they somehow manage to be both blessed and cursed with only half of the bipolar diagnosis, and so we call them unipolar, a condition that many of them love, even as they irritate to pieces all the people around them and make terrible messes of their lives.

But by far the most common conclusion to mania is the aftermath of depression, which for me did not come slowly or with subtlety. It was like having the turf pulled out from under me; a *whisk* and a *whoa* and all of a sudden, in a single and terrible second, I recognised that I was a forty-something female standing amidst stones that were scattered everywhere in her study and, worse, stored everywhere in her house, so that when you opened the cupboard, stones came tumbling out on to your toes. I had no energy, certainly not enough to clear away the stones, and besides that, I was embarrassed. I suddenly saw myself in a whole new light, or darkness may be the better word, a weird crazy old lady collecting pebbles and in some cases serious slabs that weighed as much as 4.5 or 9 kilograms (10 or 20 lb). What had come over me? And what was coming over me now, this dread, this fear, this gulf, this grief, this terrible understanding of time, which moved so slowly I could see it, that cruel second hand inching its way around the surface of an equally cruel clock with filigreed numbering on an otherwise blank white face, a huge moon face that mocked me from its place on the wall in the hall.

I backed up. I backed away. I wanted to cry, and I remembered Rosemary, who'd had such unrestrained grief. Crying would have been a real release for me, and it would have also shown, to others, something of what I was now feeling inside; words could not do it justice but wetness would, or could. But I had no tears. My eyes were little scorched sockets, two holes in my head, that's all. So I closed them and tried to go to sleep but I felt the heaviness of the house all around me, what with all these stones. I managed to call a contractor to come take them away. 'What were you using them for?' he asked me as he whisked the last batch out the door. 'I had this idea,' I said to him, but then I could not finish the sentence. There was no way to explain the ridiculousness of my collecting obsession, so instead I shoved money into his hand and turned away.

Now, without the mania, the nights were terrible. Sleep evaded me or, worse, came over me for only seconds at a time, the drift of a dream and the sudden snatch back into the blackness. I went driving then. I'd wake up and stuff my feet into dirty slippers and get into my car and drive the roads flanked with trees tremulous in the wind, the moon a sliver so small it threatened to disappear. I had a recurring thought: that one day the sun would never set. It would burn on and on, past five o'clock, past six o'clock, past nine and then ten o'clock, the sky stubbornly bright as our yellow star flared on and on, the heat high and the night-time driven down and out. A world in which there was no darkness, not even dusk, no crisp coolness, the lawns parched and everyone trapped in a white hysterical light.

I dreaded the daylight because it provided too clear a contrast to the black ooze that was inside me. The nights, even though they rarely offered me the relief of sleep, were somewhat soothing, and so I cruised the empty roads, past darkened shopfronts and houses with every window snuffed. Sometimes I heard things: the yowl of a cat, the whir of wings, the coyotes as they exited the forest. I became confused as to what sounds were real and what were imaginary. Had I hallucinated a fox whisking over moss with a mouse in his mouth? I drove deep into the countryside, where there were no street lights, and yet still, somehow, I saw a black hat, like a magician's hat, roll slowly across the road and disappear down an embankment.

I stopped the car, stepped out. I wanted to catch that hat but it was gone. Even though the darkness was dense I had seen it specifically, perfectly, a tall black hat full of endless silver scarves, a hat I'd put on my head for an instantaneous cure. Above me circled a large hawk, and my eyes were suddenly so sharp I could see the rabbit clasped in its beak; I could see the blood on the rabbit's hide, its paws pedalling the air in a frantic motion. Frightened, I stepped back into the car and resumed driving, fast, and it happened in just a shaving of a second, this shadow whipping across the road, the stick-thin legs of a little girl who carried, in each of her upturned palms, toads that glowed from within. I swerved but it was too late. I hit her anyway. When my car made contact, though, she did not go down. This ghost girl merely melted and the toads became winged things that went as high as the sky, until they too were gone.

I had hit a girl, or so it seemed, but she was nowhere on the road; she had disappeared into droplets and risen up. I kept going. Now the girl was following my car on a carpet that flew and she was singing a song so mournful and accusatory that my heart burbled and seemed to claw at my chest. After some time, her song turned to tears and then the night was over and the sun climbed a vine high in the sky. I heard that girl all that day and all the next day and then the days turned to weeks and still she wept in my ear.

My psychiatrist, meanwhile, was writing me prescriptions:

ziprasidone, aripiprazole, risperidone. I was desperate enough to try anything. And then one day my doctor suggested a drug called Zyprexa (olanzapine), the name of which sounded to me like a musical instrument, an accordion from which you could gently squeeze a song. Zyprexa, a prescription I filled. I took the first tablet in the evening, the second tablet the following morning, and within a mere three days something clicked inside me and suddenly I was back in balance again. I remembered everything that had happened, the mania of stones, the grief and the girl's high cry, but primarily I was grateful, as I always am, whenever I come through a psychiatric event – or let's call it what it is: a breakdown. I've had many in my life, and one of their side effects, so to speak, is gratitude, because there is nothing so sweet after a breakdown as returning to the normal world and tasting curry or asparagus or buttered corn on the cob. In the case of olanzapine, the drug increases your appetite while simultaneously slowing down your metabolism, so in short order I got fat, but this seemed a small price to pay for my sanity. Then I got diabetes, another potential side effect of olanzapine, but even this seemed a price worth paying.

I don't want to go back. I know, however, that sooner or later I will. My adulthood has been marked – marred – by periodic depressions preceded by stupid, inane manias. This is who I am, like it or not.

An Element Becomes a Twentieth-Century Drug

Cade's patients were worse than I am but only by degrees. The reason I have not been hospitalised in over thirty years is that I have learned how to have breakdowns in the comfort of my own home. Many of Cade's patients, by contrast, were long-term residents of the asylum, and these chronic cases were the ones that most interested him for lithium experimentation, because he believed that 'in them spontaneous remission is far less likely to occur'.

It remains unclear whether Cade was familiar with any of the published reports from doctors like the Lange brothers of Denmark and Sir Alfred Garrod, all of whom had used lithium to treat madness with some success in the previous century. His notes suggest that he was, and that he also had awareness of the potential deleterious effects of the drug and of the dosing instructions in the literature of the nineteenth and early twentieth centuries. Nevertheless, 'How to proceed?' Cade wrote in his notebook. '*Primum non nocere*. The older pharmacopoeias did not describe any toxic effects of lithium salts but was that good enough? There is always the number one experimental animal, oneself.' That conclusion didn't really please Cade's family. As one of his sons recalled, 'Our kitchen refrigerator usually had jars of manic patients' urine and racks of blood samples in it, always on the top shelf and much to my mother's consternation. Her greatest distress was when Dad started taking lithium carbonate himself for a few weeks before giving it to patients.'

We can consider it a great relief that Cade felt no ill effects whatsoever from the lithium, because if he had, the history of psychiatry and the fate of millions of men and women would likely have been completely altered, and for the worse. Instead, having deemed the drug safe, he brought it to his patients, deciding the dose on the basis not of prior medical evidence but of his own experience. In total he treated nineteen patients, ten with mania. Of those ten, three had chronic mania and seven had recurrent mania. He also dosed several schizophrenic patients and three patients with deep depressions.

W. B. was possibly the patient who meant the most to Cade. His was a chronic case of severe and unremitting mania that rendered the patient, long regarded as 'the most troublesome in the ward', utterly disabled and confused. W. B. was fifty-one years old at the time Cade gave him his first dose of lithium and had been 'in a state of typical manic excitement for five years, restless, dirty, destructive, mischievous, and interfering'. Cade started W. B. on lithium on 29 March 1948, and watched the metamorphosis unfold as this pest, this dirty and dishevelled man who had 'enjoyed preeminent nuisance value in a back ward for all those years and bid fair to remain there for the rest of his life', slowly settled down. Ever the cautious scientist, Cade was not sure he could credit the change to lithium, wondering if W. B.'s convalescence was due to Cade's own 'expectant imagination', noting three days after treatment had begun that it was April Fools' Day.

Within a mere three weeks, however, W. B.'s trajectory towards mental health became obvious to everyone. He ceased making life so difficult for others on the ward. He was polite and to the point. That W. B.'s brain was still intact was noteworthy, as his illness had been so long and so persistent that he might have been a candidate for lobotomy. Once Cade was sure of lithium's efficacy, he pointed out that the drug could and should be used in place of that severing scalpel.

A calmer, more reasoned W. B. eventually moved from the chronic ward to the convalescent ward, where he took in the new surroundings and tried to accustom himself to the slower tempo. 'He had been ill for so long', wrote Cade, that 'he found normal surroundings and liberty of movement strange at first'. But on 9 July 1948, a little over three months after treatment had begun, this apparently hopeless case was well enough to be released from the asylum with instructions to take five grains of lithium twice a day. Cade considered the transformation 'highly gratifying'. W. B. was now back at his old job and settling into a steady life – so steady, in fact, that over time he became lax about his lithium, at first just skipping a dose here and there and then, over a period of time, letting days slide by without the drug, until he finally ceased taking it altogether. Thus, on 30 January 1949, W. B. was readmitted to the asylum. In his private notes Cade wrote that it was with 'the most abject disappointment that I readmitted him to the hospital six months later as manic as ever'. W. B. was dirty and chattering and completely erratic, just as before. Once again he was started on a lithium regime and, once again, the illness receded and the person emerged from behind a set of scrambled symptoms, a little like a photograph in fluid, with the span of obliterating white slowly giving way to shape and form and detail.

Cade's original paper in which he reports on the effects of lithium on his cadre of patients is, in total, four pages long. It was titled simply 'Lithium Salts in the Treatment of Psychotic Excitement', and was published unassumingly, in September 1949, in the *Medical Journal of Australia*. Cade's writing is spare and decidedly undramatic, consistent with the man's modesty and his attachment to the scientific argot. Psychiatrist Barry Blackwell wrote, 'Cade's research ... is remarkable because it is the very first scientific evidence of a biological cause leading to drug treatment for a major psychiatric disorder, made almost three years before the discovery of chlorpromazine for schizophrenia.'

Cade's paper gives only hints of the thrill and the sense of mystery he must have felt as he watched patient after patient emerge from a manic twilight. Of his second subject, Cade wrote:

> E. A., a male, aged forty-six years, had been in a chronic manic state for five years. He commenced taking lithium citrate, 20 grains three times a day, on May 5, 1948. In a fortnight he had settled down, was transferred to the convalescent ward in another week, and a month later, having continued well, was permitted to go on indefinite trial leave whilst taking lithium citrate 10 grains three times a day. This was reduced in one month to 10 grains twice a day, and two months later to 10 grains once a day. Seen on February 13, 1949, he remained well and had been in full employment for three months.

All of the published case studies in Cade's first lithium paper read as above, bare-boned and almost, if not entirely, emotionless. But while the paper reads like a book report, the case notes make it clear that Cade was an empathic clinician as well as an objective scientist. His case notes give glints of his character, his heart, his hopes. After all, while grounded in reality always, he was also the man who had spent years in captivity, a man with a muscular mind that had built hypotheses which allowed him to survive the incarceration and torture that many others did not.

The Dark Side of Lithium

It was the scientist in Cade, however, who noted which patients lithium did and did not help. The schizophrenic patients, for instance, responded to lithium, but much differently than did the manic patients. While the manic patients who took the lithium got better, and got better fast, the schizophrenic patients who took lithium ceased their uproar but were as mad as ever, their hallucinations and delusions continuing unabated. This suggests something highly significant: unlike chlorpromazine (then unknown), which wiped out psychosis but acted, at the same time, as a major tranquilliser, making it unclear whether the drug was treating a specific set of symptoms or was simply subduing those who took it, lithium seemed much more selective in its actions. It appeared, therefore, that the drug targeted specific neural networks rather than blanketing the whole brain. Cade hypothesised that in manic patients there might be a deficiency of lithium ions which the drug was now restoring, allowing those so afflicted to return at long last to normalcy.

The one group of people who were not helped by lithium were Cade's depressed patients, and subsequent studies by other researchers confirmed that outcome. R. M. Young, deputy medical superintendent of Parkside Hospital in Macclesfield, England, near Manchester, actually found, in 1949, that lithium salts could aggravate 'endogenous depressive states', but like Cade, he also found that the effects on patients suffering from mania were stellar.

In time, however, some of lithium's darker, dangerous aspects were revealed. W. B., for instance, experienced severe nausea while being treated with lithium, and after his second release his side effects became so severe he had to be readmitted to the hospital with a frank case of lithium poisoning: dyspepsia, fever, nocturnal vomiting, diarrhoea and bradycardia, an abnormal slowing of the heart rate. After the bradycardia persisted for a month, his dosage was lowered, and then he was taken off lithium altogether. Two months later, Cade wrote, W. B. was 'back to his old form again – restless, dirty, mischievous, destructive and thoroughly pleased with himself'. According to historian F. Neil Johnson, 'he remained in this state for just over a week, becoming emaciated and developing infected self-inflicted sores'. Hence, once again, W. B. was started back on his lithium regime and, once again, he calmed down considerably. But as it turned out, he would tolerate the lithium treatment for only one more week, at the end of which his body started to seize as he faded into semiconsciousness. Once more the lithium was withdrawn, but this time too late. On 22 May 1950, Cade reported that W. B.'s skin was 'breaking down everywhere'; he was 'in extremis', with 'continuous myoclonic twitching'. The following day, Cade wrote in his case notes that W. B. had died from 'toxaemia due to lithium salts therapeutically administered'. Thus his first lithium patient – the one who had responded to the drug with such stunning success, emerging from a five-year mania to become in all respects a solid citizen, holding down a job and engaging appropriately with family and friends – was killed by the very drug that had given him back his life.

No One Listened

Cade did not discuss the dangerous side of lithium in his 1949 paper. After all, despite the fact that lithium could be toxic, it was also, clearly, a kind of miracle drug, yanking insane people back into the quotidian world and doing so quickly, eradicating the

seething and spectacular fantasies of those made mad by their
manias. Cade hoped the world would recognise what he had discovered. A four-page compendium of miniature biographies in
which one ordinary citizen after another was saved the same way –
by salt from a stone – was without doubt a revolutionary treatise.
And yet, at least in the beginning, the paper stirred little interest.

The oversight was massive, considering that Cade's work clearly
suggested that there could very well be a cure for a crippling
psychological disorder. Beyond that, even when lithium failed to
cure completely – with depressives, for instance – it nevertheless
seemed capable of targeting specific symptoms in a way no other
medication could. In the 1940s and '50s, psychiatrists had at their
disposal very few chemical options. The barbiturates, discovered
in 1903, broadly sedated people, as did morphine and, eventually,
chlorpromazine. But these were broad-brush drugs, blanketing the
entire brain in syrupy side effects, whereas lithium, it appeared,
went straight to the site of 'excitement' and dampened it, leaving
other neural functions and their behavioural sequelae relatively
untouched. Lithium, therefore, was the first 'magic bullet', a site-
specific drug, or at least a *symptom*-specific drug, auguring what
would follow decades down the line: the selective serotonin reuptake inhibitors (SSRIs) such as fluoxetine and sertraline, hailed
because they could – supposedly – work on a single neurotransmitter system without involving the entire brain, unlike the 'dirty'
drugs that had preceded them. Lithium, it could be argued, was
psychiatry's first clean drug, modifying a discrete set of symptoms
without spread or stain.

But all this – the specificity, the lives lost and then regained, the
implications for treatment, the tale of how it had all happened with
guinea pigs in the garden and one man and his hypothesis built
bit by bit in a POW camp – fell mostly on deaf ears. If lithium had
been a synthetic drug that a chemical company could have com-
peted for, Cade might have found himself instantly famous and
potentially quite rich, but this was not the case. The drug was a

simple salt. It came from a stone; it could be found by the seaside. These facts made it all but prosaic. It didn't cost a ten pence piece. It wasn't made in a lab by spinning complex molecular constellations together. And because there was no way to patent the drug, no great profit motive existed.

There were a relatively small number of studies following up on Cade's work, including four in Australia and ten in France. And among the few who did take note was the aforementioned English doctor R. M. Young. Upon reading a summary of Cade's paper in 1949, Young 'found a supply of effervescent lithium citrate on the back shelf of the dispensary'. He wrote that, after giving the lithium citrate to his patients in a double dose, as instructed by the Australian article, he 'was immediately converted by the dramatic way in which the manic symptoms were switched off in a few days'. Otherwise Cade's paper seemed largely to disappear.

A Champion in Europe

In 1952, however, three years after Cade published his findings, Danish psychiatrist Erik Strömgren, head of Aarhus University's psychiatric clinic in Risskov, came across Cade's case histories and then turned them over to Mogens Schou, a junior psychiatrist, suggesting to Schou that here was a topic he might want to investigate. Mogens Schou claimed he had 'caught' psychiatry from his father, who practised throughout Schou's childhood at a provincial mental hospital which housed psychiatric and epileptic patients. Schou recalled how his father built what he termed a 'nervesanatorium', the purpose of which was to treat neurotic patients. It ministered mostly to those with 'light psychoses' and 'mild depressions'. Schou, immersed from his youngest days in the despair of other people, clearly remembered the 'drooping attitudes' and the 'disconsolate faces' of the men and women who wandered in a park surrounding the hospital as the trees cast their shadows on to the verdant grounds.

Schou was struck – both as a youngster and, later, as a psychiatrist himself – by the absence of effective treatment for psychological illness. Thus when he read in Cade's paper not only about W. B.'s emergence from madness but also about the eight other patients who were cured, many of them living outside the asylum and holding down regular jobs, his interest was more than piqued. Here, finally, was a compound that might be more effective than the barbiturates, which simply put patients to sleep, or opium drops, which relieved despair but replaced it with either addiction or somnolence. As Schou would say several decades later, he was convinced from the beginning that 'Cade's paper would soon have become known, and it unavoidably struck the clinical by its vivid descriptions of the patients and their responses to the treatment.'

After reading Cade's study, Schou, along with several other colleagues in the hospital where he worked, set up a clinical trial aiming to test the anti-manic action of lithium. Their methodology was quite different from Cade's and notable for its complex design. The patients with more prolonged manias participated in a double-blind design that shifted between lithium and a placebo, while those with more frequent manic episodes were treated with lithium continually. In total thirty-eight patients were treated. Schou's study was, in fact, the first placebo-controlled trial ever to occur in psychopharmacology.

In 1954 he published his findings, which were largely consistent with Cade's. Lithium had a therapeutic and specifically an anti-manic effect in patients with bipolar disorder. When the manic patients in the study were switched from lithium to the placebo, they relapsed. One patient died during the study, but Schou claimed that the death was due not to lithium toxicity but to a pre-existing heart condition. Schou's paper and his study differed from Cade's in at least two significant ways, one being the double-blind, placebo-controlled design, the second being the use of a recently invented device called a flame spectrophotometer, which allowed the Danish research team to monitor the serum blood levels of lithium in their study participants, and to correlate those levels with possible toxic side effects.

Can Lithium Cure Depression?

Over the next several years Schou continued to experiment with lithium, and by 1959 he was able to report that he had treated in total 167 manic-depressive patients with the drug and that 77 per cent of them had significantly improved. Meanwhile, scientists in other countries were beginning to take note, as Cade's paper combined with Schou's research finally began having an effect. In France there were two reports of thirty-five patients treated with lithium, with an 86 per cent improvement rate. In England researchers treated thirty-seven patients and got a 92 per cent improvement rate. Ten years after Cade's paper was originally published, there were records on 718 manic patients treated with lithium, and 64 per cent of them, according to their doctors, had shown 'discernable improvement'.

One day, in reviewing his records, Schou noted that one man had responded to lithium with a reduction not only in his manic episodes but in his depressive episodes as well. (Cade had found that lithium did not help lift depressions once they were started, while Schou hypothesised that lithium might work prophylactically, preventing a depression from occurring in the first place.) This set Schou to thinking. Might lithium be an effective prophylaxis against the depressive cycle in bipolar disorder? Mania and depression, after all, in true bipolar disorder, are hitched at the hip, one following the other with real regularity and, in doing so, suggesting that, although depression and mania might be 'symptomatically different', they also might share a common source or substrate. And if this in fact was the case, then was it not also reasonable to hypothesise that lithium would be an effective agent in treating each of the polarised mood states that constitute manic depression?

Here is where Poul Christian Baastrup, a fellow Dane who had read Schou's studies, enters the picture. In 1957 Baastrup carried out his own clinical trial at the state hospital in Vordingborg and found the same thing all the other researchers had found, namely, that lithium dampened, if not destroyed, manic excitation. As part of his trial he conducted follow-up examinations on discharged patients, all of whom had been ordered to cease taking lithium because Baastrup wanted to determine whether lithium might cause late and undesired side effects. 'The result', wrote Baastrup, 'was hair-raising'. A number of study participants had not listened to him. Instead, 'eight patients, all with a bipolar course, had continued to take lithium and two of them had even bestowed these "miracle pills" upon manic-depressive relatives. None of these people had had any kind of check-up, of course. Their reason for continuing the treatment in spite of our agreement was consistent: all of them said that continuous lithium treatment *prevented psychotic relapse.*'

Baastrup went on to do a retrospective study of patients on lithium in order to examine more closely whether the drug really did have a prophylactic effect on manic and depressive psychoses. He looked back over the three years during which his patients had been on lithium and compared their rates of relapse during this time to their rates of relapse when they had not been on lithium. When he published his results several years later, in 1964, the evidence was compelling. Lithium, according to Baastrup's findings, did indeed prevent recurrences of depressive episodes in patients suffering from bipolar disorder.

Meanwhile, Geoffrey P. Hartigan, a psychiatrist working around the same time at St Augustine's Hospital in Canterbury, England, gave lithium to twenty of his patients, most of them with chronic or intermittent manic episodes, except for a group of seven who suffered from recurrent depression only. Five of these seven, once started on lithium treatment, did not merely recover from their current depression but ceased having recurrences altogether. Hartigan did not publish his results, but he spoke about them at a meeting in 1959. While admitting there wasn't much in the published studies that was encouraging about lithium's chances of improving depressive syndromes, and cautioning against its use during an acute depressive episode, he nevertheless gave vivid accounts of five patients' struggles and successes.

The first, a man of forty-seven, had always been ineffectual and unassertive, a pale-as-plaster type with a timid and banal disposition, 'subject to spells of depression'. He occasionally attended therapy, drifting in and out of treatment, and, when his condition really worsened, submitted to courses of electroconvulsive shock. The current and concomitant seizure would relieve his mood for short periods of time, after which the dark dogs returned, again and again, and the patient found himself plodding along in an anaemic and desultory manner, his spirits sinking lower and lower each time a new bout took hold. At one point during this dreary existence, his mother and father both died within a month of each other and his symptoms became still more serious. He was admitted to the hospital, where Hartigan and the nursing staff persuaded him to try the lithium and to take it on a regular basis. 'He is now on a maintenance dose', Hartigan noted, 'and has remained symptom-free for the last eighteen months. His wife reports that during this period he has shown more self-confidence than ever before.'

Hartigan also reported on the graver case of a forty-eight-year-old man whose father had committed suicide and whose mother suffered from a 'nervous illness' of an unknown nature. In 1929 this man had tried to kill himself by slitting open his own throat with a pair of scissors. He was hospitalised and recovered from that depression, stayed well for many years, and then, in 1949, relapsed into a severe depressive episode which led to his rehospitalisation, whereupon he received thirteen electroshock treatments.

These seemed to straighten him out, and he was discharged, only to fall back into blackness five months later, when he was once again readmitted as an inpatient. This time around he underwent twelve more electroshock treatments, without success, until, in the summer of 1950, he submitted to the scalpel that severed the fibres of his brain: a prefrontal leucotomy. Even this extreme measure, however, did not bring this man peace of mind; he continued to fall back into states of dread and despair, necessitating many psychiatric hospital admissions.

It was during one of these admissions, in 1958, that Hartigan introduced him to lithium carbonate. The man developed, as a result of the drug, a tremor in his hands and a facial tic, but both patient and doctor stayed the course, lowering the dose and waiting to see what would happen. Over time, the tremors faded and the tic went away. Eventually the man was discharged from the hospital and he returned to work. Despite the severity of both his depressions and the types of treatment he had sought, Hartigan wrote that he stabilised and 'has kept very well since and says that he feels better now than he has for a long time. His present cheerful appearance at out-patients contrasts markedly with his former apprehensive and crestfallen demeanour.'

Schou heard about Hartigan's work from Hartigan himself, who wrote to Schou and subsequently sent him a copy of the talk he had given. Schou urged Hartigan to convert the speech into a publishable paper, but Hartigan, by nature a shy and self-effacing man, was hesitant. In 1961 Schou wrote to Hartigan to ask if he had any further clinical data. 'I am asking about this not only out of interest in the use of lithium in psychiatry', Schou confessed, 'but also because one of my brothers has been suffering from depressions that recur with great regularity.' Hartigan was sympathetic, but the revelation would later be used by others against Schou in a malicious way.

In fact what Schou had written to Hartigan was something of an understatement. Schou's younger brother was more or less decimated by the regular recurrence of his black moods. Schou eventually medicated his brother with lithium, and the results were dramatic, giving the man a whole new way to live a life that had previously been stunted by melancholy. Suddenly, the periodic depressions that had so plagued Schou's brother vanished. He was able to be reliable in ways that before had been impossible for him. In 1981, when Schou received an honorary degree from Aix-Marseille University, he described what his brother's depression and its disappearance had been like:

> From the age of twenty he suffered from repeated attacks of depression, which periodically made him unable, in spite of high intelligence, to carry out his chosen profession. The attacks usually lasted some months, and then disappeared, but they reappeared again and again, year after year, inevitably. Then, about fourteen years ago, he was started on a maintenance treatment with lithium, and since then he has not had a single depressive relapse. He still needs to take the medication to keep the disease under control, but functionally he is a cured man. You will understand what such a change meant to himself and to his wife and children, and how much of a miracle it appeared to us in the family. Fear of the future has been replaced by confidence and new hope.

A Promising Prescription

I have a recurrent nightmare, very simple, very stark. I dream of depression. I dream of a black hat rolling across a dark road, of a girl turning to sugar and swirling away. I dream I am hunched in a rocket roaring across space. Sometimes the images jumble. Ants are everywhere. Fish fly. Things snap. A whip. A wand. A whisper.

Once every night I dream these dreams. My sheets are wet with sweat. I dream my dreams summer, autumn, winter and spring. And always when I awaken it is with a sense of a great and grateful relief tinged with dread because I know what lies in store for me, somewhere down the line. Ever since the age of ten I have been regularly felled and then regularly resurrected, but the resurrection does not dilute the dread. Depression is so many things, but for me, primarily, it is the loss of love – my people falling away – and the loss of language, my words dwindling so low that my thought seems to move without rhythm or reason.

I had been on lithium before and hadn't found it helpful. The drug had never relieved my depressions or stabilised my mood. Furthermore, the white salt caused a tremor in my hands – just as with Hartigan's patient – a very slight, almost imperceptible tremble that became apparent only in my handwriting, which got shaky under the influence of the drug. The tablets are huge, fat white oblongs that leave in the throat the feeling of having swallowed a stone. Prescribed to me not as an anti-manic agent but rather as an adjunct to my antidepressant – a little step stool, so to speak, allowing fluoxetine to more easily influence my neurotransmitters, specifically serotonin – lithium turned out to be a dud. The effects of my SSRI were exactly the same whether 'lifted' by lithium or not. I must confess, however, that I never stayed on lithium long enough for it to really work. I disliked the tremble in my hand, the way words slipped sideways on the page, my sentences resembling ones composed by a nursery school child, tipping downwards and skating off the paper.

My doctor's surgery is in the cellar of one of the buildings at McLean, the large mental hospital in genteel Belmont, Massachusetts. Once a month, for the past thirty years, I have been coming to this old private asylum known for the famous people it has housed – Sylvia Plath, Anne Sexton, Robert Lowell, to name a few. The buildings, mostly red brick, are bearded with ivy, the paths between them pebbled, with fountains burbling and birds' nests spilling from the rafters of gracious entryways where ancient corbels hold up cresting roofs. It feels less like an asylum than a university campus, and the only sign it is the former is the occasional patient in a stained shirt walking aimlessly and mumbling to the voices in his head.

A rickety lift takes me down to the bowels of the building holding my doctor's surgery, and I step out into a long hall painted a dirty beige, with a complex mesh of leaking pipes overhead, their corroded copper gone green, the water pooling in small puddles on the concrete floor or dripping into plastic buckets the caretakers have set out. The closed blank doors lining either side of the hall, with no names or numbers or anything else to identify them, can appear a little magical. Often I imagine they open on to rooms filled with old copper baths, or skulls with trepanned holes, or a science lab from another century, with dusty test tubes stored in rusty racks.

At the end of the hall, my doctor's door was wedged open, which meant he was expecting me. He is a funny, frumpy man with curls framing his face and a bald scalp, like a clown's, except he is not scary. He wears baggy trousers and carries a rucksack bursting with books and papers and who knows what else. His office is a world I never tire of: a massive mahogany desk, papers stacked erratically in all corners of the room, a bubbling aquarium, the small half windows at ground level, so all you ever see is speckled dirt or the feet of the occasional passerby, the room dimly lit despite the long fluorescent tubing that runs the length of the water-stained ceiling.

In his spare time, my doctor collects gems and crystals from all over the world; displayed on his shelves are huge geodes halved by blades, so you can see their swirling centres, their galaxy of specks that look like embedded stars. Gems from South America, sea-blue, deep turquoise, royal purple. A scatter of crimson pebbles that might be from Mars or the moon, strange bumpy rocks that have a haunted history – you can tell just by looking at them – rocks that were once part of meteors hurtling through the heavens, broken-off bits that fell to Earth. Because of my former manic rock obsession, I take an interest in his collection, and before we start each session we talk about his newest acquisitions, from Belize or Chile or even Antarctica, with their seemingly endless and mesmerising depths of purple or teal interiors.

Today, however, was different. Today I was a woman on a mission. I walked into his office, breezed past his sizeable display cases, took my seat in front of his desk and crossed one leg purposefully over the other. Usually my doctor starts the session with the rote 'How are you?' but not this time. This time I began, catching his bright blue gaze and holding it in my own. 'I think I should be on lithium,' I said.

'Lithium?' he said. 'I love lithium. Lithium is a wonderful drug.'

'Why's that?' I asked.

'Studies show', my doctor said, 'that lithium can stop suicidal ideation. Isn't that something? If you have a patient in danger of killing himself, pop him on to lithium and chances are that idea will just waste away.'

'I'm not in danger of killing myself,' I said, and then related the reading I'd been doing about lithium acting as a prophylactic against recurring or periodic depressions of the sort I have.

'Your Zyprexa does the same thing,' my doctor said, referring to olanzapine as he lifted both hands to his chin, smoothing the skin there as if he were stroking an invisible beard.

'It might,' I said, but countered that with the weight gain, diabetes and dangerously high triglycerides, all serious side effects. 'Why not lithium?' I asked.

'You've been on lithium before,' he reminded me. 'And you didn't like it.'

'I wasn't on it for long enough. I'm willing now to really give it a go.'

My doctor, I could tell, did not much like this idea. I asked him if he was familiar with the work of Mogens Schou, and how research from the 1950s and '60s shows that lithium can prevent depressive recurrences, especially in those with a bipolar diagnosis, and to my surprise my doctor said no, he hadn't heard of any such thing. Zyprexa, meanwhile, was a newer (and, the thinking goes, better) medication, and a blockbuster at that, earning for its maker, Eli Lilly, billions of dollars a year as one of the most prescribed psychotropics in an ever more obese America. Weighing in at just over 72.5 kilograms (11 stone 6 lb) at only 152 centimetres (5 ft) tall, I was another example.

Behind me, the aquarium bubbled patiently and persistently, and I turned to look. The blue water was filled with fish floating like ghosts in and around the exotic rocks made to resemble ancient castles. The fish flickered. I reached over and sprinkled some of their food on the surface, and they all shot upwards, their mouths forming tiny o's. The biggest and fastest fish reached the surface first. He puffed himself up and ate with gusto.

Taking inspiration, I puffed myself up as well. 'I think if you read the studies of Mogens Schou and Poul Christian Baastrup,' I told my doctor, 'you'd be convinced, as am I.'

'Going off Zyprexa,' my doctor said, 'is no easy thing.'

But I insisted I was willing to try. And I was. I knew psychotropics could be hell to get off, but the thought of finding a drug that would reliably prevent my periodic depressions from recurring and that, unlike olanzapine, would not cause me to swell like a puffer fish, until my blood was thick with sugar and grease – that was something I was willing to fight for.

In the end, I won. My doctor took out his pen and wrote me a prescription for Eskalith, the brand name for an extended-release form of lithium. 'You have to go down slowly on the Zyprexa', he advised. 'You won't feel well. After one week of being completely off the Zyprexa, you can start in on the lithium.'

That night I shook a single olanzapine tablet out of its brown bottle and held it in my palm. Tiny writing embossed on the surface announced the name of its maker: *Lilly.* My doctor had instructed me to go down in increments of an eighth, but keen as I was to start the lithium, I ignored that injunction. I snapped the tablet smartly in half and popped it into the chute of my throat.

Olanzapine is intensely sedating, and that night, with only half a dose, I had some trouble sleeping. When slumber did finally come, I dreamt of monkeys perched on balconies in a strange hot city. I woke up parched with my head full of fizz and felt unbalanced all day. The second night I broke off just a quarter of a tablet and wound up awake until dawn, the daylight a fevered pink line, like an infection, at the seam of the sky. The fact that I knew why I felt the way I did was helpful. My good mood, my balance, was all but gone and I wobbled through the world as my body tried to figure out how to function without its daily dose.

Psychiatrists hate to admit that their drugs are no different in many senses from whatever you might buy on the street. Heroin addicts need to detox from heroin the same as olanzapine users need to detox from olanzapine. Detox is difficult – it's a burden on the body – but I knew, if I could just get through, that waiting on the other side was another kind of medication that might be even better. On a Sunday, while the kids were out with my husband, I lay in bed and looked at the prescription my doctor had given me, and decided that I would fill it when I was down to a sixteenth of a tablet, essentially just some dust and crumbles that I'd bite off and swill down with water.

I was off the olanzapine completely within four days. I felt, well, despairing. I was still on my antidepressant, but on its own it wasn't doing much to prop me up. I was scared that I'd get into a rut too deep to climb out of before the lithium could kick in, or that my brain would take a sudden swerve and I'd ascend higher and higher to the beautiful dirty place of warped angels and wrecked houses and off-key singing that is the signature of my mania. When I walked I did so slowly, deliberately, one foot in front of the other, keeping a tempo in my head, *one two, one two, one two*, trying to turn my confused brain into a metronome to steady my psyche. That night, as I stood in front of my mirror, surprised to see a hint of bone beneath my skin, my ribs having put in an appearance for the first time in who knows how long, I made a fist and curled my arm up. Some strength. It was a feeling that I hoped the lithium would help me hang on to.

Lithium as a Salt Substitute

Schou continued his studies in Denmark, amassing and inter-preting data, trying to persuade Hartigan to write up and publish his own findings. Lithium, meanwhile, had already made its way to the United States, only it came to our side of the sea not as a psychiatric medicine but, rather, as a salt substitute for patients who needed a low-sodium diet because of hypertension, heart disease, kidney disease or oedema. Starting in 1948, four companies, having read that lithium has a naturally salty taste, produced this salt substitute – under the names Westal, Foodsal, Salti-salt and Milosal – and it didn't take long before doctors were encouraging their patients to use it as a way of flavouring their food.

Patients (and doctors), unaware that lithium, in excess, could be poisonous, sprinkled it liberally over their meat and potatoes, and soon a number of people either became seriously sick or died. A. M. Waldron, a doctor in Ann Arbor, Michigan, wrote to the *Journal of the American Medical Association* (*JAMA*) that he had treated four patients who had consumed the lithium salt substitute and, as a result, presented with tremors, disturbed gait, general weakness, exhaustion and blurred vision, all of which are signs of a toxic lithium reaction. Waldron, probably unaware that toxic reactions to lithium can become lethal, did not suggest that the companies which made the salt substitute should cease doing so. He merely recommended that 'practitioner[s] should be warned of its possible toxic reactions'. In the same issue of *JAMA*, however, another group of doctors reported the deaths of two patients who in both cases had been using Westal, while still another doctor described a patient severely poisoned by Westal. 'Taken together', according to historian F. Neil Johnson, 'the four reports sounded a loud and very clear warning against the continued use of lithium-based salt substitutes.'

These deaths and poisonings, not isolated cases, were eventually reported in high-profile publications such as *Time* magazine, among others, and the result was what Johnson has called 'the toxicity panic'. The FDA (the U.S. Food and Drug Administration) reacted swiftly, banning lithium from use in the United States in 1949. Once the FDA banned lithium, it became difficult to obtain legally in the country, although that didn't stop some intrepid doctors from prescribing it in the years that followed. After all, the spectrophotometer, if used correctly, could in fact monitor blood levels, thereby preventing poisonings. There were US doctors who followed the publications coming from Denmark and Australia, and, through ingenuity, found ways to access the drug. Remember that most asylums still had huge canisters of lithium left over from the nineteenth century, and thus those psychiatrists, like R. M. Young in England, who happened to have read Cade's paper often had a ready supply to try on their own flock of patients. Because manic or highly excitable patients are notoriously difficult to deal with, the temptation to administer the drug, despite the ban and despite the reports of deaths and toxicities, must still have been strong.

The toxicity panic was clearly a low point in the history of lithium but it had at least two positive impacts. First, it spurred researchers to develop ever more effective means of measuring blood levels of the drug in an effort to avoid lithium poisonings, and second, it raised the drug's profile so that more and more doctors and psychiatrists became aware of it, took note of it, and began, presumably, to read the reports from Schou and Baastrup.

The Great Clash

Schou, meanwhile, already a believer in the therapeutic benefits of lithium, began to envision it as something of a wonder drug for a certain subset of patients – namely, those with manic-depressive disorder and those with recurrent depressive disorder. Throughout the 1950s and '60s he was doing what he could to spread the word, speaking at symposia, publishing papers, collecting data, so immersed in his work that in all likelihood he was blindsided when, in 1968, an article appeared in *The Lancet* titled 'Prophylactic Lithium: Another Therapeutic Myth?'

The paper, co-authored by British psychiatrists Barry Blackwell and Michael Shepherd of London's Maudsley Hospital, was particularly fierce, critiquing Schou and Baastrup's 1967 showing that lithium could effectively prevent periodic depressions from recurring. Shepherd and Blackwell had several criticisms, the most important one being that Schou and Baastrup had not done a double-blind, placebo-controlled study this time around and thus were vulnerable to all sorts of biases, primary among them observer bias – the contention that the results of their studies were compromised by their awareness of the goals, which influenced their observations and made it impossible for them to report impartially.

Shepherd was convinced that Schou was actively avoiding the rigours of a double-blind, placebo-controlled trial. It was an impression stemming from a meeting both men had attended in Göttingen, Germany, during which Shepherd had discussed the importance of double-blind trials and later claimed that he had tried to 'point out politely' to Schou the need for further research, while Schou insisted that his evidence was compelling enough to suggest that there might be new avenues and interventions when it came to curing manic depression. Schou, in an effort to underscore how powerful lithium prophylaxis could be, told Shepherd the story of his younger brother's miraculous recovery, completely unaware that in Shepherd's eyes this was still further proof of researcher bias, an emotional overinvestment in what should be a strictly scientific question, and therefore a subjective stance that would surely stain whatever results Schou obtained in his work.

According to Schou, Shepherd 'clearly felt that when I showed gratification with my findings that I must necessarily be a "believer",
an enthusiast, naive and not to be trusted.' And indeed, in their
1968 paper, Shepherd and Blackwell did accuse Schou and Baastrup
of using 'an "open" method to evaluate a therapy for which they
have been enthusiastic advocates for several years'.

The *Lancet* paper, and the attack contained within it, caused
quite a stir in psychiatric circles, in both Europe and the United
States, as doctors divided on the question of whether lithium was
an effective prophylactic against recurrent depressive disorder,
perhaps losing sight of Shepherd and Blackwell's core argument,
which was not so much about the drug's efficacy as it was about
the researchers' methodology. Schou and Baastrup responded to
the attack one month later, but what they could not do, Schou felt,
and felt passionately, was continue to implement a double-blind,
placebo-controlled study to test the question because to do so presented Schou with a terrible ethical dilemma. Although Schou had
conducted, with lithium, a double-blind, placebo-controlled study
in the past, he had not known then about how effective lithium
could be in treating mania and depression.

Now, however, he did know, and doing a double-blind study
would mean assigning some manic-depressive patients to a placebo when there was a proven treatment for their condition. Such
patients, on a placebo, would be left to the terrible turmoil of their
own minds and, in a manic state, might spend away their savings
or do other damage, while, in a depressive state, might go so far
as to commit suicide. The fact that Schou's brother had not had a
single depressive episode since starting on lithium only intensified
the quandary for Schou. 'How', he asked, 'could I put him, or others
like him, in a clinical trial where he would face the possibility of
lithium being withdrawn?' Indeed, he went on to say, in more
forceful language: 'Could we ... expose a random sample of our
patients to a placebo ... to painful relapses and possibly suicide
in order to obtain evidence for the benefit of patients in England

and the United States? To do so would presumably be against the Helsinki Declaration, which clearly states that patients must not be exposed to risk through experiments unless these are of potential benefit to themselves.'

Shepherd and Blackwell, however, appeared to see no ethical problems in doing a double-blind, placebo-controlled study. But the debate was not relegated to the strictly scientific. Blackwell and Shepherd continually questioned Schou's motives, hinting, if not outright stating, that as a scientist he was emotionally over-involved in the subject and therefore not qualified to draw meaningful conclusions from his data. In later interviews, Shepherd went so far as to be condescending about Schou's bearing and attire:

> He was a genial man ... He wears a blazer; he speaks perfect English; he has considerable charm; he's got this Danish humour ... I realised that I was in the presence of a believer – somebody who knew ... He told me that a relative had been ill and that he was taking it and that really there ought to be a national policy in which everybody could get lithium. Because he had this jovial manner I wasn't altogether certain he was serious but then I realised he was ... Quite inadvertently we sparked off a nightmare which went on for years ... I had to restrain Blackwell; otherwise there would have been further trouble.

With the stakes so high (that is, the possibility, in their view, that patients from whom lithium was withheld might commit suicide), and with the accusations seemingly laced with personal judgement, Schou and Baastrup struggled to defend themselves. It is ironic that Shepherd and Blackwell accused Schou in particular of being overly involved with his study and thus unqualified to come to conclusions when in fact it appears that they were the ones who were personalising the debate, yanking it from the realm of science into something much more subjective by psychologising

Schou, by questioning not his data but his underlying motives, his putative 'over-involvement'. It was not the criticism per se to which Schou objected. 'Critical debate is what science thrives on and should at all times be welcomed,' he stated. 'But one does not appreciate having one's data ... and ethics rejected totally and unfairly. Conjectures about other scientists' motives are irrelevant in and should be kept out of scientific discussions.' Blackwell countered that Schou's entire professional life had been 'dominated by lithium', and that 'his persistent refusal to attempt double-blind methodology is partly determined by his strong personal convictions about the drug'.

Knowing they needed to respond to the criticism in some fashion, Schou and Baastrup decided, in the end, to do a modified double-blind, placebo-controlled study as a way of attenuating the critiques cast their way. Eighty-four patients who had been taking lithium for a year or more were involved in this study. Some of these patients continued with their lithium treatment, while others were given a placebo, but if the patients on the placebo relapsed, then the blind was broken and they were restarted on the lithium. At the end of six months, the findings, according to Schou, were 'unequivocal'. 'More than half of the patients given the placebo had relapsed,' he wrote. 'None of the lithium patients had done so. In the view of the authors of the report, the prophylactic efficacy of lithium had been conclusively demonstrated.'

Blackwell and Shepherd remained unconvinced, claiming that the study still had methodological flaws. Perhaps, they suggested, the placebo-treated patients might have been aware that their medication had been withdrawn, given the sudden absence of lithium-induced side effects, and this knowledge could in and of itself have caused a relapse. But despite the misgivings of Blackwell and Shepherd, Schou and Baastrup's second study appeared to settle the prophylaxis argument in their favour within the majority of the psychiatric community. The victory came at quite a cost to

Schou, however, both personally and professionally. The public debate – so full of vitriol and so time-consuming – and the unending criticism, at once pointed and personal, took a toll. Even as the kerfuffle raised the profile of lithium still higher, David Healy claims, so that now it was a well-known drug in every first world country, the entire debacle, with papers flying back and forth in *The Lancet* and other publications – complete with attacks, rebuttals, refusals and the like – cast a shadow over Schou's career. The controversy had been that loud and long.

And despite the fact that Schou and Baastrup prevailed in the end, even years later Shepherd was unpersuaded, eventually suggesting that, with the pharmaceutical companies not pursuing lithium development, Schou had been partially motivated by an economic incentive. 'They saw a killing here,' Shepherd claimed.

> The industry had ignored lithium because it's an element, it's cheap and suddenly they saw money ... We got involved as a sort of scapegoat in all this because we'd had the effrontery to raise the questions. Well, at least it did force them to do a more scientific study. I didn't think that the evidence from the trial justified the conclusions ... but it was never an important matter to me, whereas it was a very important matter to Schou because it challenged an article of faith and of course his reputation was built on this.

Lithium's Rising Reputation

Schou's reputation aside, the notoriety that lithium gained from the long and painful controversy surrounding it meant that more and more psychiatrists in the United States were beginning to petition the FDA to lift the ban that had followed in the wake of the great toxicity panic two decades earlier. One such enthusiast was Ronald Fieve, a psychiatrist in New York who began using lithium on his manic-depressive patients in the 1960s, touting the drug with considerable vigour. Comfortable in the public eye, perhaps even somewhat of a show-off, Fieve, who would later write the bestselling book *Moodswing*, helped lithium make headway in the American public consciousness, in part by persuading one of his famous patients – Joshua Logan, producer and director of the Broadway musicals *South Pacific* and *Camelot*, whose manic depression had been successfully treated with the salts – to appear with him on multiple national television networks in the 1970s, giving candid interviews about both the drug and the disorder it treated. Even respected textbooks such as *The Pharmacological Basis of Therapeutics* stated that 'the lithium ion has no known therapeutic applications'. But Fieve and other US psychiatrists hoped to change the drug's official status on this side of the sea, and to get the lithium ban lifted.

With the efforts of these psychiatrists to spread the word in the United States, and with the drug's profile having been raised by the charged arguments between Blackwell and Shepherd on one side and Schou and Baastrup on the other, more and more clinicians in the United States began applying to the FDA for permission to use lithium on their patients, both those with manic depression and those with periodic or recurrent depressions. Eventually the FDA became so overrun that 'many of the FDA staff were eager to grant approval simply to avoid having to process further applications'.

At the same time, Smith, Kline & French – famous for chlorpromazine – and Rowell Laboratories, perhaps at last sensing a financial opportunity, submitted new drug applications for lithium carbonate to the FDA. The pressure from the pharmaceutical companies, combined with the clamour from individual psychiatrists, went a long way towards persuading the FDA to lift its ban, which it finally did, on 6 April 1970, more than two decades after it had first outlawed the drug. Lithium was approved in the United States for the treatment of manic-depressive disorder. This, however, was the sole indication granted. Despite the research of Schou and Baastrup, the FDA did not approve lithium – and to this day has not approved lithium – for prophylactic use in the treatment of recurrent depression.

On Lithium

Still I dreamt of depression. A sheet fell over me, trapping my body beneath. A shadow, swollen, crept across a wall.

The pharmacy was overbright, with festive red notebooks, spotted headbands, lipsticks in coloured casings, false eyelashes mounted inside plastic boxes. I waited in a line of people, all with their own square script, a single piece of paper that had compressed within it a long unscrolling story. My prescription was written in a hurried, arterial scrawl, with various flourishes, the letters loopy and linked together in an idiosyncratic cursive. This turned out to be a problem.

When it was my turn I presented my prescription to a white-coated woman whose lipstick was siren red, her earrings tiny pearl points, her shirt buttoned all the way up the slender stalk of her neck so that her head appeared to hover, detached. Her hair was pulled back and coiled into a bun that perched primly on top of her head, glazed and shiny, like a pastry. Extending her hand, with its long and glossy fingernails, she picked up the script between thumb and forefinger, as though it, not me, had the disease. She scanned the prescription, her lips pursed, and gave me a long look, then very deliberately smoothed the prescription with one hand, pressing it into the counter, erasing any wrinkles, after which she picked up the prescription and held it up to the light. The people in the line behind me shifted, shuffled. In one of the aisles a child started to cry.

'I'm sorry,' the woman said at last, 'but I can't fill this for you.'

'What's wrong?' I said. 'It's from my doctor.'

'Your doctor's handwriting is exceedingly difficult to read.'

'It's for lithium,' I said, aware that everyone behind me could hear the conversation, but now I didn't care. By this point I'd been off the olanzapine for several days. My body felt as if it had hollows that were filled with shrill chirps and sharp shards. A desperation came over me, quickly and completely, a belief that lithium alone could fill the hollows with its soothing salts. 'Lithium,' I said again, a little louder this time, although my voice sounded tiny, as if it were coming from some smothered place far away.

'I can't fill a prescription I cannot read,' the pharmacist said, her lips a slender seam I wanted to reach over and rip.

A tiny stream of sweat was trickling from the nape of my neck down my back. The line of people behind me sighed and shifted once more, as if they were a single organism moving as one. 'I can read the prescription just fine,' I said. 'It says "Eskalith XR". The "XR" stands for extended release.'

'Can you read *that*?' she said to me, her finger pointing to a bit of scrawl, her voice triumphant.

'I can,' I said, throwing back my shoulders. But when I looked down at the words, I saw how worthless they were, the typical script of a rushed doctor, and I sagged inside.

'I'm sorry,' the pharmacist said, 'but I can't make heads or tails of what's on here, and my licence forbids me to fill a script I can't read.'

I left the pharmacy, stepping out into the yellow day. The people moved as if they had battery packs in their backs, everyone powered by something suspicious and inhuman. My mood was wobbly, a wall of compressed tears aching in my throat. I wanted to cry but was afraid to. After all, what else are eyes but holes in the head and who knows what might emerge? I pictured a girl with marbles sliding down her face.

On the walk home I stopped in a woody grove and pulled a slinky pink worm from the chocolate earth, watching as he coiled in the cup of my hand, his slender body as cool as the soil he'd come from. I would take my comforts wherever I could find them: a worm, the sun-warmed wood, or the trefoil feet of a sparrow on my window ledge. When I got home, I called my psychiatrist and left a message with his answering service.

Several hours later I was back, this time at a different pharmacy, after my doctor phoned in the prescription. I waited half an hour in an orange plastic chair and, when my name was called, paid, grabbed the bag and left. In my kitchen I took out the bottle, inside of which were jammed thirty lithium tablets, each one an orb with no score marks, just smooth and cool and fat against my cheek. I filled a glass with water, planning to wash one down, but instead, at the last minute, I dropped the tablet into my glass and watched as it dissolved, thinking, as my medicine turned from solid to bubbles, of long ago, of the lithia waters given for every ailment under the sun. It took time for the tablet to completely dissolve, but once it did, I drank it all down, cool and tangy on my tongue.

The next morning, when I woke up, my room seemed oddly peaceful. This, I knew, was a placebo response, but I take my cures in whatever form they come to me. Downstairs the laughter of my children sounded lovely. The shadows of the trees made lace on my walls and I watched as the lace lifted and swayed, a continuous dance of dapples. I got up and then stood on my bed, the better to see out my wide windows, which looked down on to my tiered garden growing at the base of a wetland. The soil there is so packed with nutrients and so continually drenched that everything thrives, the roses in profusion, the chocolate mint spilling from level to level, sporting tall purple spires that tangle with the masses of yellow asters and the spiky pink bee balm and the butterfly bushes' long branches topped with mounds of tiny pink flowers that attract the monarchs and the moths I could see right now. Huge orange butterflies were landing on the plants, their wings flexing as they drank, butterflies as big as books, it seemed, the pages of their wings opened to black dots and zigzags of gold. The moths were much plainer but beautiful in their alabaster flights. I had seeded this land and tilled it and cultivated it and coaxed from its willing soil every bush and flower below me.

Lithium takes at least a week to build up in the blood. One swig from a glass won't buy you your prophylaxis; the drug needs to accrue in the body. So the day after that first dose I could confidently claim my sudden spurt of joy as my own. For the next seven days I walked around tentatively, almost on tiptoes, with one ear cocked to my innards, as if listening for some click to tell me my medication would work. I was happy when I noticed a fine slight tremor in my hand, a sign that the drug was present and that it might provide me with a portal out of olanzapine. I worried not at all about lithium poisoning; I knew to get my blood levels checked once a month. More days passed. Two weeks became three. July had rounded the bend into August, which then became September. The evenings took on cooler currents and the stars seemed defined against the black backdrop of sky, each one a speck of precious salt. The kids and I took the telescope out on to the deck and peered through its lens. I had traded one of the most popular mood stabilisers psychiatry has to offer – the highly profitable olanzapine – for an old standby whose workings were mysterious. John Cade's earliest hypothesis is still as good as any – that lithium works because those with manic depression have a dearth of lithium ions in the body.

Sure enough, as the weeks passed, my mood evened out, the ground glass in my hollows went away and was replaced by a certain silky softness. Not much bothered me, but neither was I numb. There is nothing as precious as the recession of mental illness, which leaves in its wake a gorgeous clarity. The dividends of darkness, I call it. Every day when I am even is a blessed day, a banquet day, the long table set with an array of colours, the white cloth as bright as a sail walking on water. With lithium, my bones returned. My hands, no longer wrapped in fat, displayed a certain elegance, and so I wore a ring with a simple white moonstone on it. The sugar left my bloodstream, and after four weeks off olanzapine, my GP told me I was on my way to becoming non-diabetic. But it was still too early to know for sure whether lithium would work for me in the long term, whether it would do for me what it had done for Schou's brother and for many of his patients, too – which is to prevent recurrent depressions from returning while also keeping me from mania.

No Profit to Be Made

Mogens Schou died in 2005. Aside from Cade, he was probably lithium's fiercest champion. In fact, when the drug began to receive approval for psychiatric use around the world, Cade himself credited Schou as 'the person who had done the most to achieve this recognition' for lithium. Schou saw it cure countless patients and save his brother. Unlike drug researchers of today, at least some of whom are motivated by profit, Schou, and Cade before him, had a purity about their pursuits. Despite Shepherd's accusation, these men knew that lithium would never make them rich. It existed as a natural element first found on the rocky island of Utö, and was thus available for free. Yet they dedicated their lives to it anyway. What they saw in the drug was a powerful treatment for a devastating disorder, a capsule that raised some of psychiatry's most fascinating questions. Unlike chlorpromazine, lithium appears to act with unusual specificity, eradicating manic excitement while leaving other symptoms untouched. Schizophrenics who take it calm down, but their hallucinations and delusions continue unabated. According to Erik Strömgren, the Danish psychiatrist who had first suggested the compound to Schou, lithium, because it is chemically so simple, provides a potential lens into the neurocircuitry of mood much more effectively than the 'therapeutic effects of complicated compounds which had no clear preference with regard to the different disorders they were used for'.

Given lithium's specificity, one would think it would be a highly studied drug, that researchers would be probing the patients who take it in an attempt to understand what regions of the brain it affects, how it dampens or excites neurotransmission signalling, all in an attempt to better understand the extremes of human emotion – mania and despair – which, once grasped, once marked and mapped, might also shed light on their more common cousins: sadness and happiness, grief and joy. But, oddly, few scientists have spent much time looking through lithium to the brain beneath, trying to grasp the hows and whys of the drug's machinery and the delicate dance it does in the human head. 'It's done a lot for psychiatry, without question,' said Alexander Vuckovic. 'But it has never really excited neuroscientists, because there's no profit in it, no money to be made.'

Perhaps better than any other drug, lithium reveals the extent to which psychiatry is tightly tied to capitalistic corporate interests, how closely allied the field is with the major pharmaceutical houses, where millions, even billions of dollars are made in mere months. This is why, although lithium had worked so well for so many people, drug developers set about discovering new mood stabilisers that had patent and profit possibilities, whipping up in their high-tech cauldrons scores of new pharmaceuticals to treat bipolar disorder or, better yet, converting already existing medications – drugs, say, for epilepsy – into treatments.

The pharmaceutical company Abbott Laboratories, in 1983, obtained a licence for a drug called valproate, which was an anticonvulsant. Abbott then twice successfully applied for a patent to make valproate semisodium, a more stable sodium. This new compound differed from its predecessor, valproate, by just one sodium ion, and so, according to David Healy, it was 'as good a symbol of the vacuity of current patent law as any'. The next step occurred when psychiatrist Harrison Pope and his colleagues completed a study which showed that valproate semisodium was an effective treatment for mania, an outcome that guaranteed Abbott financial success.

The Abbott example is but one of many. Numerous anticonvulsants – drugs used to treat epilepsy – were repurposed in the

1980s and '90s as drugs to treat manic depression, now known as bipolar disorder. This came about when doctors became aware that a drug called carbamazepine could suppress seizures kindled by the amygdala, a part of the brain's limbic system that detects fear. Psychiatrists then went on to study carbamazepine in mania and found it effective. Perhaps, psychiatrists thought, mood disorders could be seen as a kind of psychological convulsant, as if the bipolar brain was flipping from despair to euphoria in a kind of seizure-esque way.

Once bipolar disorder was refashioned as a convulsive equivalent, all sorts of drugs previously used only for epilepsy became not just possible but relevant, and pharmaceutical houses, smelling potential profit in this new paradigm, began offering up their antiepileptics with new labels hastily applied to the bottle. The term 'mood stabiliser' came into wide use around this time, and drugs that before had been confined only to treating epilepsy now saw a broader and more profitable purpose. One of these, gabapentin, grossed $1.3 billion a year once it became a mood stabiliser. This new class of drugs seized the field and went some way towards eradicating the use of lithium, to the point where, in the 1990s, newly minted psychiatrists going through or just emerging from their residencies usually had far less experience with lithium than they did with anticonvulsants – this despite the fact that there existed no evidence that the 'new' mood stabilisers worked any better than lithium did. More significantly, there was virtually no evidence that bipolar disorder actually *was* the moody equivalent of epilepsy. It was simply one possibility, one model, but it created the paradigm that justified the newfound 'mania' for anticonvulsants, especially in the United States.

The Magic Fades

On lithium, I no longer dreamt of depression returning. I was, literally, lighter than before, when I had been weighed down by olanzapine's side effects. I would not go so far as to say I was cured of my cycling moods; there were days here and there when I could sense a slippage, a sudden slit in the air and a sense of dropping down. I tried not to flail as I fell, because experience has shown me that only makes it worse. I have learned how to still myself as I tumble through that rent and go down, down, to an empty beach below, with black rocks jutting up, seagulls screaming, bloated boats overturned and the carcasses of crabs on the sand. I don't want to land there, and after starting lithium I didn't, although there were days I came so close I could feel the sand skim the soles of my feet, could smell the salt in the rotten air and the matted tangles of seaweed decomposing in the dampness, could hear the scuttle of some bug as it made its way towards the waves, with a lone lighthouse off in the fog, its single beam too anaemic to pierce the muffled mist.

In the long run, however, despite my expectations, the drug did not work as well as I had hoped. Sometime that winter, to my dismay, when the skies were darkening in the afternoon, when light leaked out and disappeared, when the wind bit into the back of my neck, my depression returned and, frightened, I reached for my olanzapine, trading my body for my mind. For many people, though, lithium, that salt from a stone, is enough, is in fact all they need. I envy them. And when Alexander Vuckovic said, 'I use lithium with many of my depressed patients and I've found it to be as effective as an antidepressant as it is for bipolar disorder', I wish I were one of the ones he is talking about.

I don't think there exists any drug that can totally seal the ruptures I so often sense around me. But sometimes I wonder: do I even want a drug that could set me solid on some shelf, where I could pose, all pretty? Perhaps there is a part of me that likes my madness, in measured drips, the dreams of rocks and black hats and girls of swirling sugar. Perhaps I like my drugs too. Perhaps I like the act of taking them, which I did each evening, always dropping the fat lithium tablet into a tall glass of cool water, watching as it bubbled white and frothy, like some kind of magical concoction. In the moments after I'd swallowed it, a syrupy lethargy came over me, a lethargy not unlike the one Cade observed in his guinea pigs, a lethargy that was almost enough to induce bromide dreams of springs and spas, of bottled waters we once believed in, of vast salt plains dazzling in the strong sunlight.

3

Early Antidepressants

The Three-Ringed Molecule and the Psychic Energiser

The Beginning

No, I don't know when it started. I could have been ten, or two. I could have been unborn, a fleck and then a foetus with the haze of my new heart visible beneath translucent skin. When does the brain first form? It could have started then, whenever that is, or it could have been that God, if you believe in him, accidentally nicked my corrugated cortex with his silver chisel, and from that dent darkness poured and poured until I was covered in it, complete. I don't know how I was held in my earliest days, or even if I was held, although my mother has told me that, as an infant, I cried so wretchedly, so continuously, that she put me in a wind-up swing and let me scream as I careened back and forth. Unable to be comforted, I was not, as they say, an easy baby. So perhaps it started when I started, and has been with me ever since. I'm speaking of depression – the night without a moon.

I remember a stifling day, when I was six or seven, in a dead-quiet July, the roses on their stalks brown balls of burn, the street almost fluorescent with light from a white-hot sun in a white sky, the gardens gone limp and the trees shifting with the barest hint of a breeze. My older sister and I were sitting outside on the steps, two little girls in pinafores and Mary Janes, our white ankle socks edged with frills. We were going somewhere special, although now, at the age of fifty-four, I cannot recall where. What I recall is the heat, heat, heat and the black tarmac on the road turning taffy-soft and my skin beginning to crisp. I recall seeing, from the steps, far down the road, a figure coming towards us, his outline resolving as the distance diminished, a man dressed in a dark suit with his jacket buttoned up and fastened by two golden pins glaring in the summer day. His face perspired heavily as he knelt by my sister and me and asked if we would like to see his monkey dance. He was so close I could smell his cinder breath and then I saw his hand, or rather his lack of a hand, how one empty cuff just hung down, the skin at the knob of his bony wrist marbled and seamed. A monkey, a little creature with fur the colour of driftwood and a tiny triangular hat on his tiny head, leapt from I know not where and began to jig on the smoking pavement. Then the man sang and the monkey danced to the sound of the song and my sister laughed and laughed. But I felt horrified – by this man, this monkey, this absent hand, this heat everywhere over me and in me as the creature shimmied and spun. I can't recall the song the man sang or how it ended, only that he and his monkey were there one moment and gone the next, seemingly sucked up into the sky by the enormous force of the golden heat, or the crooked magic of midsummer itself.

That night I dreamt I was trying to call someone but despite looking everywhere could not find my hand and thus could not complete the call. I woke up, drank from a paper cup by my bedside, the water warm, the cup damp and close to collapsing. I fell back asleep and when I awoke again the night was gone and my room was filled with a blinding whiteness that obliterated everything. It was the whiteness of a blizzard except the air was heavy with heat and when I tried to call for help my voice got lost in the particles, fine as flour, that had dusted everything out of existence. I lay awake, alarmed, surrounded by a terrible dazzle and unable to speak or move. How or why it ended I do not know, but somehow, eventually, the regular world resumed its rightful place and my bedroom furniture came back into being and my body came back into being and I held up my hands – two of them, ten fingers, each one working and complete. Something, however, was wrong. There was a weight in my limbs, a stone in my stomach. I looked out my window, afraid the monkey man might return. But very early in the morning the streets were empty and quiet except for Mr Slotnick in his back garden, cleaning his pool with a large net filled with green and gleaming leaves.

I had in many ways (but not all ways) a terrible childhood. My mother did not know what to do with me. In reality there was nothing so special about me, but for whatever reason I frustrated her and seemed to be a blot on her existence. She dealt with me as an infant by stowing me in a wind-up swing and when I got older by sometimes grabbing a clump of my hair and dragging me across the floor, a few times to the sink, where she washed out my mouth with soap, although I never swore. My mother herself was depressed and thus there's a reasonable chance I learned depression from her, just as I learned from her the alphabet and how to ride a bike. That's a theory – depression as something you acquire, even master, like an instrument with all sorts of strings. Another theory: that I was born with a broken brain and thus the blinding white dazzle that choked me the summer I was six or seven was simply the inevitable manifestation of an illness beginning, an illness I'd harboured if not since conception then soon after. There is some convincing evidence that depression, especially the bipolar sort that I have, is inherited via the genes, and there's also speculation that mothers who are depressed during pregnancy may pass those dark dogs on to their offspring as the mother's stress hormones, which accompany melancholy, seep into the body of her unborn baby and cause a second syndrome.

At the age of ten I started psychotherapy with a very tall woman named Dr Sugarman. This was because by year five I'd become so bereft and terrified that I skipped school most days. I lived with a horror of many things, most especially the supermarket with its clean, antiseptic aisles and bloody meats packaged in parts – here a thigh, there a breast. The chicken parts appeared to swim in anaemic-looking blood and the butcher waved a blade, his apron flecked with scarlet, his wares spread out in display cases on beds of crushed ice, long fillets of pale fish and, in a case of water, living lobsters with black blind eyes, their antennae wavering as they crawled over one another's carapaces.

For me, ever since I was young (how young, and when, and why, I don't know), the world has been a weird place, a surprisingly surreal stage on which little monkeys and handless men dance to jigs no one wants to hear. Chequerboard floors rolled out endlessly and sometimes my mother slapped me so hard her hand left an imprint on my face. Was this nature or nurture, the depression that came to claim me completely by the time I was thirteen and old enough to act out, which I did by using my mother's razor to rend my skin, watching intently as blood bubbled up and astonished at how easy it was to do this?

By then Dr Sugarman was a thing of the past, but when the school saw my skin and the craziness of the cuts they persuaded my mother to find me a second psychiatrist. Dr Miriam Mazor was a psychiatrist in her mid-thirties who lived in the Orthodox Jewish section of Brookline, Massachusetts. I went to her office three times a week after school, transporting myself there by tram. I would drop my dime into the collection box and step down the stairs into a world where men wore what looked like black top hats and had coils of curls swinging at the sides of their faces, which were often buried in books they read even as they walked. Springs and summers the doors to the synagogues were often open and the haunting sound of Hebrew chanting often spilled into the street while I made my way to my doctor's office. Behind the large plate glass windows of kosher delicatessens and shops, bakers kneaded their dough, stretching and softening it, shaping it, finally, into bundles they slathered with vegetable fat before sliding them into brick ovens.

I saw Dr Miriam Mazor from the time I was thirteen until I was in my mid-twenties, more than a decade of thrice-weekly appointments, and yet I cannot recall much of what we discussed. What mattered was not what I said or what she said. What mattered was that *something* was said, that conversation coursed between us like a river beneath whose currents ran a clear assumption: that whatever was wrong with me could be fixed by language, if only because it had been caused by language, or a lack thereof, words of love or affection never uttered in my household growing up. The idea of a chemical depression back then, in the mid-1970s, was almost unheard of among people with no special medical expertise. Nor was I in psychoanalysis. There was no leather divan on which I could fling myself down to free-associate. I sat upright in a chair and often looked at the pattern in her rug, seeing in it, on some days, friendly faces, and on other days sneers and stares.

While we rarely discussed the underlying assumptions of treatment, it became terrifically clear to both of us, as suggested by Dr Mazor, that I had repressed feelings, probably of anger, towards my less-than-nurturing mother, and that if I could just *get in touch with these feelings* and spit them out on to Dr Mazor's rug or into her hands, I'd be cured of the dark mood, of my fear of the terrible white night-time snow and the monkey man, of the sensation of limblessness. Thus I spent a lot of time during my fifty-minute sessions trying in vain to locate certain feelings, trying to talk myself into rage, for instance, when all I felt was dead. Meanwhile, my symptoms kept getting worse and worse throughout my adolescence. The cutting continued, each slice a little closer to the tributaries of veins that forked at the rim of my wrist, and by the time I was eighteen I was swallowing promethazine and pseudoephedrine and afterwards having charcoal shoved down my throat in the A&E department as I retched into a blue bowl.

The 1970s passed; I went to university and acquired an eating disorder, bingeing and purging, the bones of my body now very visible. It was 1981, 1982, 1983 and I was vomiting into bin bags and then tossing the whole hot mess into skips at the fringes of the campus. I would force the food back up with my fingers or, when that failed to work, shove the handles of hairbrushes down my throat, scraping the tender lining of the oesophagus, until one day my throat started to swell with infection. My whole neck bulged. Swallowing was excruciating and it was hard to get my breath. I wound up in the campus infirmary, drinking the thick pink of liquid penicillin from a tiny cup four times a day. The medicine coated my blistered throat as my fever soared and I saw winged things and snowflakes, huge wheels of white lace falling all around me.

All through these years I had continued to cut, and to bleed out my arms even as my menstrual period dried up and went away. Three times a week I still saw Dr Mazor, who had witnessed my weight fall, my bones jut out, my throat collapse and then puff. When I was well enough to make my way from the infirmary back to her Brookline office, something shifted in the treatment. This was a time when electric typewriters were being replaced by primitive computers and daisy wheel printers that clattered as they worked. The World Wide Web was less than a decade away and some especially savvy people even knew how to email. Computer 'memory' could be stored on a chip. Humans, too, began to be viewed in machine-like terms. Our axons and dendrites were visible now on imaging devices, and the brain became a compendium of pieces and parts, of bleeps and flashes and chemicals we could replicate in test tubes.

This did not mean there was a quick fix for me, but I clearly recall the first session after my stint in the infirmary, a Friday afternoon. Dr Mazor watched me with an attentiveness – a thoughtfulness – that made me fidget in my seat. Now in her forties, she wore bifocals. Her eyes were large and luminous, a velvet brown rimmed with a fringe of thick black lashes. With her hands folded in a bundle on her lap, she sat at her desk and studied me for quite some time, the silence in the room growing denser by the moment, until at last she sighed and said, 'I've been thinking you might respond well to drug treatment.'

It was a statement as banal as could possibly be today, when we chat about our chemical imbalances, our low serotonin, our site-specific drugs, all with the ease of people knocking back a few beers at the bar. But it wasn't always this way. Even with the advances of chlorpromazine and lithium and other psychotropic drugs, during the decade I was in psychotherapy the prevailing belief among many psychiatrists was still that language and the insights it spawned could be profoundly curative. Psychiatric medication, to my mind and the minds of most of the general public, was for madmen and women locked up behind metal bars in stone-cold asylums set high up on hills.

'Imipramine,' Dr Mazor continued. 'I think you might respond well to it.'

'Imipra what?' I said, encircling my knobby wrist with my fingers and feeling the throb of my pulse patter away.

'Imipramine,' she repeated. 'An antidepressant.'

It was 1982 and I had no idea what an antidepressant was. I also had a firm-as-fact notion that taking anything that might tamper with my brain seemed sacrilegious, seemed extreme beyond language. I resisted the argot itself, unable, literally, even to pronounce this drug's name, while on a deeper level, I also resisted the idea that my problem was biological as opposed to psychological. For me it was rooted in deficiencies of nurture as opposed to nature. I believed, furthermore, that there was a deep division between psyche (the psychological) and brain (the biological), in which case cutting corners by taking drugs was tantamount to sin, a dangerous shortcut that eclipsed the insight of language and embraced quick chemistry in its stead. As I sat there, profoundly ashamed, thrashing this out in my nineteen-year-old mind, observing the rug as if it held the answer, my psychiatrist continued to study me as though I were a spectacle, her gaze sad, suggesting that we had come to the end of some road, that I had failed the calling of psychodynamic psychotherapy, in which I had placed all my faith and effort, arriving three times a week for half a dozen years so far and each session trying to fashion feelings my doctor would see as correct, obedient, cathartic.

At last, having no response from me, Dr Mazor picked up her pen and wrote me a prescription, which I took tentatively. I exited her office and walked out on to the street. It was mid-December and lights festooned the bushes and trees lining her lane. My breath was visible in the frosty air, each exhale a small ghost birthed from my body, floating by my face briefly before atomising into the wintry blue. There it was – my breath – unable to be captured. It was made of oxygen and carbon and could be described, even drawn in molecular terms, but that didn't alter the fact that it drifted from my mouth and vaporised before I could catch it in my ready hands. When I was nineteen, all the ways that we did not, and could not, yield to science's scalpel soothed me. I didn't necessarily believe in ghosts or God, but I firmly believed the human mind was bigger than the brain that boxed it, that we would never be able to fully articulate that mass of corrugated matter because, in order to do so, we would need to rise above it with a keener, purer intelligence than we humans currently possessed. And that was as it should be. Human misery and mirth, I was convinced, had at least one limb in some heavenly sphere beyond language and touch.

Standing at the end of Dr Mazor's street, several streets from the tram that would lead me to the train that would deposit me back on my university campus, I took the prescription from my coat pocket and tried to interpret the cryptic writing. I folded the piece of paper into the shape of a tiny plane and then put it on my palm and waited for the wind to take it. The wind did not come. When nothing happened I refolded the script into the shape of a swan – origami was something I was good at – and again placed it on my palm, an offering to the sky, but the bird would not fly. Snow began to fall, little icy flecks of it, almost like sleet. I opened up the bird and smoothed the paper flat, the creases still visible, then folded it into a small cube I put back into my pocket. Darkness was falling fast and the store windows glowed, huge orange squares of ambient light. The baker was making his Jewish bread known as challah, plaiting the dough with dusty expert hands.

The apothecary's door jingled when I opened it. Down the end of a long aisle stood the pharmacist himself, in his white coat, counting tablets that seemed to glow preternaturally in the winter's night. The shop must have been bright but in my memory the aisles are dim. Behind me, out the shop window, the snow had started in earnest, the tiny icy flecks having turned into fat flakes spinning lazily through the air and sticking to the streets, which were whitening fast.

'Can I help you?' the pharmacist asked and I said nothing, just reached for the cube in my pocket and tried to flatten it out on the counter between us. The pharmacist took the prescription and, glancing down through his bifocals, read it, then gave me a long look. I shrugged. 'Give me ten minutes,' he said, and that was that. In ten quick minutes I had sixty red tablets that were smaller than pick-and-mix sweeties, each of them with tiny indecipherable writing across their equators.

Back in my dorm room, right before bed, I took two, per the instructions on the bottle. I was unprepared for the effect. Sleep hit me like a wall of water. I didn't merely go to bed. I fell into it, on to it, through it, under it, pounding away the hours in a deep slumber of densest black. When my alarm went off the next morning, I had to struggle up from unfathomable depths just to find the snooze button and then went down again, down and down to the bottom of some private sea.

Finding the Drug

It was March 1949 when 23-year-old Alan Broadhurst disembarked at a sagging train station in Rhodes, England, a small mill town outside Manchester that one imagines as a sooty place with crooked streets and a perpetual drizzle glazing everything with a dull gleam. The idealistic Broadhurst had come at the behest of the Swiss pharmaceutical firm Geigy, which had hired him to help establish its British branch. Broadhurst walked the town's cobblestone pavements, looking for the company he had agreed to join, and finally found it, not in some impressive high-rise or esteemed brick structure with ivy lapping the sides, but in a tiny house with a film of filth over the windows and sunken stairs that increased his alarm with each step he took, until at last he stood before a door.

The interior of the Geigy office was cluttered. Broadhurst walked through tiny tilted rooms with cardboard boxes heaped everywhere and folders scattered on metal desks. In the laboratory, which was crammed into a back lavatory, test tubes lined the sink and the shower stall. It is difficult to imagine this abode as one that could give birth to the tricyclics in general and to imipramine in particular – and indeed the actual work of invention would be done back in Geigy's Basel office – but it was here, with Broadhurst and other colleagues, that imipramine, a drug that psychiatry hails as its first antidepressant, and one that would help hundreds of thousands, perhaps millions, of people to overcome depression, got its notional start.

Broadhurst would certainly have known about the famous experiment performed by the German chemist Friedrich Wöhler, in 1828, in which Wöhler successfully demonstrated that urea, a substance found in mammalian urine, could be synthesised in a laboratory, the first evidence that the human body and its biological substrates could be made by man. In hindsight, according to David Healy, this was the first time we were confronted with the truth that there is 'nothing intrinsically special about human life.' Contrary to what many scientists had previously believed, the synthesising of urea revealed that 'making life did not require a divine or other mysterious intervention.' Had I known, at the age of nineteen, about Wöhler's experiment, perhaps I would have been less ambivalent about seeing my disorder as biochemical. Whereas I, along with millions of others in both the nineteenth and twentieth centuries, saw human life as a transcendent, even spiritual phenomenon, firmly separated from test tubes and Bunsen burners, Broadhurst was prepared to use just this kind of equipment to make some new drug, in some new way.

But where to begin? For whom would this drug be intended? Broadhurst started by looking at the antihistamines. He and the executives at Geigy were aware of the exciting new developments at Rhône-Poulenc, particularly the phenothiazine nucleus that lay at the centre of the dye methylene blue. What would emerge in the end is imipramine, called a tricyclic because of its three-ringed molecular structure. Like its cousin chlorpromazine, this drug, the first antidepressant, was also developed from a dye, not methylene blue but summer blue, sometimes called sky blue. In the years before its psychiatric properties were understood, however, Geigy was hoping merely to discover another medication that could perhaps be employed in heart surgery, and as a sedative or analgesic, much as promazine (the precursor of chlorpromazine) initially had been. But they would have to do it without using the phenothiazine nucleus, which Rhône-Poulenc had been working from. Broadhurst wondered whether there might be more to mine from antihistamines, while at the same time he and Geigy wanted to avoid creating what the field calls a 'me too' concoction, a drug that is basically the same as its source with maybe a few side molecules tweaked. (An example would be valproate semisodium, the anticonvulsant that I discussed in the last chapter, which was the same as its predecessor, valproate, with the exception of a single ion.) Taking antihistamines and the desire to create a heterocyclic compound as their starting point, Broadhurst and his team wanted to create a truly unique drug.

In general, psychiatric drug development in the middle of the last century worked this way, and still to a considerable degree works this way today, with the drug preceding the knowledge of the exact disease it will treat. Drug research proceeds by seren-dipity, by hunches and building discoveries deductively, without a definite goal. Pieces of information drift in and are sifted and sorted, suggesting the next step, until at last a novel compound emerges, although what it might treat and whom it might help are questions to which the answers are still often unknown.

Remember, chlorpromazine started its life as an anaesthetic potentiator, lauded for its mood-altering properties, its ability to cool patients down, to slow the blood supply to the limbs and, in so doing, to make surgery easier to perform. Chlorpromazine as we know it was born not when chemists Paul Charpentier and Simone Courvoisier chlorinated the antihistamine promazine, but rather before that, when Henri Laborit observed the indifference in his surgery patients who were under the influence of promethazine, a similar antihistamine, and thus suggested it for psychiatric use. The drug came into being because someone saw it in a new way and dared to dream about uses that were not immediately obvious. In some senses all drug discovery, while clearly the work of scien-tists, is really done deep in dream, in vision, and proceeds more like the making of a novel than the compounding of chemicals for a clear purpose.

In their casting about, young Broadhurst and the group of sci-entists he oversaw gravitated towards the antihistamines because the French, in chlorpromazine, had given them a big, bright clue. 'Eventually', wrote Broadhurst in his recollection of those times, 'the spotlight fell on iminodibenzyl', a tricyclic substance that, like chlorpromazine, was descended from a dye – summer blue rather than methylene blue – but was 'actually very different in chemical terms'.

Once the scientists made the choice to focus on iminodibenzyl, they had effectively narrowed their search. At the company's request, Geigy's organic chemists created derivatives of the substance, forty-two in all, by making minor alterations in iminodibenzyl's molecular side chains. The scientists next began testing these derivatives on lab animals – rats, mice and rabbits – with the goal of discovering which compounds were toxic. Broadhurst, like Cade before him, even went so far as to ingest one of the compounds himself. Eventually the team narrowed in on G22150, the code number given to the least toxic and most sedative of the compounds. Even when administered in heaping doses to the smallest of the animals, the chemical remained non-toxic and efficiently sedating. The thought at Geigy was that it might be developed for clinical use as a hypnotic. Again and again in these accounts one is struck by the arbitrary nature of the entire endeavour of drug research. Insomnia was not a problem the Geigy scientists had set out to treat. They had no specific interest in it. But as often continues to be the case, drugs came first, diseases second.

Testing the Drug

In 1950, a year into their efforts, the chemists at Geigy approached a number of psychiatrists, asking if they would be willing to try Geigy's new substance on some of their insomniac patients. One of these doctors was Roland Kuhn, an esteemed and self-assured psychiatrist at Münsterlingen Hospital, in Switzerland, on the shores of Lake Constance. After considering the proposal, Kuhn, though he was formal and somewhat stern, agreed to test the drug on his sleepless patients.

Nowadays no drug is tested in the way the Geigy scientists sought to test G22150. A drug developer does not home in on a derivative that might have some use and then find a doctor willing to give it a whirl, using his or her patients as subjects. The process has become highly regulated, with clinical trials and a double-blind design and an institutional review board overseeing the process. Moreover, a new product is always tested against a placebo, which takes years and years and a lot of money. The story of imipramine's development, like chlorpromazine's, has an almost fairy-tale quality to it, in a time and a country in which there were no agencies such as the Medicines & Healthcare products Regulatory Agency (MHRA) or the US's Food and Drug Administration (FDA) – or institutional review boards. On the one hand, drug development has probably gained from its much stricter surveillance, as patients are at the very least protected by ethical guidelines. Psychiatrists such as Kuhn, however, believed that the best way to test a drug was not through clinical trials that proceed in excruciatingly slow and expensive stages, but rather through careful clinical observation that arises only in the context of an empathic and understanding relationship between patient and practitioner.

After agreeing to give it a try, Kuhn dutifully dispensed G22150 to Münsterlingen's insomniac patients, and thus the chemical began its life as a sleeping tablet. It was a failure. Some patients slept well; others seemed entirely unaffected. Geigy abandoned G22150 and with it the fleeting desire to help those afflicted with insomnia.

Their scientists, however, soon identified a new focus, G22355, which shared many chemical similarities with chlorpromazine. Broadhurst and others at Geigy were becoming aware that chlorpromazine had slipped from surgery into psychiatry in France, and that Jean Delay and Pierre Deniker were getting outstanding results in treating schizophrenics. Even though Geigy's scientists did not want to develop a 'me too' drug, they could not help but wonder if their new darling might also be a successful treatment for psychosis. 'The road to Münsterlingen was already well trodden,'

Broadhurst recalled, 'and soon we were retracing our steps to the psychiatric hospital there to ask Dr Kuhn if he would try out our new drug in schizophrenia.'

Despite the failure of G22150, Kuhn was willing to give this new drug a chance. Schizophrenic patients who were currently on chlorpromazine, which was growing too expensive for regular use, were pulled off, and Kuhn assembled a group of drug-free schizophrenics as well. All were administered G22355. Despite their scant knowledge of the compound, the Geigy scientists, the staff at Münsterlingen and Kuhn himself all thought that this drug, so similar in structure to chlorpromazine, would work, and that when it did, there would be a second antipsychotic to add to the arsenal.

Thus the whole team – everyone involved with the trial except the patients themselves – waited expectantly, hoping that this time would be an arrow straight into the bullseye of their patients' intense suffering. As the drug flowed through the patients' veins, the nurses watched closely for just a flicker of change, although they knew that no drug, not even chlorpromazine, could instantly alter an illness as severe and static as schizophrenia. A silence descended over Münsterlingen in the days during which this new drug was being transmitted to patients – the silence of suspension, of something held aloft.

Eventually, in a period ranging from a few days to several weeks, the patients who had been given the new drug began to show some behavioural changes that 'were not only fascinating,' according to Broadhurst, but also, 'in some patients, quite alarming.' What happened is this: a group of usually quiet, sedate schizophrenic patients began to pace, showing increasing agitation. Some became energised, but the energy was disorganised and senseless. They skipped in small circles, or sang nonsense songs. *Row, row, row your boat. Down the dock. Made of rock. Hackensack. Believe your back. Life is but a dream.* One patient, charged up with insane energy, managed to get hold of a bicycle and, one night, with the stars wheeling over the mountaintops, pedalled over to an adjacent village in his nightclothes, singing at the top of his voice. The sleeping denizens rose from their beds and parted their curtains to see a sweating man speeding down the street with his head tipped back and his voice tumbling and trembling as the songs spewed forth and billowed into the air like smoke.

The Geigy scientists, the nursing staff, even Kuhn himself – all were crestfallen. Clearly the drug had had an effect, but it surely did not organise schizophrenics. There were a few patients, those with a depressive streak in their illness, in whom some improvement was noted. But only *some* improvement. Nothing like the huge hits that had been happening with chlorpromazine in France. 'Our disappointment was intense,' wrote Broadhurst. In dismay, they abandoned the clinical trial and 'spent many agonising hours trying to find an explanation as to what might have happened to precipitate such a reaction in certain patients. We stumbled around, examining a number of unlikely hypotheses and mechanisms.'

These stumbling sessions took place at Geigy's headquarters in Basel, where the scientists cast about for an answer. But they were all ambition, no vision. They had not even an inkling of what it was they might want to try next. As they huddled around a table one day, trying to make sense of why it was that their antipsychotic had failed so miserably while chlorpromazine, so similar, was such a spectacular success, an idea crystallised. Who spoke it first is unclear – Broadhurst believes it may have been his colleague Paul Schmidlin – but the scientists began to speculate on the reasons for the drug's tremendous *energising* effect. Those pacing schizophrenics had acted as though they were wearing battery packs. And that bicycle man, the one with his song streaming out of him beneath a starry sky – he was a man without an orbit, wavering and wobbling, but *happy*. Yes, some of the patients had seemed oddly happy on G22355, had they not, or if not happy, then at least endowed with an intention that made them circle and pace. The drug had bestowed on almost every patient who took it some sort of motivation, and thus … could it be, might it be … an antidepressant?

In hindsight, when everything appears so obvious, it seems incredible that the scientists took so long coming to their conclusion. But as Healy points out, the word 'antidepressant' was not really in existence when imipramine was first discovered, a lack of language that may shed some light on why the insight that was finally wrought from their tortured speculations did not occur to them earlier. According to Broadhurst, 'In retrospect, it all seems so naive, so preposterous, so mechanistic and yet so simple, but we wondered if the apparent mood elevation seen in the schizophrenic patients might also occur in depressed individuals, but in this case with a beneficial outcome.'

So it was that the scientists returned to Münsterlingen for the third time, asking Kuhn once again if he would be willing to try G22355, only this time on his depressed patients. 'I well remember the look of suspicious disbelief on his face,' wrote Broadhurst. But eventually Kuhn was persuaded to undertake a new clinical trial, which began in late 1955. First intramuscularly and then orally, G22355 was administered to a group of asylum patients with severe vegetative depression. Forty patients altogether were given the drug, after which came, once again, the waiting game, the empty silence, the staring, with no evidence of effect as the days dripped by and everyone waited – most especially the patients, who had the most to gain and the most to lose. Unlike the previous patients who had taken the drug, these were not the walking wounded. Nor were they schizophrenics lost to the world. They were cognisant of their condition, trapped in a terrible paralysis. Patients hospitalised for depression in the 1950s tended to be seriously stuck, immobilised by their relentless pain, entirely unable to cope but nevertheless harbouring clear memories of who and what they had been prior to their descent, the knowledge of the cruel contrast difficult to bear.

As with the earlier trial of G22355, this one was also entirely uncontrolled. The scientists simply gave some samples to Kuhn, who in turn administered those samples to the patients he picked. But the simplicity that may appear distressing or careless was not necessarily so. While Kuhn had never employed a double-blind study, placebos, a statistical treatment of data or any of the other accoutrements of clinical trials that today are paramount, he 'examined each patient individually, often every day, on several occasions, and questioned each patient again and again'.

The first patient to show a change was 49-year-old Paula J. F., who had been depressed and deluded for years. She began treatment with G22355 on 12 January 1956, and only days later appeared completely well. About three weeks after the start of the trial, both the scientists and Kuhn were able to see incredible results in many other patients as well. 'It was clear that G22355 was producing a dramatic, and this time beneficial, response,' wrote Broadhurst. 'About two-thirds of the patients showed marked reduction in their depressive symptoms. Individuals with biological – or as Dr Kuhn described them, "vegetative" – symptoms tended to do best.'

Resistance

Like chlorpromazine, which found success through large public mental health hospitals, G22355 was slow to make inroads into the psychiatric community, again at least in part because the 1950s were the heyday of psychoanalysis and psychodynamic therapies, an era in which depression was seen as internalised rage, sublimated sexual distress or even the externalisation of a psychological snarl the patient had yet to work through. It was one thing to calm a psychotic person through chemical means, but treating depression with drugs was antithetical to the zeitgeist. Drug treatment, it was widely believed, would slow down or short-circuit the patient's effort to get to the heart of his trouble and was therefore to be avoided at all costs.

Certainly I harboured these notions as I stood on the street outside the apothecary that snowy night, rolling my just-filled bottle of imipramine back and forth in my ungloved hand, watching the flakes form on its curved surface, until the bottle was furred with snow and the ink ran black, staining the pristine white. I clearly remember later on, back at my dorm, placing two of the tiny candy-coated tablets on the pad of my tongue and washing them down with water, followed by a sweet aftertaste and then the swale of sleep drenched in contorted dreams full of clowns with melting mouths and clouds rolling on the ground, the red scream of a siren, a swan in full flight, bones in a bag, the dagger of an icicle with a drop of water trembling at its tip. My hesitations and the extreme side effects of the drug that set in the very next morning – fuzziness, sweating, a tacky mouth and tongue – did not, however, stop me from taking it, because I had already tried, unsuccessfully, to dredge up my rotten rage, to blame my mother, to deeply weep, and it had all come to naught. So what other choice did I have, exactly? I have to think that, twenty years earlier, just as G22355 was being tested, the patients taking it must have felt similarly.

And it may be that some psychiatrists felt similarly too. Broadhurst recalls Hilda Abraham, one of psychiatry's distinguished psychoanalysts, 'the last person [he] would have expected to be interested in the drug treatment of depression', contacting him about getting G22355 so she could begin a trial of it. Abraham was known for doing what my psychiatrist did, namely, trying to transform patients using insight and catharsis alone. One of Abraham's colleagues set her up with a real trial, using a control group and a double-blind design. 'I remember how amazed Abraham was', wrote Broadhurst, 'when nearly two-thirds of her depressed patients recovered with the drug.'

Credit

Who gets credit for scientific discoveries is always a complex question. In the case of chlorpromazine – the first psychiatric drug ever created, the drug that moved the field from the mere management of severe and persistent mental illness to, in many cases, at least partial remissions so long as the drug was continued – it was unclear, in large part because no one could figure out who had held the crucial key. Was it Paul Charpentier, who, in his laboratory at Rhône-Poulenc, first chlorinated promazine and came up with chlorpromazine? Or was it his colleague Simone Courvoisier, who, in her experiments with lab rats, first noted chlorpromazine's central effects? Was it Henri Laborit, who, perhaps more significantly, not only noted the indifference that his surgery patients displayed when under the influence of both promethazine and later chlorpromazine, but also avidly pushed psychiatrists at the Val-de-Grâce military hospital to try chlorpromazine on their patients? Or was it Delay and Deniker, the first psychiatrists to use chlorpromazine widely and without additional drugs or ice, thereby discovering that chlorpromazine was in its own right and by virtue of its own actions a steadfast antipsychotic?

Similarly, G22355, which became imipramine, was another huge breakthrough and, as in the case of chlorpromazine, it is difficult to assess who should get credit for what. Without a doubt Broadhurst and his colleagues at Geigy, including the chemists who concocted those forty-two derivatives of iminodibenzyl, played a pivotal role. Yet they have more or less dropped out of view, their names seldom mentioned when the topic of the discovery of antidepressants is broached. Instead it is Kuhn who is usually credited with single-handedly discovering imipramine, which is not at all the case, though it is true that at this point in our story, once the very first clinical trials have been run, the Geigy team recedes and Kuhn steps forward to play a bigger part.

He was not well liked, by his colleagues at least. Some found him curmudgeonly, others tightfisted. He published broadly but sometimes failed to put others' names on the papers, despite the fact that they were clearly collaborative. He sought recognition and was consistently disappointed that more did not come his way. He was not always invited to crucial conferences.

Kuhn had been born on 4 March 1912, in the small town of Biel, Switzerland, north-west of Bern, where he would later train in psychiatry at the university, with the great Jakob Klaesi, who pioneered deep-sleep therapy, a treatment that relied primarily on the notion that in states of prolonged rest accomplished with hypnotics and barbiturates, patients' nervous systems would have the chance to recalibrate and right themselves. (Deep-sleep therapy swept Europe in the early to mid-twentieth century, though it never really caught on in the United States.) Kuhn apprenticed himself to Klaesi for some years. When he was done with his training, he left Klaesi's practice and went to work at Münsterlingen, a state hospital which housed seven hundred inpatients along with an expanding outpatient population.

Klaesi understood some forms of mental illness to be a biological phenomenon, and when one looks closely at Kuhn, Klaesi's fingerprints become apparent, as Kuhn took on his mentor's views concerning the biological basis of depression. Nevertheless, Kuhn's proclivities as a clinician, despite the fact that he would later achieve renown for the imipramine drug trials, were more psychodynamic and existential, probably because he was also heavily influenced by Ludwig Binswanger, a Swiss psychoanalyst and existential philosopher whom he considered 'a genius in his understanding of mood disorder'. Like Binswanger, Kuhn probed his patients for the psychological paradigms that might have caused or contributed to their mental illnesses. In his work he stressed empathic listening with existential insight into the profoundly problematic human condition, as his patients struggled, as we all do, with the knowledge that ultimately we live and die alone.

When it comes to G22355, Kuhn tells a somewhat different

tale than does Broadhurst. In Broadhurst's story, he and his fellow scientists approached Kuhn, asking if he would be willing to try their derivative, but in Kuhn's version it was he who approached the Geigy team, asking to try G22355 in the hopes that it might, like Thorazine, help schizophrenic patients. When it failed in this regard, Kuhn claims that it was his idea to refashion it as an anti-depressant. Despite these discrepancies, there are several points of convergence. All agree that there was the first alarming trial on more than three hundred schizophrenic patients, some of whom badly deteriorated, including the one who bicycled into town in his nightshirt, singing lustily. And all agree that the study was abruptly discontinued.

In any event, once the efficacy of G22355 as an antidepressant was established, Kuhn went on to publish his findings in a Swiss medical journal, in August 1957. The following month he attended the Second World Congress of Psychiatry, held that year in Zurich, where he reported his results during a session in which there were just twelve or thirteen people in the audience. The biology of depression and the treatment of mood disorders were very much out of vogue.

Vital Depression

Kuhn, however, was undeterred. By 1958 he had treated more than five hundred depressed patients with G22355, taking the initial input from the Geigy scientists and then extending the research broadly. Here is where the role of Geigy – of Broadhurst and Schmidlin and the other scientists – fades into the background while Kuhn steps forward as an essential protagonist in this story of the early antidepressants. Despite being somewhat disliked by his colleagues, Kuhn was sensitive and attentive to his patients, both empathic and observant, so much so that he was able to ascertain what types of depression would most likely respond to G22355 and to describe to Geigy the drug's effects in a nuanced fashion, explaining that, while it was an antidepressant, it was not a euphoriant, a critical distinction for the field in particular and for the public in general.

Euphoriants – cocaine, for instance – are not drugs that treat a discrete disease, while an antidepressant, according to Kuhn, would be able to do that. Moreover, in Kuhn's view, an antidepressant would work only on someone suffering from a particular kind of despair, one that he called a 'vital depression', a state marked by reduced appetite, psychomotor retardation, a worsening of mood in the morning with some relief granted as the day went on. Those with vital depression tended to sleep poorly, were gripped by guilt and hopelessness, and either wept copiously or stared dry-eyed out into a world without colour. These were the patients who responded best to G22355. Patients without vital depression tended to experience no effect or a negative effect. Kuhn explained in the papers he published that it was possible those suffering from vital depression might not show any overt sadness at all. The depression might, he claimed, instead take on the guise of a phobia or an obsession. Thus he used G22355 on patients with phobias and obsessions as well, and got good results.

Meanwhile, as Kuhn was conducting his trials of G22355 between 1954 and 1957, Geigy knew they had a useful compound on their hands, but the firm was slow to bring it to market. It wasn't that there was no other interest. The Canadian doctor Heinz Lehmann – one of the first, you'll recall, to prescribe chlorpromazine in North America – had been at the Second World Congress of Psychiatry, where Kuhn gave his poorly attended talk. Lehmann read Kuhn's lecture on his flight back to Montreal and, intrigued, contacted the Geigy offices in Canada once he was home to ask for some samples. The Canadian branch of Geigy had never even heard of G22355. Nevertheless, Lehmann managed to get his hands on some samples and immediately started a trial at his own asylum, using the drug on eighty-four depressed patients and reporting, in 1958, that two-thirds of them responded positively. But despite its stellar success in treating a devastating condition, still G22355 did not catch on.

Is There a Market?

For fretful Geigy, the overarching question was whether there would ever really be a market for the drug. In a post-fluoxetine era this concern seems astounding. A market for an effective anti-depressant, and safe to boot? Of course. Without a doubt. But this was well before fluoxetine had made depression into a superstar syndrome. By emphasising for Geigy that G22355 was not a stimulant, Kuhn forced company executives to tussle with a paradoxical phenomenon – a compound that eradicated the creep and crawl of severe depression, a compound that allowed its users to feel joy, vitality, *energy*, but that was not a stimulant or a euphoriant? Then what *was* it? Kuhn couldn't say but he was quite sure the drug would be most useful for patients who were appropriate candidates for electroconvulsive therapy; in other words, for seriously ill patients, which, from Geigy's point of view, made for a very small market indeed.

Studies by the World Health Organization to determine the range and reach of depression indicate that, on any given day, up to 350 million people worldwide are suffering from the disorder. Had Geigy been able to see into a future in which fluoxetine would one day so saturate our culture that it has literally leaked into our waterways, they might not have dallied in marketing their new product. But they were operating in a cultural milieu in which 'depression' was not yet a household word, not by a long shot. In their milieu, one suffered in silence, and often got treatment only if or when the depression became so severe that the ability to function was lost.

By late 1958, more than a year after Kuhn's presentation at the Second World Congress of Psychiatry, Geigy did finally throw its weight behind G22355, but not because the company came to a clearer understanding of how or why it worked, or of what class of drug it was precisely, or, indeed, of whether there was really a market for it. What happened is this: the wife of one of the company's top shareholders, Robert Böhringer, had become depressed. In a move that echoes Mogens Schou's concern for his brother, Böhringer, who was made aware of Geigy's work on G22355 by Kuhn, asked for some samples, brought them home and within a week his wife recovered. After that Böhringer became insistent, and since he was one of the owners of Geigy, his vote counted.

But there was more. The previous year another antidepressant, iproniazid, had been announced on the front page of the *New York Times*. Now there was competition. Geigy shot forward. Given the name imipramine, G22355 was brought to market first in Switzerland, and then in other European countries under the name Tofranil, by which it was also known in the United States, when it was finally released here, in 1959, a full eight years after Geigy had first patented the drug.

Rocket Fuel

Meanwhile, back in the United States, a charismatic figure named Nathan Kline, who was the research director at Rockland State Hospital, an asylum in New York on the western bank of the Hudson River, had his hands on the competition, a class of drugs called monoamine oxidase inhibitors (MAO inhibitors, or MAOIs, for short). A monoamine oxidase is an enzyme that interacts with neurotransmitters such as serotonin, dopamine, and noradrenaline, removing them from the brain. Scientists had begun to wonder if an MAO imbalance in a person – too little or especially too much of the stuff – could cause schizophrenia or depression. Perhaps the MAO inhibitor could restore the balance of monoamine neurotransmitters in the brain by preventing the enzyme from removing them, thereby making them more available for use.

Unlike tricyclics such as imipramine, a three-ringed chemical structure, the MAOIs were made of much different stuff, specifically hydrazine, a toxic liquid better known as rocket fuel – the same fuel, in fact, that the Germans had used during the Second World War to launch their V-2 missiles. Once the war was over, Germany found itself in possession of excess hydrazine, useless with the imposition of the new military limitations. With no need for hydrazine any longer, the country passed it off cheaply to different chemical companies keen to experiment with it.

Both of our two earliest antidepressants, then, have lyrical links. The first, like chlorpromazine, our original antipsychotic, has its roots in the dye industry, springing from summer blue, treating the blues with the blues. The second, birthed from the fuel that propelled rockets into the sky, was rediscovered for the purpose of propelling people, launching them upwards and forwards to a place from which they could shed their misery. The MAO inhibitors were as celebrated as imipramine was ignored, at least initially, and they caused a major hubbub in the United States, with pictures in the press and great claims made and prizes awarded. Would there be a market? Geigy had asked. The answer was an emphatic yes.

Hydrazine. Rocket fuel. In 1951 scientists discovered that it had anti-tubercular effects. The following year one of the compounds cooked up from hydrazine, iproniazid, turned out to do something else in addition to being effective against tuberculosis. Scientists noted that patients treated with it manifested not only an improvement in their primary disease but also a greater vitality overall, a sense of extreme well-being along with a marked increase in social activity. An Associated Press photograph from the time, taken at Sea View, a hospital on Staten Island for tubercular patients, shows the patients in a party mood. The caption reads, *A few months ago the only sound here was the sound of victims of tuberculosis, coughing up their lives*. In another photo, patients waltz in the dayroom above the caption *Dancing in the halls tho' there were holes in their lungs*. Well before iproniazid became a bona fide antidepressant, then, its euphoriant effects were noted. The road it travelled, from a tuberculosis drug that put a smile on sufferers' faces to an approved 'psychic energiser' for the treatment of depression, is long and twisty, with a number of years between the first observations of its mood effects and its proper packaging as an antidepressant.

But how did Nathan Kline become the primary discoverer of the MAOIs? The 1950s and '60s, sometimes called the 'golden era of psychopharmacology', were a time when it seemed the doors to understanding human suffering, previously sealed, were being flung open, as the brain yielded up its harvest of secrets and paths, and new neurotransmitters were discovered one after the other. Noradrenaline. Serotonin. Dopamine. If you listened closely you could almost hear the click of axons and dendrites, the stutter of cognitive sparks, the sound of neurons nicking one another as they jostled inside the circle of the skull.

This was the world in which Nathan Kline moved and worked, circling the New York psychiatry circuit lit with enthusiasm and spark. He seemed to know everyone who was anyone. And if Roland Kuhn, his contemporary, was slow, steady, strict and regimented, then Kline, who a decade later would appear on the cover of *Fortune* magazine as one of the ten best-known men in America, was his polar opposite: flashy, magnetic, keen and malleable, easily adopting new ideas. Kline was ambitious, too, and had every intention of discovering a drug. Interest in iproniazid was beginning to develop, and he wondered what would happen if it was systematically dispensed to depressed patients. But before he tried doing that, he appeared before Congress in July 1955 to discuss the new drugs just cresting the horizon and the need for proper evaluation tools. Because of Kline's passionate and convincing presentation, Congress awarded $2 million for the study of the new mental health drugs, a vast sum at that time, so much money, Healy wrote, 'that those charged with administering it found it difficult to give it away'.

Part of the reason why Kline could get such significant backing is that he was already well known for a 1953 study that demonstrated the effects of reserpine, an alkaloid, on 710 psychiatric patients, finding that it was an efficacious antipsychotic. (For this he was later awarded the first of his two Lasker prizes, sometimes called the 'American Nobel', sharing it with Henri Laborit, Heinz Lehmann, Pierre Deniker and Robert H. Noce for the contributions that each had made to the treatment of schizophrenia.) Reserpine did not cause the big bang that chlorpromazine did, in part because it tended not to cause the same kind of dramatic awakenings that Delay and Deniker witnessed in Paris. And eventually Kline abandoned it entirely, once he realised that although it managed his most troubled patients' psychoses, it had the unintended side effect of sometimes inducing depression.

Reserpine, however, did become an indispensable research tool, perhaps *the* most significant research tool of that era. Remember those reserpine rabbits? In Bernard Brodie's laboratory at the US's National Institutes of Health, researchers demonstrated that reserpine caused a lowering of serotonin in rabbits' brains while simultaneously making the animals lethargic, thereby providing researchers with their first animal model of depression, along with its neurochemical signature – low serotonin. Interestingly, rabbits pretreated with either imipramine or an MAOI were protected from 'the reserpine effect'. And when the pretreated rabbits' brains were sliced and studied, their synapses were found to be loaded with serotonin, suggesting, for the first time, that depression, and its cure, were closely allied with this neurotransmitter.

Kline knew about the animal studies done using iproniazid and reserpine, and he needed to make only the littlest leap to conceive of using the MAOIs for depression in his own patients. In November 1956 Kline began to test his hypothesis, treating seventeen inpatients with iproniazid while also giving the drug to some of his melancholic outpatients as well. Two-thirds of the patients showed marked improvement.

The pharmaceutical firm Roche produced iproniazid. Kline alerted company executives to his findings only to discover that Roche did not much care. Nevertheless, iproniazid was already on the market as a tuberculosis drug, so Kline's hurdle was not that high. As a means of swaying Roche executives, and because of his general love of publicity, Kline reported his study results to the *New York Times* and various articles were written about this new old drug that could produce 'remarkable mood improvement'. The public took note, and thanks in large part to Kline's expert public relation efforts, the drug took off. Within the first year 400,000 people were treated with iproniazid, usually with positive results.

A Psychic Energiser

Kline, for his part, did not call the drug an antidepressant. He preferred the term 'psychic energiser', a concocted category which feels very different from the term 'antidepressant'. A psychic energiser has a whiff of magic to it. It feels more closely allied to a vitamin than to a drug. It calls to mind the ephemeral, immeasurable psyche, with a little fizz now added, as opposed to the plodding and stern term 'antidepressant'. Would iproniazid have caught on so widely had Kline labelled it an antidepressant? After all, who *can't* use a little psychic energy?

In the end, however, despite Kline's efforts, the serious and stodgy won out. The term 'psychic energiser' faded away, and MAOIs are now called antidepressants. But let's consider what would have happened if we had gone Klineian instead of Kuhnian; if we had decided to call the new drugs psychic energisers rather than antidepressants; if when you went to see your psychophar-macologist, he agreed to write you a prescription for a psychic energiser; if you said to friends that you were on a psychic ener-giser. Would we have been as quick to pathologise depression if the tablets to treat it didn't suggest sickness? A psychic energiser is Everyman's medication, while an antidepressant seems destined for the sickest of souls. One can only conjecture, of course, but the question underscores the weight of the labels we give and how, in our quest to define things, the things we name in turn name us.

The public popularity of the MAOIs with the thousands upon thousands of people who were getting psychically energised foreshadowed the offshoot drug that was still decades away: fluoxetine, that green-and-ivory orb hailed as a breakthrough. The story of the MAOIs first revealed to us that we have long been clamouring for a cure, that we want to be believers, and that we are quick to embrace and be swayed by the offerings of pharmaceutical companies. Our belief can seem astounding when one considers the facts, which, depending on your perspective, were either nil or simultaneously abundant and contradictory. As with the drugs that had presaged them, no one really had any idea how imipramine worked, or how the MAOIs worked, only that for many people they did. True, when it came to the MAOIs, we had some inchoate theories about the level of neurotransmitters. And yes, the research of Bernard Brodie's NIH laboratory on reserpine had shed significant light on the link between levels of brain serotonin and depression, suggesting that low serotonin leads to low mood. That light vanishes, however, when we face yet another fact: reserpine itself, which *lowers* serotonin, supposedly the opposite of what we want for a depressed person, has been shown in other studies to be an effective *anti*depressant. So the facts tell us this: reserpine causes *and* cures depression, a statement that cancels out understanding in one swift swipe.

We know that reserpine causes lethargy in animals and that when the reserpine rabbits' brains were analysed they showed a depletion of serotonin, leading one to think that low serotonin is a culprit in depression and that the new antidepressants must have been somehow 'raising' levels of this neurotransmitter, especially because when the rabbits were pretreated with either imipramine or an MAOI, they did not show lethargy after imbibing reserpine. The same is true for rats. Rats treated with reserpine and then fed a tricyclic, in this case desipramine, a close cousin of imipramine, not only shrugged off the reserpine cloud but also became *more* active. The brains of these can-do rats were swimming in serotonin. The only explanation, then, was that their zeal and zest had to be a by-product of the antidepressants they were on. And yet – and in this story of drugs and neurotransmitters there is almost always an 'and yet' – when researchers have measured serotonin levels in actual depressed human beings and compared them to controls, they have found that some depressed people have low serotonin, some have normal levels of serotonin and some have high levels of serotonin, a statement that makes you swing your head dizzily around, or better yet duck so as to miss the facts flying every which way.

As we have seen with virtually all psychotropic medications, when it comes to drugs and the complex chemical soup of the brain, the only shred of certainty is this: there was, and still is, no real understanding of how and why our drugs work. The public continues to clamour for them, imbibing them in continually increasing doses, keen to believe the pharmaceutical companies' simplistic pictorial explanations, which tend to show a synaptic cleft drained of its serotonin along with the ever-present phrase 'chemical imbalance'. The roots of this understanding, or mis-understanding, are planted firmly in Kuhn and Kline, or, more fairly, in the pharmaceutical factories that manufactured not only the two men's drugs but also the necessary 'explanations' that would sell these drugs to the public. There is a sense in which one becomes converted to the antidepressant narrative spun by pharmaceutical firms. It may not be psychologically possible for some people to take a substance that alters their psyche at its most precious points and at the same time admit to themselves that the substance is mired in contradictory evidence that effectively cancels out the possibility of certainty. Thus, when one agrees to take an antidepressant, one may also be agreeing, to some extent, to adhere to a certain story about how the drug works.

Side Effects

It should not be surprising to us, given what we know about chlor-promazine and lithium, that the side effects of the tricyclics and the MAOIs turned out to be not insignificant. Imipramine, for example, can leave the mouth so dry that the teeth start to rot, deprived of saliva's sealants. One also gets groggy on the tricyclics, and emerging from slumber can be like coming up from under a pool of sludge with your eyes tarred shut. As for the MAOIs, they cannot be mixed with any food substance, such as cheese and red wine, that contains the compound tyramine. In the event that an MAOI is combined with tyramine, the patient risks dangerously high blood pressure, haemorrhaging and other possibly toxic events.

Novelist and essayist David Foster Wallace has been one of our more famous public figures to take an MAOI. Wallace lived with the side effects of his MAOI, phenelzine, for many years before finally deciding to go off the drug. His decision was spurred by a dining episode. One night, after eating at a Persian restaurant he frequented, Wallace became seriously ill. It wasn't food poisoning but rather an interaction of his phenelzine with tyramine, which, unbeknownst to Wallace, had been in his food. Wallace experienced heart palpitations and was felled by terrible stomach pains that laid him low for days. After he recovered he decided he wanted off, he wanted out; he had been on the drug for more than two decades and it was time to see if he could transition to an antidepressant without the MAOI side effect profile. His psychiatrist agreed.

They did a slow taper that took months, and for a time, at his own insistence, Wallace even tried to go without medication entirely. It didn't work, and he was hospitalised for severe depression. After his release, he cycled through many different antidepressants, not always staying on them long enough for them to take effect, and each time his dark mood returned, coming in as a series of grey days that eventually darkened dangerously, sapping him of strength and vigour. His depression was deep, and had teeth. According to his biographer D. T. Max, in the spring of 2008, almost a year after the initial event, 'a new combination of antidepressants seemed to stabilise Wallace'. But the reprieve turned out to be short-lived, and in June of that year he made a suicide attempt.

Following that episode, Wallace underwent twelve rounds of ECT, and returned to his old standby, the MAOI phenelzine, which had worked so well for him before. Surely it would work again, as it was the same drug and he was the same man. He had hope. He took the phenelzine tablets. But now, for reasons neither he nor anyone else in his circle could really understand, it no longer worked for him. Days turned to weeks turned to months. Something was terribly, cruelly wrong. He was getting no relief this time. No one knows why a drug that once worked well ceases to have any effect at all after a patient tries it again, but this is a documented phenomenon that makes relinquishing a well-working drug very risky. That his psychopharmacologist could not explain to Wallace why the phenelzine was so spectacularly ineffective this time around when before it had held him aloft for over two decades must have made his suffering that much worse.

Depression is a disorder of desire in which the world, stripped of its meaning, becomes absurd. The naked trees look like upright forks spearing the skin of the sky. A smile is a split in the skin, a red rip, each tooth a tiny tombstone. Your dreams are drenched in dark, all the figures faceless, blurred by an inky sludge. How long can a person survive in this mindset? Wallace made it more than a year, which is, when one really thinks about it, a heroic achievement. At last, however, with the phenelzine no longer working, and with Wallace's profound depression remaining unyielding to any other pharmaceutical intervention, he ran out of hope. One evening his wife left him alone for just a little while, to set up an art show at her gallery nearby, and when she came back home he was hanging from his belt, which he'd nailed into a rafter on their patio, the lawn chair he'd used kicked over beneath him.

The suicide of Wallace underscores the seriousness of depression, the lethality of it and why its steady rise – the increase in diagnoses – is a phenomenon we need to understand from as many angles as are available to us. As said, psychiatrists have little understanding of why a drug that once worked well for a person ceases to have any effect. All we know, in the case of David Foster Wallace and hundreds of thousands of others, is that the MAOIs have provided stepping stones out of terrible depressions. But the MAOIs, despite their efficaciousness, have all but disappeared from the current antidepressant landscape. Given how potent they are, why are they so rarely prescribed any more? Is it because we do not want to be psychically energised? Is it because we have realised that researchers know really nothing about what the drug does once it's absorbed into our bloodstream and circulated to our inner and outer extremities, ferried on the backs of cells into the sacred chamber of the brain, where it ... where it ... and here words run dry. We can fall back on hypotheses for depression – the catecholamine hypothesis, for instance, which states that depression is due to a deficiency of noradrenaline, or the serotonin hypothesis – but a hypothesis doesn't do us much good when we're talking about putting tablets into the vault of our one and only body. We'd like to know. We *should* know. And yet, even so, the lack of knowledge does not explain why MAOIs went from being homecoming queen to beggar under a bridge, in what seems like a snap.

It had something to do with cheese. Cheese? Yes, yellow cheese, white cheese, stringy cheese, aged cheese. At first, everything appeared to be delightful for the several hundred thousand people who went on the drug. Previously mad or morose people were suddenly social and socialising, as the world took on a positive tint. For some, however, that tint became jaundiced. In 1957, there were 127 cases of jaundice reported in those taking iproniazid. It was hard to know for sure whether the MAOI was causing the jaundice; it could have merely been a correlation. Perhaps people prone to depression were also prone to jaundice. And 127 cases represented just 0.03 per cent of the people who had been prescribed the drug. If it had been one hundred, just twenty-seven fewer, it would have been the same amount that occurs in the normal population. Kline shrugged his shoulders and waved away the whiff of something wrong. Roche, however, withdrew the drug.

That could have been the end of the whole story, but by this time other pharmaceutical houses had developed their own MAOIs, which were now on the market. In 1961 *The Lancet* reported on a patient who died from a sudden haemorrhage while taking the MAOI tranylcypromine, available in the United States under the brand name Parnate. Between 1961 and 1963 there were, all told, six more cases reported of people on MAOIs spontaneously haemorrhaging. The problem was that because these patients were all on other medications as well, you couldn't point the finger at the MAOIs. Perhaps the problem had been due to one of those other medications, or perhaps simply to chance. But that possibility seemed less and less likely when GPs began to report occurrences of headaches in patients taking an MAOI. Some of these patients, it turned out, also had elevated blood pressure, which can contribute to spontaneous haemorrhaging. Still, no one was sure.

The first inkling of understanding came through a hospital pharmacist from Nottingham who wrote to researcher and doctor Barry Blackwell (one of the famous antagonists of Mogens Schou in the battle over lithium) that his wife, while taking an MAOI, had experienced headaches and hypertension after eating cheese. *Could cheese be the culprit?* the pharmacist wondered. Blackwell and associates laughed that off. Cheese! Everyone loved cheese. Just to show that people taking an MAOI could safely and serenely eat their cheese, Blackwell and a colleague ingested an MAOI for one whole week, after which they ate cheese. Nothing happened.

That should have shut down the whole issue but it didn't. Hundreds of thousands of people in the United States, and thousands more in Europe, were now launched on MAOIs, and some subset of them seemed to be getting sick in dangerous ways. Soon after Blackwell had demonstrated the innocence of cheese, in fact, he noted that a patient who haemorrhaged had eaten a cheese flan for supper, an incident that was shortly followed by Blackwell being called out to see a woman who was on an MAOI and had developed a crushing headache and high blood pressure after eating a cheese sandwich.

It is unclear exactly how many people died from the MAOIs, although Blackwell claims that forty deaths attributable to this particular side effect of hypertension were recorded in the first eight years of the drug's existence. Eventually scientists figured out that cheese – along with other foods such as beans and beverages such as wine and beer – contains a substance called tyramine, which the MAOIs were increasing, an increase that resulted in escalating blood pressure and headaches and haemorrhaging. It became apparent that certain foods had to be avoided if a person was on the drug. Chocolate, for example. Olives, too. Pickles and cured meats. All of them contain tyramine and must be renounced if a person is taking an MAOI. These revelations are what ultimately sounded the death knell for what had heretofore been a very potent and useful antidepressant. The drug's usage was vastly curtailed not because no one knew how it worked or what it did once it entered our bodies – not, in other words, because patients realised they were swallowing a mystery – but because of the dietary restrictions patients would have to follow lest they lose their lives.

Despite the fatalities, the drug was not actually taken off the market. Instead, MAOIs were repackaged with black box warnings. To many psychiatrists, then, the tricyclics emanating from imipramine seemed so much simpler and certainly safer to prescribe. After all, could a doctor trust his patient to follow the food guidelines? One small slip and a burst of blood. At the same time, there was the fortuitous appearance of a prominent study from the UK which concluded that the tricyclics were the new gold standard in the treatment of depression. Gradually doctors began prescribing MAOIs less and less frequently, until finally they became what they are today – last-ditch drugs that you try when there's nothing else left. By the time Dr Mazor suggested I try a psychotropic medication, imipramine and other tricyclics had survived the intervening decades, while the MAOIs largely had not.

Thought Leaders

The MAOIs are a mini-drama showing the rise and fall of a superstar drug in a compressed fashion. When we watch the mini-drama, we come to understand how it is that drugs gain popularity and how it is that they lose it. Behind the tricyclics stood stodgy Roland Kuhn. Behind the MAOIs stood the dynamic Nathan Kline, who literally called the *New York Times* to report his study results, who culled from Congress $2 million, riding the crest of his charm and cheer.

We have probably all heard stories of the aggressive marketing strategies of pharmaceutical firms, which pay charismatic 'thought leaders' to tout their newest concoction, and we fret over the handouts, the gifts, the lavish lunches, and wonder how the process can possibly be impartial and accurate. Drugs, we like to think, are the product of science and, as such, rotate in pure spheres, but this is hardly the case. Charisma, the preen and polish of the thought leader who lends his or her light to whatever the product is, plays a huge role in drug development and dissemination. While this behaviour is perhaps more extreme now than it was then, we can see that back in the 1950s Nathan Kline all but fed rocket fuel from the palm of his gilded hand to hundreds of thousands of Americans. Beyond that, every drug is mired in a marketing campaign that colours the way we understand them. In the case of the MAOIs, they were advertised as peppy tablets in the *New York Times*, and as energisers by Nathan Kline, who sang a better song than Kuhn could ever hope to.

When the MAOIs disappeared from view, they did so not because they were ineffective but because one had to follow certain dietary restrictions. Not eating cheese or even chocolate seems a small price to pay for the recession of a debilitating depression. And yet the cheese, the olives, the peanuts – together they put a taint on the MAOIs, a sort of scarlet letter, something that, in the end, burnt brighter than anything even the charming Kline could say or do to counteract it, and the public rejected a potent antidepressant in favour of the delicatessen and chocolate bars. How does one make sense of that? As much as drugs define us, capturing us – our moods, our minds – in their chemical complexities, we also define drugs, deciding which capsule we'll endorse, and doing our crucial part to create the currents by which drugs move in and out of culture.

The Shape of a Swan

Imipramine never worked for me. I gave it a good go, staying on it for several years. I had every side effect noted, or so it seems: a continuously tacky tongue, a dry mouth that eventually caused massive cavities, a tendency to perspire profusely even when sitting still. The drug also caused my heart to stutter – arrhythmia – and gave me enormous dreams that clung to me like mud each morning. On imipramine I dreamt of golden loons and screaming monkeys hunched on parapets, parrots of every conceivable colour repeating nonsense words in a green and gleaming jungle, a river thick with bones and bodies strewn along its bank in torn translucent garments. In my dreams I was washed away again and again, sometimes in the river full of ribs, other times in the ocean, as the tides pulled me out to the satin scar of the horizon while tiny unreachable houses perched on rocky promontories in the distance. In the beginning, every month or so my doctor upped my dose, hoping for a response, and each time she did I dreamt in the daylight. The drug gave me hallucinations such that sounds became colours – a scream like a red siren – and scents became visible in the air like tendrils of filmy smoke.

Although imipramine is an antidepressant, it had an opposite effect on me, at least for the first few weeks after a dosage adjustment, when I'd weep and weep – skinned, it felt like; without defence. All my griefs came calling, all my losses, some small and some severe, each one honed to a piercing point. I cried for rabbits and books and broken eggs, for the scarf I'd loved and accidentally left behind on a train trip years earlier, for my mother and the mask she wore, for our faces, every one of which, it seemed to me, was full of holes. I don't know why Dr Mazor chose to keep me on the drug when all it did was make me weep and sweat, but this was the early 1980s and there were not many alternatives, certainly not the cornucopia of antidepressants we have now. It's reasonable to ask why, other than out of a deference to authority, I myself didn't stop when the prescription didn't help me at all. I can only say that after a while, although the drug offered no relief, I worried that if I went off it I'd get even worse.

At one point, likely at her wits' end, Dr Mazor sent me for a consultation with a colleague at Mass Mental, a Dr Carl Salzman, who offered me an MAOI to try instead. But first, he said, if I was interested, there was actually a new drug just come around the corner and he thought it might be even more helpful to me. Prozac, he said. Prozac? The brand name for fluoxetine to me sounded dull, dead and on that basis alone I doubted it would help me, but given the severity of my mood and the ineffectuality of imipramine, I was game to try.

I didn't know then that this new drug, this fluoxetine, would lift my symptoms off me as if they were mere mist, and that I would stay on a serotonin booster not for six years, and not for sixteen years, but for almost thirty years, swallowing it down each night with a tall glass of water while around me debates raged about the safety of the medication, especially for long-term use, with some critics saying it causes irreversible damage to the brain. Still I stayed on it because, for me, I didn't see any other option. Without the drug I could not properly function. Prior to fluoxetine in particular, and the SSRIs and SNRIs in general, I had been hospitalised five times and many mornings could not make it out of bed. Fluoxetine made of me a functioning individual on the one hand, while it also turned me into something of an addict on the other hand. Psychiatrists are quick to distinguish their drugs from 'street drugs', but in fact I see very little difference between the legal tablets that prop me up and the illegal tablets you can buy in that back alley somewhere in the city. Just like an opiate addict I have experienced tolerance (needing to raise my dose over and over again to get the same effect), dependence and withdrawal effects if I try to cease taking the medication. I identify myself as a highly functioning addict and I tell myself that, God knows, there are worse things I could be. Yet on many days I wish it were not so.

In the end psychiatry has sickened me even as it has saved me. I know the bind I'm in is not unique to me. Think of all those patients awakened to the world by chlorpromazine, a deeply restorative drug that then turned around and bit back hard, causing tardive dyskinesia. Psychiatry has yet to find a drug that does not exact a physical price. Everything in the psychopharmacological arsenal gives and takes. Sometimes the price is uncertainty itself, because no one knows what chronic use of any of these medicines really does to the brain. There are scant studies of the brains of people who have been chronically exposed to imipramine, the MAOIs, fluoxetine or chlorpromazine, in part because few long-term users give their brain to science upon their death, preferring to go to the grave intact.

If I touch my temple I can feel the thread of a pattering pulse. But the actual brain itself has no nerves, no pain receptors whatsoever, which I find odd: the seat of all emotion, all sensation, is itself purely numb. Before neuroscience stepped in, there was phrenology, reading the person by the telltale lumps and bumps on the human head. The phrenologist would close his eyes and move his hands around your skull, maybe muttering to himself as he went. Here a rise, there a small swell, here a dent downwards, all of it suggesting something, but what? What?

We have supposedly progressed far from that, with our fMRIs and PET scans glowing gold and green. But still today, when it comes to the persistent use of these chemicals cooked up by men who hope to help (and reap the rewards of that help), we ask, *What? What?* It's the same question I ask of my psychopharmacologist as he scrawls my next prescription, the handwriting, as always, illegible and full of signs and symbols that mean nothing to me. Even all these years later, I take each prescription and make of it an origami plane or plant, or, my favourite, a tiny white swan with wings enfolded, with a miniature beak, perched gracefully on my palm and delivered to the pharmacist, who, seemingly with a snap of his fingers, a wave of his wand, turns my bird into a bottle of tablets.

4

SSRIs

The Birth of Fluoxetine

The First SSRI

In the 1950s and '60s, scientists were beginning at last to unpack the black box of the brain. The post-mortem studies of those rabbits that had been given reserpine continued to be an important benchmark, showing as they did that reserpine lowered serotonin while the tricyclics raised it. In the mid-1960s, Joseph Schildkraut, a psychiatrist and researcher at Harvard University in Massachusetts, cemented the theory that evolved into the monoamine hypothesis of depression. Monoamines, remember, are neurotransmitters such as dopamine, noradrenaline, epinephrine and serotonin. Schildkraut, building from a growing consensus among scientists, theorised that depression was the result of a deficit of some or all of these neurotransmitters. Noradrenaline, he thought, was related to alertness and energy as well as to anxiety, attention and interest in life, lack of serotonin to anxiety, obsessions and compulsions, and dopamine to attention, motivation, pleasure and reward. Schildkraut and other proponents of the monoamine hypothesis recommended that psychopharmacologists choose the antidepressant on the basis of the patient's most prominent symptoms. Anxious or irritable patients should be treated with noradrenaline reuptake inhibitors, while those patients displaying loss of energy or lack of enjoyment in life would do best on drugs that increase dopamine.

This theory predominated for roughly a decade and then was further refined by Swedish researcher Arvid Carlsson, an eventual Nobel winner. In 1972 Carlsson, funded by the pharmaceutical firm Astra, patented zimelidine, the world's first selective serotonin reuptake inhibitor (SSRI), a class of drugs that increase the amount of serotonin in the synaptic cleft – the space across which nerve impulses are transmitted – by hindering its absorption, or reuptake. Carlsson's Zelmid, born in Sweden and disseminated throughout Europe, suggested that the critical monoamine in depression was serotonin. Months after it had been on the market, however, Zelmid started making some people ill with strange flu-like symptoms and, still more worrisome, Guillain-Barré syndrome, a neurological condition that can be fatal.

Astra quickly pulled its drug from the pharmacies, but not so fast that pharmaceutical giant Eli Lilly failed to get a glimpse of all the sunniness and smiles, prompting its researchers to take another look at their own serotonin compound, which had been stalled for several years with nothing more than a numerical label, LY-110140, a drug they had created but had not even bothered to name because they hadn't yet decided what to do with it. Serotonin, after all, is present outside the brain. In fact it's omnipresent in the body, playing a role in sleep, digestion and blood pressure, among other things. Given this potentially wide range of application for LY-110140, Lilly had solicited the opinions of leading scientists as to its possible uses. Perhaps it could be a weight-loss drug, or an anti-hypertensive, both of which seemed more lucrative to Lilly, at that time, than a drug for depression, which one scientist had suggested. Initially, Lilly executives were quick to shoot down that idea because they were not convinced that their compound would actually work as an antidepressant, or that there would be a significant market for it. With no decision made, LY-110140 had languished in the shadows until zimelidine came along, proving that serotonin-specific drugs could definitely improve and regulate mood, if only their unfortunate side effects could be curtailed.

Eli Lilly is located in Indianapolis, on a gracious campus with gleaming buildings of steel and stone. It was here, in the 1970s, that Ray Fuller, Bryan Molloy and David T. Wong, working from the compound LY-110140, created fluoxetine. After the success of zimelidine in treating depression, they were aware in every instance that what they were seeking was a chemical that would increase the amount of serotonin in the brain. The antidepressants that preceded fluoxetine came to be considered 'dirty drugs' because they worked on multiple neurotransmitter systems at once and therefore caused a host of unpleasant somatic side effects. By selecting only serotonin, the inventors of fluoxetine sought to cure depression while sparing patients the blurred vision, the dry mouth, the excessive sweating, the sluggishness and the weight gain that were part and parcel of prior antidepressant treatment. In 1975 the manufacturer finally gave its creation a name, fluoxetine, which would eventually also be known by its brand name Prozac, especially in the United States.

From Nerves to Tears

Drugs, however, are not mere chemical concoctions. They are capsules, tablets, liquids, what have you, released into a culture that will, inevitably, bestow meaning on them. In the 1930s, '40s, '50s and beyond, the culture was largely one of anxiety. When people suffered, they attributed it to their 'nerves', while psychoanalysis posited anxiety to be the root cause of almost all neurotic problems. Depression was seen as a fringe condition, and a deadly serious one to boot. The *Diagnostic and Statistical Manual of Mental*

Disorders for the 1950s lists four kinds of depression, three of which include psychotic features. The depressed were often patients of the back ward who were lost to light and hope. This doesn't mean that there weren't milder forms of the disorder; it's just that people were far more prone then than now to understand their wayward moods as a bad case of the jitters.

Then along came Roland Kuhn and Nathan Kline. Kline wasn't merely a show-off. He also made it his mission to educate the public about depression, visiting family doctors and counselling them to diagnose the disorder when presented with a patient who had psychosomatic complaints. Slowly word spread that the country was suffering not from nerves but from numbness. What had been a fringe illness very gradually became commonplace as the culture let go of Freud and his theories. There is no definitive point at which this occurred; it was a slow process, with the new antidepressants and their inventors contributing to the change. When Kline won the much-coveted Lasker Prize again for his discovery of the MAOIs (he is the only person ever to win it twice), he declared that 'more human suffering has resulted from depression than from any other single disease.'

Not long after that, Freudian adherent Aaron T. Beck broke with psychoanalytic tradition and created what is called cognitive behavioural therapy (CBT), which taught patients to identify flawed or maladaptive patterns in their behaviour or their thinking, and to replace these defective ways of behaving and thinking with patterns that were more prudent and conducive to avoiding despair. It was a mode of treatment especially suited to dealing with disorders of mood. Nervous illness waned as patients learned, through CBT, that their depressions were borne on the back of self-critical thinking and that, by reframing negative self-talk, they could lift their sunken spirits. The therapy grew and grew in popularity, until it now has millions of adherents.

Some might say that the MAOIs and the tricyclics caused the interest in and the awareness of depression, that Kline and Kuhn manufactured a disorder for the new drugs to treat. The anti-depressants of the 1950s and '60s, however, were never superstar chemicals, partly because, unlike the antipsychotic chlorproma-zine, which was pushed for a multitude of off-label uses, they were never directly advertised to consumers. Their range was narrower from the beginning. Furthermore, they had whole rafts of side effects other than tardive dyskinesia, some of which were merely extremely unpleasant, while others were downright dangerous. An advertisement in a medical journal for the tricyclic amitriptyline in 1965 suggests that the drug might replace electroconvulsive therapy, underscoring the seriousness of the condition it was meant to treat. But although the first antidepressants may not have been household names, they nevertheless started a subterranean cultural shift in our understanding of ourselves, priming us for fluoxetine, so that when the drug was finally approved for release in 1987, we were at last really ready to see ourselves as sad.

Specificity?

In the US mass-marketing campaign that accompanied fluoxetine's eventual release, Lilly touted the supposed specificity of its drug, likening it to a magic bullet, or a Scud missile that lands with pro-grammed precision on millimetres of neural tissue. This, however, is misleading. Although fluoxetine is called an SSRI, in reality the phrase 'selective serotonin reuptake inhibitor' does more to conceal than to reveal. The truth is that there is really no way to have a serotonin-specific drug because the chemical serotonin casts a wide net over the whole of the human brain, is intricately tied up with our other neurotransmitter systems, is furthermore found through-out the human corpus – especially in the gut – and beyond that, as noted earlier, is implicated in dozens of physiological functions, from sleep and appetite to pain perception and sensory integra-tion, to name just a few. Indeed, serotonin is one of the oldest neurotransmitters on the planet. It was present on Earth millions of years ago and is found in myriad other life forms as diverse as birds, lizards, wasps, jellyfish, molluscs and earthworms. Given serotonin's wide net, not just across species but within the human body and brain, it is virtually impossible to create a drug that acts directly on it, because serotonin not only has so many systems but also is so intimately tied up with dopamine and noradrenaline and acetylcholine and all sorts of other neurotransmitters that flicker inside our skulls.

Still, this didn't stop Lilly from celebrating its brand-new compound as a site-specific drug that, given its putative ability to home in on a tiny target, would cause few to no side effects. In the United States, within six months of releasing fluoxetine under the brand name Prozac in January 1988, doctors had written more than a million prescriptions for it in that country alone. Annual sales reached $350 million in the first year. Two years later it appeared on the covers of both *Time* and *Newsweek* as the long-coveted cure for depression. It seemed like everyone was either talking about Prozac or taking it and, indeed, feeling fine.

Depression on the Rise

And yet something strange was happening. If fluoxetine was really the cure for depression, then why did the numbers of depressed patients suddenly start to rise in concert with the drug's release? When anti-tubercular drugs were discovered, tuberculosis rates dropped off sharply and then finally almost disappeared altogether. When antibiotics were invented deaths from infections became less frequent. Vaccinations wiped out dreaded illnesses like measles and tetanus. Each of these treatments undoubtedly and clearly contributed to a healthier society. The opposite happened with fluoxetine. The drug was offered to society and society just got sicker, and with precisely the illness the drug was created to treat. In 1955, one in 468 Americans was hospitalised for mental illness. By 1987, however, one in every 184 Americans was receiving disability payments for mental illness. Two decades after fluoxetine's release, there were almost 4 million disabled mentally ill US citizens receiving financial support through government programmes. In fact, reported incidences of depression in the United States have increased a thousandfold since the introduction of antidepressants. Depression on the rise isn't an American phenomenon: a 2016 study by the Royal College of Psychiatrists found that mental health disorders have become the main reason for receiving benefits in the UK. Between 1995 to 2014 claimants increased by 103 per cent to 1.1 million, and by 2014 almost half of benefit claims were for a mental health problem. A cynic might say the tablet to cure depression was in fact causing it.

There are multiple theories to account for the astounding rise in the diagnosis of depression and its odd timing with the release of a supposedly superior antidepressant designed to treat it. The most obvious explanation is that depression has always been as terribly common as it is now, but that in past decades it was also terribly stigmatised, and that it took fluoxetine to lift that stigma and allow floods of people to come forward and claim their cure. This theory, however, cannot explain why now, thirty years after fluoxetine's release, the rates of depression have only continued to rise. Surely the stigma is gone by now, and depression is a disorder that is almost hip to have.

Perhaps it makes more sense to look first at the society into which fluoxetine was released. The drug debuted in the United States as Prozac in the late 1980s during the end of Ronald Reagan's presidency and became a blockbuster even before 1993, when Peter Kramer published his popular book *Listening to Prozac*, claiming that the drug made us better than well and that cosmetic psychopharmacology had finally arrived. The 1980s were a time of fierce individuality in a country that had always prided itself on autonomy, and now even more so. President Reagan was something of a Marlboro Man who cut funding to social service agencies and admonished American citizens to get off their sofas and earn a living, acquire a skill, do something, anything, with the ultimate goal of creating a self who is capable of surviving in a bubble. Money for benefits such as 'welfare' was slashed, mothers with young children were told to find day care and a job, or if not a job, then job skills training at centres set up for such a purpose. Nursing homes, day care centres, after-school programmes, homeless shelters – all these institutions that were geared towards maintaining the fabric of a cohesive and helpful society – lost their federal funds and dwindled in size.

I remember it well. In my mid-twenties, I was the director of a small community mental health centre serving SPMI patients, those with 'severe and persistent mental illness', schizophrenic people felled not only by this dread disease but also by the added burdens of poverty and homelessness, the kind of street people you find muttering in alleys or talking to invisible angels. I watched as our agency's state and federal support was halved, and then quartered, as therapy sessions that had been unlimited were reduced under Reagan's rule to just six, as though that were adequate for penniless patients haunted by visions and voices. But meanwhile Wall Street boomed and the stock market more than doubled during Reagan's two terms. The images of the 1980s were sleek black limousines and sleek silver skyscrapers, with the money pooling at the upper end of the social spectrum while the rest lost what little they had.

'What does this have to do with Prozac?' you might wonder. Everything, really, if you take a sociological view of what is usually understood as a deeply individualistic experience: depression. For a moment, step back and scan the horizon. Study after study has shown that rates of depression rise in concert with isolative societies. For the upper class, the Reagan years may have been lucrative, but for those who depended on a web of social services, Reagan's presidency was difficult, if not destructive. Help went away. There were no more handouts, and thus, for some people, no more helping hands. Schizophrenics and others with mental illness lost their access to treatment providers.

I remember my patient Amy Wilson, a 31-year-old woman with a red seam of a scar across her face where a boyfriend had broken her nose with a baseball bat and left her beautiful features slightly askew. She had glitter-green eyes, her lashes coated with mascara thick as tar, her tapered nails painted a carmine red. Despite a stunning facade, Amy struggled with devastating depression and relied on her twice-weekly therapy sessions for succour and perspective. When her government-funded medical insurance was cut and our six sessions ran out, there was nothing I could do. I met her by accident in the supermarket one day, her three toddlers jammed into a trolley filled with cheese puffs and cheese dip, her face as pale as a pillow. Amy is just one of the thousands, maybe millions of people who suffered in the avid 'do-it-yourself' society that marked the Reagan years.

It would be overly simplistic, however, if not absurd to target Reagan as the sole cause of social breakdown and the rise in depression that may have resulted from it. Reagan, after all, inherited a presidency in a culture that had been steadily moving towards the sort of isolative individualism that breeds widespread depression. He accelerated the process, but its provenance lies in the history of that country, as far back, perhaps, as the nineteenth century, when Tocqueville, coming from France to watch Americans at work and play, remarked on the rampant and insistent autonomy that undergirds so much of what we strive for. In Asia and Africa it is not unusual for whole families to share a bedroom and a bed, while in the United States we fetishise Richard Ferber, who admonishes us to let our children cry it out in their own cots in dark rooms, a method that is also practised in the UK. We know that infant animals separated from their mothers secrete the stress hormone cortisol and that high levels of cortisol, while not causative, are implicated in depression.

In 1897 the Frenchman Émile Durkheim, whom some call the father of sociology, published *Suicide*, the classic text based on a study he did of suicide rates among Catholics, Protestants and Jews. His basic question was this: 'Which religious group had the most suicides, which had the fewest, and why?' What Durkheim discovered was that Protestants were the most likely to kill themselves and Jews the least likely, a finding that was surprising because in Judaism, as opposed to Christianity, there is no eternal punishment for killing yourself. Under church law, a person who commits suicide not only suffers the eternal fires of hell but also brings upon his surviving family shame and, in past times, even punishment; in the seventeenth and eighteenth centuries, for instance, the church regularly confiscated the entire estates of suicide victims, leaving their brethren destitute. The remaining family members had to forfeit their cows, their farming implements and all other items necessary to survival, much less prosperity. In England in the seventeenth century, a miller inflicted upon himself a fatal wound and was reported to have cried out, 'I have forfeited my estate to the king, beggared my wife and children!' Compare this to the Jewish response to suicide, in which the victim still gets a proper burial and a full-scale shiva, the traditional seven-day prescribed period of mourning.

Durkheim posited that the higher rate of suicide in Protestantism than in any other Western religious group had something to do with the essence of the religion itself. Protestantism developed in the sixteenth century as a response to the suffocating nature of Catholicism. In Catholicism one must rely on a priest to talk to God. One must go to confession and pour forth one's venial sins. The religion is full of pageantry. Those who began to oppose it sought something simpler and purer. Most importantly, they wanted a direct, autonomous route to the divine, a God they could access entirely on their own. Eternity would no longer be the business of a priest with his incense and myrrh. Durkheim proposed that the highly individualised nature of Protestantism, the do-it-yourself emphasis, the loss of clergy in whom to confide one's transgressions, created an ultimate loneliness that made Protestants more vulnerable to ending their own lives. That

Americans live in a primarily Protestant country and that their suicide rates are among the highest in the industrial world may not, therefore, be a coincidence.

More than a century after Durkheim wrote *Suicide*, another sociologist set out on a similar but opposite quest, seeking this time the rates and reasons not for misery but for its antithesis – happiness. Roko Belic was a 34-year-old documentary film-maker when his friend and colleague Tom Shadyac read a *New York Times* article that reported the United States as only the twenty-third happiest country in the world. Given that the country's gross domestic product is the highest in the world and their medical hospitals are staffed with unsurpassed experts, Shadyac, a successful film-maker who lived alone in a 1,580-metre-square (17,000-square-foot) mansion in Los Angeles and was himself struggling with depression, thought it interesting that they were, as a country, so unhappy. Shadyac, offering to fund the project, told Belic to go out and find out why and make a film. Thus began Belic's four-year journey winding around the globe, into and out of fourteen different countries, seeking the source of happiness or, as he put it, 'the secret of life's greatest mystery'.

In the course of making his film, *Happy*, Belic interviewed a beauty queen who had been run over by a lorry and lost her good looks as a result, and who was happy nevertheless. He interviewed a rickshaw driver living in the slums of Kolkata where sludge and sewer waste ran in rivulets through the streets, a man whose hut was made of bamboo sticks and plastic tarps which did not keep out the rain during monsoon season, and who was happy nonetheless. He interviewed a Cajun fisherman in a Louisiana bayou and several centenarians in Okinawa in Japan, the island with the longest-lived residents in the world. What Belic learned was that, in every instance, happiness depended on a strong and supple social fabric, and an interdependence of family and friends. In Denmark, rated the happiest country in the world, Belic found co-housing projects where families lived together, dined together, celebrated

and mourned together. Co-housing offered a salve against loneliness and the modern-day pressures on the nuclear family, in
which, at least in the United States and in the UK, two working
parents are somehow supposed to raise their children while giving
forty hours a week to their jobs.

Ann Bolo

Ann Bolo was thirty-five years old, struggling with postnatal
depression, living in a suburb of Boston in Massachusetts with
her husband and their new baby when she saw Belic's film on
happiness. Her house, a single-storey style flanking a motorway,
was beset by the whir and wheeze of cars, audible in every room.
It was pervaded by a damp odour as well, and the lawn was
studded with giant weeds bearing platter-sized leaves and spiky
purple petals. A painter and a social worker, Bolo was taking time
off from work – a six-week maternity leave – in order to care for
her newborn.

'Six weeks,' she said, and shrugged, leaning over and looking
at Emily who was swaddled in a bassinet, only the tiny disc of
her face visible above the striped baby blankets. 'If I lived in a
European country I'd get six months off,' Bolo said. 'If I lived in
Denmark I'd have a whole community of caretakers and wouldn't
have to worry about paying for health care'. She also mentioned
she wouldn't have to worry about paying for university – both of
which is correct. The Danish government endows every citizen
with lifetime health care and free university education. Bolo,
when she first spoke with me, had given birth a month earlier, by
Caesarean section; her wound still hurt, she reported, and until
starting fluoxetine – which for her, unusually, worked within
days – she had felt tired and low. In those first two weeks after
Emily's birth, isolated in her small house by the side of a buzzing
motorway her only daytime company an infant, Bolo had quickly
grown despondent, and then depressed.

'At first I lost my appetite,' she said, 'and when that happened I knew something was wrong, because I love food. But nothing looked good to me.' Bolo was sitting in a padded gliding chair. As she spoke she pushed the chair back and forth with her feet. 'After my appetite went, my sleep followed. I still have to get up every few hours to feed the baby, but before, when she was done and back in her crib [cot], I would just lie awake, staring at nothing.'

When her appetite went, in addition to having trouble sleeping Bolo started crying for reasons she could not articulate. 'The strangest things made me sad', she said. A crack in the plaster on the wall of the hall. The polished brightness inside their brand-new freezer. The supermarket, where packed chicken pieces floated in fluid, where marbled meat hung off hooks in the butcher section.

'I didn't hear voices or see visions,' Bolo said, 'but I began to think I was going crazy. The morning was the worst. I'd wake up seized with terror. But it wasn't tied to anything; it was free-floating, it was everywhere. I'd lie in the bed and think, *All I need to do is swing one leg over the edge and put my foot on the floor*, but that action seemed insurmountable to me. The smallest things were completely overwhelming. I was scared all the time, even in the shower. I felt like I was moving through jam, or sludge. Then Emily started to seem' – and here Bolo's voice dropped, as if in shame – 'demonic to me. It's odd how depression can do that, can so alter your perceptions. When I first saw my baby, when they lifted her out of the slit in my stomach and held her up, this pudgy ball with blue eyes, I thought she was adorable. But two weeks later when I looked at her, I thought her eyes seemed possessed and her crying was like nails on a blackboard. It caused my whole self to shrivel up.'

Alarmed, Bolo called the 800 telephone number at the bottom of her health insurance card. She got what most insured citizens in the United States would have gotten in her situation: one fifty-minute session with a psychopharmacologist, whose sole mission is to dole out drugs and to provide monthly fifteen-minute follow-up sessions called 'med checks', the purpose of which is to assess the efficacy of the antidepressant prescribed in the initial consultation. Bolo was lucky. Neither she nor her doctor could have predicted just how swiftly she would respond to her initial fluoxetine doses. Within four days, her symptoms began to abate.

Bolo's brief first encounter with her psychopharmacologist is the norm in the United States, where the still briefer follow-up sessions are also the norm. 'Most people are under the misconception that an appointment with a psychiatrist will involve counselling, probing questions and digging into the psychological meanings of one's distress', wrote psychiatrist Daniel Carlat, of the Tufts University School of Medicine. 'But the psychiatrist as psychotherapist is an endangered species.' Carlat goes on to offer this frank observation about what has happened to the profession in that country: 'Doing psychotherapy doesn't pay well enough. I can see three or four patients per hour if I focus on medications . . . but only one patient in that time period if I do therapy. The income differential is a powerful incentive to drop therapy from our repertoire of skills, and psychiatrists have generally followed the money.'

Should it be any surprise that when I asked Bolo if she felt listened to, her response was 'No, not at all'? But she was quick to add, 'I left with a prescription for twenty milligrams of Prozac and I'll tell you, just having that prescription in my hand, just the fact of it being there, gave me some hope and lifted my spirits.'

Here Bolo is alluding to the much-discussed placebo effect that psychiatric medications must outperform in clinical trials in order to be approved by the US Food and Drug Administration (FDA). When fluoxetine, in particular, was tested, it needed to outperform the placebo in six-to-eight-week double-blind trials. ('Double-blind', you'll remember, means that neither the researchers nor the patients know who is swallowing the sugar tablet and who the real deal.) But even in Eli Lilly's published research, any difference between fluoxetine and earlier antidepressants was inconsequential, and two-thirds of the people in its trials would have fared just as well or better on a placebo.

Pharmaceutical companies, in testing a new antidepressant drug, need only come up with two studies that demonstrate their drug's efficacy. And when scientists and doctors looked into the unpublished research on approved SSRIs through the Freedom of Information Act, they discovered some pretty unfavourable data. Consider that of the forty-seven trials that were conducted for the country's six major antidepressants (citalopram, venlafaxine, paroxetine, nefazodone and sertraline, in addition to fluoxetine), the drug beat the placebo only twenty of those times – fewer than half. Second, the FDA does not mandate exactly *how much* more effective than the placebo the drug must be. In those same forty-seven clinical trials, when measured on the Hamilton Depression Rating Scale, the tool most clinicians use to measure a person's depression, the average patient improved on the drug only two points better than on the placebo, a difference that Irving Kirsch, a Harvard psychologist and associate director of the Program in Placebo Studies, has called 'trivial' and 'clinically meaningless'.

These lax requirements, in and of themselves, are disturbing. Now add in the fact that the FDA approved fluoxetine after just six to eight weeks of clinical trials. But virtually no one, in actuality, takes these drugs for just six to eight weeks. The vast majority of patients taking fluoxetine – perhaps all of them – use the drug for far longer periods of time. In fact many psychiatrists believe that patients who have had a depressive episode should stay on the drug indefinitely in order to prevent relapses, since each relapse, the theory goes, makes the brain that much more vulnerable to future episodes and thus justifies a lifetime of antidepressant use. But despite the fact that the original six-to-eight-week trials did not, and do not, reflect real life, and despite the millions of people to date who have ingested, and continue to ingest, these drugs for years on end, there have been very few studies on the long-term side effects of serotonin boosters. There have been some long-term studies on the drugs themselves, yes, and some mid-term studies (after a period of months or a couple of years) on patients' rates of remission and relapse, but not when it comes to the side effects that serotonin boosters produce. Why have so few long-term studies been done? The answer, said Donald Klein, former head of the American Society of Clinical Psychopharmacology, is plain: 'I think the industry is concerned about the possibility of finding long-term risks.'

Like most depressed patients, Bolo was informed she had a chemical imbalance that a serotonin booster would fix. She was not made aware that there is, in actuality, a paucity of evidence to support the view that depression – or, for that matter, any other psychiatric disorder – is tied to a chemical imbalance in the brain. Instead, the offices of psychopharmacologists in the United States often display laminated posters from the various drug companies showing how SSRIs, by inhibiting the reuptake of serotonin, keep higher levels of this crucial neurotransmitter available in the synaptic cleft, thereby boosting serotonin throughout the brain. 'I was told,' said Bolo, when I spoke to her for the second time, six months after the birth of her baby, 'that I had low serotonin and that my symptoms were classic and would likely respond to a drug. I had some hesitations, but the doctor told me that if I was diabetic I would take insulin, and that there really was no difference.'

Bolo had no way of knowing that the all-pervasive diabetes metaphor which some psychopharmacologists use in order to persuade their patients to take drugs has no merit. Diabetes is a disease for which we absolutely know the cause. We know that in diabetes the pancreas stops producing insulin and that, as a result, blood sugar gets dangerously high. We do not know, in the case of depression, why suffering starts and why it continues, whether it is the result of an excess of the stress hormone cortisol, hereditary gene expression, neurotransmitters run amok, an overly individualistic society, all of these things or none of these things. We do know, however, that it is not the consequence of something as simplistic as low serotonin alone. When it comes to diabetes, a doctor can diagnose or screen for the disease via a patient's blood or urine, using valid and reliable tests. But we have no such tests for diagnosing depression. We cannot use the fluids of the body to tell us why a patient's mood has plunged.

Medication is dispensed on the basis of a patient's report and the degree to which the patient's symptoms fit with the symptom checklist in the *Diagnostic and Statistical Manual of Mental Disorders*. The *DSM*, what some call the bible of psychiatry, was first published in 1952. It's a book that lists all the psychiatric syndromes decided upon by committee, a list that has been updated seven times over the last half century. To give you a sense of the evolution, the first *DSM*, in 1952, included 106 diagnoses; in the 2015 edition of the *DSM* there are more than 300 diagnoses. In every case the committees reaching these decisions are made up of mental health professionals, many of them psychiatrists, deciding in a fairly random manner what the diagnoses will be. For instance, up until 1974, homosexuality still appeared in the *DSM* as a disorder. In the 2015 edition we have the diagnosis 'social anxiety disorder', a diagnosis that did not exist until 1994. The *DSM* reflects the consensus of the committees that conjure it and is not rooted in real biological phenomena such as tissue samples or blood and urine tests, because to date we have no known physiological substrates for any psychiatric disorder.

Bolo was never told this. She was told, in essence, a lie: that her suffering was the mental equivalent of diabetes and that a drug would make things right. The good news for Bolo, in the short term, was that soon after starting fluoxetine, she was a changed woman. Her appetite was back. She slept soundly between feedings of her infant daughter, whose wail no longer irritated her but rather called forth an urge to comfort, to console.

In the first couple of weeks of her daughter's life, Bolo had tried joining a new mothers' group, but at the time the group's discussions focusing on types of pushchairs and car seats had quickly left her feeling unfulfilled, and she stopped going. 'The strangest thing,' she said, 'is that when I started going again to my new mothers' group, I actually enjoyed the conversations which before had sounded so stupid and superficial to me.' She paused, shifted in her chair and studied her pearlescent nails, then sighed the sigh of someone weighted with worry. Outside the window the motorway hummed and hummed as cars shot past in a blur of sun-blasted chrome. 'In that mothers' group,' Bolo continued, 'it's like I can hear the conversation on two levels. On one level it's just a conversation about Graco strollers [pushchairs] versus who knows what, and I contribute and enjoy it. On another level, though, there I am, sort of hovering above it all and wondering what's gotten into me that I find something so banal suddenly so enjoyable. There have been other things that bothered me too. I have my master's in social work and have always been bookish. But on Prozac I notice that I read less and shop more. I suddenly have a thing for scarves. Scarves', Bolo repeated, and stopped to finger a scarf she was wearing, frothy white and dotted with the palest pastilles. She pulled the scarf off over her head and, holding it between thumb and forefinger, dangled it above the floor before letting it fall, which it did, floating slowly to the carpet and collapsing in an impossibly soft heap. 'So much for that', she said.

The Little Libido Problem

Eli Lilly's sales force touted Prozac, their brand name for fluoxetine, as a clean medicine designed to provide rapid relief. For Bolo, relief did come relatively swiftly. But while she did not have the dry mouth or blurred vision associated with the older antidepressants, she began to have other side effects. Bolo's libido disappeared, and she became anorgasmic during the sex she and her husband, Ryan, did have. When one takes a closer look at the literature, it becomes clear that Bolo's experience is not unusual. In the initial Lilly package insert for fluoxetine, sexual dysfunction is listed as occurring in 2 to 5 per cent of patients, but researchers estimate that it occurs, in actuality, in 60 to 75 per cent of patients and perhaps at an even higher rate. Why the enormous discrepancy? Was Lilly truly unaware that its medication made both men and women sexually dysfunctional? Was its estimate of 2 to 5 per cent made in good faith? Or was the company, having observed the sharp downwards turn in prescriptions of MAOIs resulting from the dietary restrictions imposed on that class of drugs, trying to downplay, or even hide, a very significant problem?

The aforementioned six-to-eight-week period of the clinical trials isn't the only problem. Adding to that shortcoming is the fact that researchers performing the trials did not ask patients specifically about sexual side effects; it was only when a patient spontaneously complained that the side effect was noted and logged. Sex, by its very nature, exists in a private realm. Many people are naturally hesitant to tell researchers they hardly know that their genitals don't seem to be working.

In 1979, almost a decade before fluoxetine was approved for the general public, Herbert Meltzer of the University of Chicago's Pritzker School of Medicine had performed an important study of the drug funded by Lilly. Meltzer measured levels of both dopamine and the protein hormone prolactin (which can cause lactation even in men if levels are too high) in patients before and after starting fluoxetine. What he found was that after patients started fluoxetine, their prolactin levels increased sevenfold while their levels of dopamine dropped off precipitously, leading to sexual dysfunction. Dopamine is the neurotransmitter specifically responsible for motor movement and for sexual arousal and orgasm. Laboratory rats with impaired dopamine systems are unable to mate. Studies also show that one way to impair the dopamine system is to raise levels of serotonin in the brain; as serotonin rises, dopamine decreases.

Meltzer's study confirmed this correlation between serotonin and dopamine. In fact, the dopamine level of one of his patients on fluoxetine fell so far that the patient developed a rigid, spasming neck, a clenched jaw and an unbalanced gait, similar to symptoms seen in sufferers of Parkinson's, who are also known to have severe dopamine deficiencies. He suggested that the company's new serotonin booster shared similarities with the old antipsychotics such as chlorpromazine, which also depleted the brain of dopamine. (You may remember that an excess of dopamine is one theory as to the cause of schizophrenia, and hence one reason – the lowering of dopamine – why the antipsychotics were thought to calm mania.)

For Bolo, the sexual side effects kicked in almost in tempo with her improved mood. 'If I were a guy,' she said, 'I'd describe it as having intercourse with a sock on. I don't think I'm a 100 per cent numb, but I'll bet I'm 75 per cent numb. I just can't feel much of anything. There's two issues. Number one, my desire for sex has diminished to almost zero. Two, if Ryan or I manage to whip up a drop of desire, I can't have an orgasm. There's no way. No amount of stimulation – soft, slow, hard, fast – will do it. I can't reach that peak.'

Bolo and her husband were deeply different in their personalities and proclivities. Ryan worked as a banker. He was a man of numbers, a man who solved problems by breaking them down into their component parts, while Bolo, as a painter and a social worker, looked for the emotional undertones, the current beneath the current, and used her intuitive skills to come to comprehension and to solutions. This radically different problem-solving style often strained the relationship, and when conflicts came up, they either escalated into fights or were simply left dangling. The bedroom had always been the one place the two of them could join together in some sort of shared language. Sex was one of the few areas where they could communicate effectively, wordlessly. It bridged gaps in the relationship and acted as a salve. That language was gone now and the relationship was suffering because of it.

'If he touches me,' Bolo said, 'I feel something jump inside of me. I'm scared because his touch does nothing for me at all any more. I turn away from him. Hurt gets heaped on to hurt, and our fights fester.'

Numbness

For many patients, Bolo among them, the feeling of numbness isn't just sexual. 'On Prozac, far fewer things bother me,' Bolo said. 'I'm like a Teflon-coated pan. What would have stuck to me before now just falls off me. I'm more superficial than I was before. I saw a movie the other day with a friend. Off Prozac, I would have cried at the end. On Prozac, I'm dry-eyed.' She said that everyone else in the cinema except for her was weeping. 'I call it the "so what" side effect,' she said. 'It worries me a little, but on the other hand, I'm so relieved not to be depressed that I'm willing to live with what I call my "Martha Stewart self".' (She was referring to the American 'domestic goddess' television personality popular for her recipes, hand-made crafts and home decorating ideas.)

Bolo is far from unique in her experience of the 'so what' side effect of fluoxetine. Many patients either comment on or complain about the way fluoxetine and other serotonin boosters lacquer their world, blunting their responses and putting them at a remove from the intensity of living. No one knows for sure why this occurs, but some theorise that it is the result of damage done to the serotonin system itself, leaving the patient with a restricted range of emotions to express. Psychiatrist Joseph Glenmullen, a clinical instructor in psychiatry at Harvard Medical School, compares fluoxetine to the now off-the-market diet drug dexfenfluramine, which was also a serotonin booster and on which, unlike fluoxetine, many studies of side effects have been done. Dexfenfluramine, when fed to laboratory rats, damaged the serotonin neurons, burning away their axons and, according to Glenmullen, 'destroy[ing] the elaborately branching tentacles of serotonin neurons as they reach[ed] out to communicate with other neurons.'

Yet some researchers have hypothesised that this pruning effect of the serotonin boosters may in part be the very thing responsible for their efficacy. The frontal lobes of the brain, in their size and circuitry, distinguish the human brain from those of other animals. These lobes govern cognitive and emotional processes of a higher order, processes related to one's moral sense and one's capacity for judgement and compassion. Patients on fluoxetine are sometimes so dulled that they resemble, in their indifference, people who have been lobotomised. Rudolf Hoehn-Saric, for instance, a researcher at Johns Hopkins University in Maryland, reported on a 23-year-old man with obsessive-compulsive disorder who was put on a very high dose of fluoxetine: 100 milligrams, which is 20 milligrams higher than the highest FDA-approved dose. This patient, after taking the 100 milligrams daily for four months, developed what appeared to be frontal-lobe syndrome, displaying extreme apathy and indifference.

For every example, however, there are always counterexamples. Some patients appreciate the dulling effect of fluoxetine and experience it not as a numbing force but as a welcome de-amplification of what was previously a chaotic and operatic existence. Ella Rose, an 83-year-old woman who had been hospitalised eight times in her adult life for severe depression and obsessive-compulsive disorder before going on fluoxetine, describes struggling each day with a weight in her limbs. 'There was so much darkness,' she said, 'so much difficulty. I couldn't cry even though I longed for the release of tears. I worried about everything and had to compulsively check that the stove was off, off, off. I dragged myself through days. On Prozac, that weight and worry are gone. And in their place I have access to a full range of emotion, and I can cry, which is a gift to me. Depression and obsession clog up the pathways in my brain, so other normal emotions can't come through. Prozac clears the mental plumbing.'

After getting that initial prescription from Dr Salzman, I myself took fluoxetine for seventeen years before its effect finally wore off and I had to switch to another serotonin booster, venlafaxine, which acts on noradrenaline as well and so is called an SNRI – serotonin and noradrenaline reuptake inhibitor. Prior to my taking fluoxetine, both before and while I was on imipramine, my emotions were wild and I was whipped between states of utter despair, whirling anxiety and unstable ecstasy that allowed me to pull all-nighters writing lengthy tomes that later, in the sober light of another day, lacked what I felt at the time of composition had been a pure poetic essence. I was also a revolving-door mental patient, in and out of the hospital, admitted and discharged five times between the ages of thirteen and twenty-four, with not much hope for a full future. I cut my arms compulsively and many days did not make it beyond the bed. As with Ann Bolo, the world for me felt impossible to negotiate. I would lie beneath unwashed blankets and think, *I have to take a shower*, but I utterly lacked the ability to initiate the task. Even the effort of setting my feet on the floor seemed insuperable, a problem of deep and complex dimensions.

Fluoxetine turned my life around and did it fast, *one, two*. It was as if my world had been washed with a window cleaner and everything had an elfin sparkle at its edges. Delightful, joyful, joyous. With my psychiatric symptoms removed, there was suddenly room in my mind for a whole range of new feelings, and thus fluoxetine did not blunt me at all. Like Ella Rose, I wept easily and copiously and enjoyed this simple feeling of sadness, which had a sort of purity. During my early years on the drug, I was alternately sad, happy, angry, excited, curious and confused, which is another way of saying I was getting my bearings as a healthy person, learning to let go of sickness and all its symptoms. These were heady, incredible times. Ice cream tasted purer. Lychees were so aromatic. There was something sweet in the sadness I was now able to experience, so different from the deadness of depression.

I did fret, however, over my sudden inability to write. It was as if fluoxetine had dried up the well from which my deepest dreams and images sprang. For the first eighteen months on the drug I didn't set pen to paper, but gradually, eventually, I decided to try a short story or two, a brief essay about an animal I had loved long ago. I found that while words came more slowly to me on the drug, and that fluoxetine prevented the high I had sometimes felt when composing drug-free, or on imipramine, I could indeed still write, although to this day I still sometimes worry that I have forever lost some wattage to the tablet.

Sex Addicts

Because fluoxetine dampens the sex drive, US psychiatrists often use it to treat compulsive masturbators and others with heightened libido or sexual-addiction disorders that leave their lives in shreds. Martin Kafka, a psychiatrist at McLean Hospital in Massachusetts, the same place I go for my monthly medical checks, has an entire practice comprising men who are addicted to sex. These are largely married men who nevertheless seek out prostitutes and pornography, not once a day, not twice a day, but twenty or thirty times in a twenty-four-hour period, men haunted and ravaged by their own internal fires, men eaten alive by uncontrollable desire, men whose brains are likely damp with dopamine coursing down dendrites and being sucked up by axons in a never-ending obsessive circuit. Kafka treats these men with what you could call a chemical castration. High doses of fluoxetine make it difficult, if not impossible, for his patients to maintain an erection, never mind to bed multiple partners. Kafka is not the only psychopharmacologist who uses fluoxetine and its chemical cousins in this manner. The literature is rife with cases of excessive masturbation, fetishes, compulsive staring at crotches, ungovernable promiscuity, all trained and tamed by serotonin-boosting drugs. Kafka has seen these drugs turn men around, has seen his patients go from the far fringes of fantasy, pornography and prostitution to surprisingly conventional existences, tidy front garden and all.

Sex addicts for whom fluoxetine allows a normal life, most of whom are men, generally tend to be grateful for the gate the drug has placed in front of them. With their genitals mostly offline, they're permitted to remain in their marriages. And even if these marriages are all but sexless, most sex addicts report being happy to accept erectile dysfunction in exchange for freedom from a relentless and driving need – so happy that few appear to reflect on the disturbing fact that they are now dependent on a drug that could be causing damage to the dopamine systems in their brains, damage that may make them more vulnerable to developing Parkinson's disease later in life. It's a risk they're willing to live with.

Unable to Fall in Love

The vast majority of patients who take fluoxetine, however, are not men but women. For example, the Health Survey for England 2013 found that 11 per cent of women were taking antidepressants compared to 6 per cent of men. And according to data compiled by the US Centers for Disease Control and Prevention, researchers estimate that in the United States women are two and a half times more likely to take an antidepressant than men, and that 23 per cent of women aged forty to fifty-nine are on an antidepressant. Thus, if sexual dysfunction affects up to 75 per cent of them, a staggering number of British and American women are walking around without libido or desire or the ability to have an orgasm, women who used to notice a nick in the chin or a certain smell of sweat, but who are now numb to all that in their happy, cocooned state.

Anthropologist Helen Fisher, a researcher at the Kinsey Institute in Indiana, and psychiatrist J. Anderson Thomson Jr, a trustee for the Richard Dawkins Foundation for Reason and Science in Colorado, have asked a disturbing question and put forth a disturbing theory relating to fluoxetine's dulling effect on female libido. What might it mean to have millions of women indifferent to sex? Fisher and Thomson worry that as generic forms of the serotonin boosters become available and cheap, only more women will have their sexuality dulled. After all, it has been well established, they write, that these medications can be responsible for 'emotional blunting' and dysfunction in sexual desire, arousal and performance in as many as three of every four patients. The human brain has essentially three sexual systems within it, one for courtship, one for mating, and one for reproduction and parenting. A healthy sex drive motivates a woman to seek out a range of partners even as her capability for romantic attraction prunes the partners back, helping her, according to Fisher and Thomson, in 'conserving mating time and metabolic energy' by ultimately focusing on one person. The capacity for attachment, in turn, allows human beings to stay in a relationship ideally long enough to complete parenting duties.

But fluoxetine and other serotonin boosters, Fisher and Thomson suggest, put a deep dent in the neural substrates that underlie romantic attraction, courtship, mating and maybe even parenting. Studies using fMRI scanning of the brain show that romantic attraction and courtship are mediated via the dopamine system, the very system that fluoxetine in particular and the serotonin boosters in general suppress. 'Hence,' wrote Fisher and Thomson, 'serotonin-enhancing antidepressants can jeopardise one's ability to fall in love.' They further hypothesise that because of fluoxetine's widespread effect on the sex drive, the medication can also interfere with mate assessment, mate choice and partner attachment.

The reason is that while the male orgasm serves an obvious evolutionary role, the female orgasm, a more subtle phenomenon, also has a critical purpose in the evolution of our species. Not only does the female orgasm aid in sperm retention, but also it allows women to better differentiate between self-centred versus compassionate partners. A man who cannot bring his partner to orgasm, for instance, likely lacks the necessary sensitivity and skill that promote female sexual pleasure. But a woman whose libido has been suppressed by fluoxetine loses the ability to discriminate between partners who can take the time and effort to please her versus those who can't or won't. In some sense, then, the drug wipes out a critical monitoring device built in to the female brain. Stoked on fluoxetine, women are at higher risk for choosing men who lack the capacity to care about their needs and wants, and may therefore fall into a relationship that is stale – or, worse, incompatible – from the start, a relationship that, furthermore, puts her future progeny at risk because the bond with her mate lacks the stability and solidity it will need to make it through the early years of parenting.

Studies also show that women will be more orgasmic with men who have symmetrical body features, given that outward symmetry is a sign of inward sanguinity and health. Therefore an orgasmic woman will be naturally drawn to male symmetry while a woman who has a suppressed libido has a sort of sexual blindness. With her dopamine systems blunted and her serotonin surging, such a woman is cut off from the critical currents that suggest a 'good catch'. If Fisher and Thomson are correct, then currently, worldwide, there are millions and millions of women whose sexual detection systems are askew, women who are more vulnerable to making poor choices, which will then have a damaging domino effect that can go on for generations, as unhappy unions lead, perhaps, to divorce and children bear the brunt of the familial collapse.

Beyond that, sexual relationships are likely not the only type of bonding that fluoxetine affects. Or, to put it another way, almost all adult relationships have a sexual/erotic component of some kind, albeit usually an unconscious one. This component adds energy and gives synergy to twosomes. Studies show that touch stimulates the release, in our bodies and brains, of oxytocin, sometimes called 'the love hormone', which helps us bond with everything from pets to cousins to husbands and wives. Oxytocin is tightly tied to the dopamine system, which fluoxetine suppresses, so there's a reasonable chance that, fuelled by a serotonin booster, we will deprive ourselves of the benefits of this important bonding hormone as well.

One could claim that Fisher and Thomson's evolutionary theory is hogwash – that sperm do just fine whether or not the female has an orgasm, and that symmetrical facial features are an entirely subjective phenomenon and do not point towards a robust mate with a complementary immune system. But even if Fisher and Thomson were entirely wrong, they would still, in essence, be right. We have, by now, enough anecdotal reports to be able to say with certainty that in a large number of users, fluoxetine and its chemical cousins create a more blasé attitude towards the slings and arrows of life. The drug allows you to glide over serrated surfaces, unaware that you are tearing your tender soles. Evolutionary theory aside, we know that fluoxetine makes people feel good enough to tolerate compromised or even outright dysfunctional relationships that, in an unmedicated state, one would simply be unable to adapt to. There are, of course, far-reaching political ramifications to this, but even on a very micro scale it looks creepy. A wife adjusting to her husband's serial affairs. A husband adjusting to his wife's compulsive spending. Children adjusting to poor teachers. The high gloss and shiny polish that fluoxetine puts on the surface of life is not a warning or a maybe. For millions of people it is the total truth.

By 1993, five years after fluoxetine was released for public consumption, it was the top-selling antidepressant in the world, with doctors writing millions of prescriptions for the drug per year. The release of fluoxetine in the United States dovetailed with the rise of managed care provided by their health-insurance companies, so it was not at all unusual for a patient to see a psychopharmacologist once, maybe twice, and, like Ann Bolo, walk away with a year's worth of prescriptions for the drug and no substantial follow-up in place. By all appearances Lilly had done well with its new drug. The public clamour for fluoxetine that followed in the wake of the *Newsweek* cover feature and the myriad articles written about it in the mainstream press resulted in the company's grossing well over $1 billion in sales of Prozac in 1993. The drug was even sold on the street, where it was crushed up and snorted for what some dubiously claimed was an immediate high.

An AK-47

Despite the stellar success of the drug in the treatment of depression, from early on there was a dark undercurrent to the fluoxetine story. Martin Teicher and Jonathan Cole, a pair of Harvard psychiatrists, along with a registered nurse named Carol Glod, noted in 1990 that a group of six patients, all of whom had been free of any suicidal ideation when they commenced the drug, became acutely suicidal while on it, experiencing 'intense, violent suicidal preoccupation'. One patient said she 'felt like jumping out of her skin' and that 'death would be a welcome result'. Another escaped from the hospital, was caught by security guards and, upon her return, banged her head repeatedly against the floor while trying to mutilate herself, until physical restraint was the only option. It appeared to the treating psychiatrists that fluoxetine, far from making their patients well, had unleashed monstrous and deeply dangerous urges. Suddenly stories began cropping up in other medical journals as well. Some depressed patients, it appeared, had a paradoxical response to fluoxetine: the drug agitated them to the point of extreme violence. There were reports of patients pacing backwards and forwards, pounding walls and becoming paranoid.

Shortly after the deadly shootings at Columbine High School in April 1999, it was reported that one of the young gunmen had been taking an SSRI. In the widely read and highly acclaimed novel *We Need to Talk about Kevin*, which was later made into a film, author Lionel Shriver creates an adolescent male character who is put on fluoxetine and who then, using a bow and arrow, shoots a group of students, along with a canteen worker and a teacher, in the high school gym, which he barricades so no one can get in, killing his victims slowly, first an arrow in the foot, pinning the victim in place, then a half hour later another arrow to the chest and so on, all eleven of his victims dying excruciatingly, bleeding out on the burnished gymnasium floor while the killer, spiked on serotonin, coldly watches their lives ebb away in a tide of total red.

The fluoxetine-linked shooting that perhaps most caught the public's attention involved a 47-year-old man named Joseph Wesbecker, who had worked at the Standard Gravure printing press in Louisville in Kentucky for seventeen years until August 1988, when he left the company, after having filed a complaint the previous year regarding discrimination against him for his manic depression. Subsequently he reached a settlement with the company and was put on disability leave in 1989, with the understanding that he could return to work once he was better.

But Wesbecker, who had a significant history of psychological problems and had been on an array of different psychiatric drugs, was not destined to improve. Soon after his psychiatrist started him on fluoxetine in August 1989, a year after he'd left his job, Wesbecker took a sharp turn for the worse. He became irritable, restless and paranoid. The following month, when his psychiatrist saw how psychologically unbalanced his patient had become, he told Wesbecker to stop taking the drug. Wesbecker, however, insisted he did not want to because he believed the drug was helping him to remember. 'Remember what?' his psychiatrist wanted to know. On fluoxetine, Wesbecker falsely believed he was recalling how his foreman at Standard Gravure had forced him into fellatio in front of all the other workers, a 'memory' that only served to fuel the rage boiling within him. Again his psychiatrist told him to stop taking the drug, but Wesbecker did not heed his advice.

Three days later, on the morning of 14 September, Wesbecker loaded an AK-47 semiautomatic rifle and a German-made pistol, and packed into a duffel bag two other semiautomatic pistols and a revolver, along with back-up rounds of ammunition. He went to work and took the lift to the second floor, where the Standard Gravure executive offices were located. When the lift door opened, Wesbecker walked out into the reception area with the rifle pointed straight ahead and opened fire, in what became, according to journalist Mark Ames, 'the first modern private workplace massacre in American history.' Wesbecker moved through the Standard

Gravure offices and plant 'like a zombie, an automaton', ultimately killing eight co-workers and wounding another twelve before turning the loaded gun on himself, as his final act.

It took five more years, in the autumn of 1994, before the survivors and the families of the slain victims were able to bring Eli Lilly to court. Some of them came to the trial leaning on canes or in wheelchairs. Their claim: Lilly had mutilated their bodies and traumatised their minds by making fluoxetine – which to them was a deadly drug – available to a man they had once counted as a friend, whom they had nicknamed 'Rocky'. Lilly's defence: given Wesbecker's long history of psychiatric problems, fluoxetine could not be blamed for the horror that had occurred. This had become Lilly's standard defence to accusations that fluoxetine caused violence or suicidality. (The Wesbecker case was not the first fluoxetine-related legal action brought against the drug manufacturer. Within two years of fluoxetine's release, there were already fifty-four suits pending, and in the mid-1990s, 160 suits would be consolidated into one large class action against Lilly.) The company maintained that the drug was entirely safe – why else would the FDA have approved it? – and that when bad things happened, it was because the people taking the drug had pre-existing proclivities towards self-destruction or murder. In the case of Wesbecker, getting to the truth was complicated because he had in fact tried to commit suicide five years before his rampage, and had purchased a number of the firearms before going on fluoxetine.

Thus, in the courtroom, Lilly's lawyers claimed that Wesbecker had been a train wreck long before fluoxetine entered his life. Attorneys for the survivors and the families of the victims, for their part, brought in experts, such as Wesbecker's psychiatrists, who claimed that although Wesbecker had a history of psychiatric problems, he had never displayed any violent tendencies towards others until being started on fluoxetine. A turning point in the trial came when the judge ruled that lawyers for the survivors could introduce evidence of a painkiller called benoxaprofen that

Lilly had manufactured, marketed as Oraflex in the United States and Opren in Europe. The drug had been responsible for at least 150 deaths in the UK and the United States, and Lilly had been forced not only to withdraw the drug from the market but also to pay penalties and settlements in the millions of dollars related to 1,500 lawsuits. But then a strange thing happened. Just a day after plaintiffs won the right to include the benoxaprofen evidence, and with arguments ongoing, attorneys for the survivors abruptly informed the judge that in order to get the case to the jury as soon as possible, they had elected not to introduce any new evidence and instead would wait until the second phase of the trial, which covered punitive damages.

Unbeknownst to the judge, Lilly, panicked at the thought of how the benoxaprofen evidence could turn the trial, had reached a secret settlement with the plaintiffs. Under a 'high/low' arrangement, Lilly agreed to pay to the survivors and the family members of victims what an attorney for one of the claimants later referred to as 'a tremendous amount of money', a sum so huge 'it boggles the mind'. (Because the amount of the settlement is sealed, it remains unknown, though pretrial estimates for a Lilly loss had been in the range of $150 million to $500 million.) According to the agreement, which came to light only years afterwards when the judge in the case himself sued to have it disclosed, if the survivors won their case, Lilly would pay on the high side of its offer; if the jury found in favour of the defendants, Lilly would pay out the lower, though still enormous, figure. Payment was contingent, however, on the jury reaching a verdict. Because of that stipulation, there was a huge disincentive for the survivors' attorneys to really press their case, since if they fell short and wound up with a hung jury, their clients would get nothing. 'The incentives,' wrote Joseph Glenmullen, 'shifted in favor of "losing" to be sure the victims and their attorneys went home well compensated.' In addition, as part of the agreement the plaintiffs had also conceded that, regardless of the outcome, they would not appeal. What followed was an utter charade. The two sides went back into the courtroom, and as the lawyers acted out their parts, a trial that had been tense from the beginning was suddenly placid. Objections were desultory or entirely overlooked.

The entire deal raised profound concerns about the justice system and underscores the questions that have been part and parcel of the development of fluoxetine from its inception – a drug that appears to be one thing (site-specific) but that is really something else (far-reaching in its neural effects over the entire sprawl of the serotonin system, a system that is furthermore intimately tied to other neurotransmitters); a drug that was marketed as basically safe, despite the fact that, at the very least, it depresses the dopamine system and thus causes all sorts of troubling side effects; a drug Americans accepted as their darling, unable or unwilling to ask the difficult questions that ought to have been asked: where are the studies on long-term side effects? Why has Eli Lilly not pursued them? Is it justifiable to start patients on a path to taking a drug for years, for decades, when we know so little about its long-term effects? What does it mean that drugs with similar profiles, such as dexfenfluramine, show disturbing brain damage in animal studies? If you depress your dopamine neurons, does that make you more vulnerable to developing dopamine-related disorders such as Parkinson's disease, either now or later in life?

But for a whole host of reasons, these are questions that very few people are asking. In both its clinical trials and this legal trial, Lilly managed to come out looking clean despite challenges to its due diligence. In the end, the company 'won' the Wesbecker case, by a margin of 9–3 on the jury, the minimum number of votes it could receive and prevail, though the company's CEO presented it as nothing less than a complete vindication, claiming, in a *New York Times* article under the headline 'Jury Rules Out Drug as Factor in Killings', that Eli Lilly had 'proven in a court of law ... that Prozac is safe and effective'. And how did it achieve this victory? By effectively placating the survivors with what may be the world's best, albeit short-term, antidepressant – cash.

The Myth of Low Serotonin

But the question of why depression is on the rise when we putatively have a chemical cure has not yet been answered. Psychopharmacology celebrated the serotonin boosters as clean, safe and highly effective drugs to treat depression. Then the field went one step beyond that by claiming that at last it had the science and the knowledge to treat human despair, a belief exemplified by Jeffrey A. Lieberman, chair of the psychiatry department at Columbia University in New York and former president of the American Psychiatric Association, who wrote, 'My profession now practices an enlightened and effective medicine of mental health, giving rise to the most gratifying moments in a psychiatrist's career: bearing witness to clinical triumphs.'

One of these triumphs is certainly fluoxetine. But how do psychiatrists square their enlightened and effective medicine with the fact that the number of people with mental illness just keeps going up? Earlier in this chapter we considered a couple of possible sociological explanations for the rise of depression and other affective disorders: first, that the increase in diagnoses is due to the lowering of stigma associated with depression, meaning that people suffering from the disease these days are more willing to admit their struggles and seek treatment, and secondly, that the rise in depression is the result of our becoming a more individualistic and less communal society.

Robert Whitaker, a finalist for the Pulitzer Prize for public service journalism and a Polk Award winner for his writing on medicine and science, proposes another scenario, which is that serotonin boosters, rather than treating a chemical imbalance, may instead be causing one. For starters, despite drug company advertisements and the prevailing 'neuro-speak', there is, as we've seen, little evidence that mental illness is the result of a chemical imbalance. Scientists have searched and searched for evidence of this imbalance and have not been able to find it. Perhaps more to the point, when researchers have compared serotonin levels in depressed versus non-depressed subjects, they have found that the happy subjects do not necessarily have more serotonin than their depressed counterparts. In fact, sometimes the happy subjects have *less* serotonin than the depressed research subjects. Because of the hypothesis about schizophrenia being the result of excess dopamine in the brain, scientists have also compared dopamine levels in schizophrenic versus non-schizophrenic subjects. But in a similar result to the serotonin studies, the schizophrenic subjects did not have any more dopamine than their non-schizophrenic counterparts. In some instances they even had less.

The results of these studies and others like them have turned psychiatry's dominant narrative of mental illness on its head. After all, if there is no proof that a depressed person has a chemical imbalance, and you choose nevertheless to put that person on a medication that will alter neurotransmitter levels in his or her brain, then in effect you are causing a chemical imbalance rather than curing one. According to Steven Hyman, a neuroscientist and former director of the US National Institute of Mental Health, all psychotropic drugs cause 'perturbations in neurotransmitter functions'. And this is Whitaker's main point. We are subjecting millions of brains to drugs that change natural neurotransmission, sometimes radically, disturbing and upsetting the complex interplay inside our heads, clogging neural pathways with excess chemicals and sometimes causing the entire brain, which is intricately interlinked, to malfunction in ways we do not yet understand. An unmedicated depressed patient does not have a known chemical imbalance in his brain, but once he ingests fluoxetine, he will. The drug crosses the blood-brain barrier and gets to work, jamming serotonin into the synaptic cleft. Whitaker explains the result this way: 'Several weeks later the serotonergic pathway is operating in a decidedly *abnormal* manner. The presynaptic neuron is putting out more serotonin than usual. Its serotonin reuptake channels are blocked by the drug. The system's feedback loop is partially disabled. The postsynaptic neurons are "desensitised" to serotonin. Mechanically speaking, the serotonergic system is now rather mucked up.'

As far as Whitaker, Glenmullen, and other critics are concerned, the bewildering rise in mental illness is due not to social pressures but to the fact that so many people are drugged on serotonin boosters among other psychiatric medications and are therefore walking around with abnormal brain functioning that, in the long term, exacerbates the very symptoms the drugs are trying to treat. In other words, our antidepressants are making us increasingly depressed; thus we turn to them still more keenly, upping the dose, which causes still more neural perturbations and abnormal functioning, and so we go round and round, down and down. While, as we've seen, we have very little in the way of studies on long-term side effects for antidepressants or other psychotropics, we do have studies comparing the fates of medicated versus unmedicated patients. These have found that 23 per cent of adults, if they have never been psychiatrically medicated, will experience remission of a depressive episode without treatment in one month, 67 per cent in six months and 85 per cent in a year, while medicated patients tend only to get sicker, with the intervals between their depressive episodes shortening as time goes on.

The picture looks especially glum for depressed patients who 'recovered' on an antidepressant and then went off it. A whole range of studies has demonstrated that when patients begin taking an antidepressant and then go off it, they are likely to have a relapse of their depression within eighteen months at a rate of anywhere from 50 to 70 per cent. 'Everywhere, the message was the same,' Whitaker wrote. 'Depressed people who were treated with an antidepressant and then stopped taking it regularly got sick again.' And to make matters worse, a person who is on an antidepressant for a long period of time can expect to relapse faster, more furiously, than he would if treated for a shorter period. In a sense the drug becomes, over time, so intertwined with the user's physiology that he or she simply cannot do without it as the years tick on. This conclusion is buttressed by another study in which large doses of fluoxetine were fed to rats, whose brains were then examined post-mortem, whereupon the scientists conducting the study found that the rats' neurons were 'swollen' and 'twisted like corkscrews'.

Examination of these studies is disturbing, and one can well understand why the field of psychiatry might want to marginalise Whitaker's reportage and the arguments he has culled. But because psychiatry highly values, or is supposed to value, honest self-assessment, all who work within the field are called upon to address the issues that this research has raised, and to do so with a steady and serious concern that has thus far not been evident. Instead, mainstream psychiatry has largely ignored the studies Whitaker cites, clumping him with the 'antipsychiatry establishment' as a kind of modern-day Thomas Szasz, a radical incapable of thinking beyond his own bias. This is a shame, because the hypotheses put forward by thinkers like Whitaker and Glenmullen are entirely plausible. In attempting to exile such critics, the field has lost a chance to examine itself and learn something important in the process. If the studies that Whitaker cites are correct and we are in fact causing brain damage with our antidepressants, then, at the very least, we ought to know. Were this the case, patients would deserve to be told. Many might opt for the medication anyway, the same as many in the middle of the last century, in pursuit of mental serenity, opted for lobotomies despite the danger of neural destruction involved, so pervasive and severe was their suffering.

As psychopharmacology gains a tighter and tighter grip on psy-chiatry, with drug companies luring psychiatrists to ghostwrite papers or represent medications in a positive light in exchange for handsome fees, psychiatry seems to grow more and more unstable, less and less likely, or *able*, to address the questions, controversies and contradictions at its core. These questions are moral as well as neurological or biochemical. On the one hand, is it right to put patients on a drug that may be making their brain behave in an abnormal fashion, especially when there is no definitive evidence of chemical imbalance in the first place? On the other hand, is it right to do nothing in the face of severe suffering?

Does Depression Damage the Brain?

Helen Mayberg, a neurologist and leading depression researcher at Emory University in Atlanta, reported in 2013 that psychotherapy, specifically cognitive behavioural therapy, is just as effective, statistically, as antidepressants are in reversing depression. But what about those patients who are too sick to tolerate the rigours of reflection? Beyond that, just because we have not found a chemical imbalance in the brains of mental patients does not mean there isn't something terribly askew in those brains, something that antidepressants could be treating, albeit in indirect or not entirely detectable ways. Perhaps, for those with a depressive disorder, raising the amount of serotonin available in the synaptic cleft triggers the DNA to make a new protein, and this altered gene expression allows a patient to recover.

Suppose we do nothing for the depressive except watch and wait for him to recover? The trouble is that myriad researchers and practitioners have suggested that depression is at least as toxic to the brain as the drugs we use to treat it. Untreated depression bathes the brain in the stress hormone cortisol, and long-term exposure to cortisol can cause the brain's prefrontal cortex to waste. Thomas Frodl, a neurobiology researcher at Trinity College in Dublin, found that depressive episodes may result in neuroplastic changes to the brain. Frodl looked at inpatients with major depression alongside controls recruited from the community, studying their brains with fMRI technology both at baseline and three years later. 'Compared with controls,' he observed, 'patients showed significantly more decline in grey matter density.' In other words, contra Whitaker, untreated depression may cause brain damage too. Furthermore, other research shows that the more episodes of depression a person has, the more vulnerable he or she is to future relapse. Each episode, if left untreated, damages our grey matter, quite literally shrinking our hippocampus (a ridge in the brain responsible for memory), torquing our amygdala (an almond-shaped mass in the temporal lobe that handles the emotions) and sending our neurons into chaos.

But if it is not about correcting a chemical imbalance, how else might psychotropic drugs help our brains? There is some research which posits that the reason why antidepressants take weeks to work, even though they almost immediately raise neurotrans-mitter levels, is that the medications, far from being toxic, are actually neurotrophic, meaning they spawn the cranial conditions that allow fresh neurons and new neuronal connections to be born. Drugs like fluoxetine, this research suggests, might increase branching of the dendrites in the neuron, a process that is the substrate of how we learn and feel and play. So it could be that the way antidepressants make us feel better is by helping the brain grow a richer, thicker forest of connections, which enable us to think faster and with more acuity. This line of reasoning stands in absolute contrast to what Whitaker and Glenmullen have found in their analyses of many outcome studies which all seem to show antidepressants burning the brain. That there can be two such utterly opposing views points to the fledgling science that psychi-atry is shows we have a long way to go before even beginning to understand the interplay of people and their medicines.

Diagnostic Drift

In addition to the lowering of stigma associated with mental illness, the move towards a more individualistic and less commu-nal society, and the possibility that antidepressants are irrevocably altering the interplay of our neurotransmitters, another possible reason for the sharp rise in depression in our time could be the phenomenon called 'diagnostic drift'. This term refers to a particular diagnosis coming untethered from its initial conceptual moorings, so that a category of illness once tightly tied to very specific behaviours is suddenly relevant to everyone and his aunt, with the result that the disorder in question – in this case depression – becomes so watered down, so deeply diluted, that it almost ceases to have any medical meaning at all.

Psychiatry as a profession has been through several cases of diagnostic drift. Post-traumatic stress disorder, now as common as crisps, was once reserved for war-ravaged veterans trying to reintegrate back into a society hardened against them. Then, as a result of cultural shifts and the rise of feminism, 'trauma' became a household word, and it wasn't long before patients were suddenly releasing repressed 'memories' of heinous acts perpetrated by people dressed as devils. Memories, for a time, got so out of hand, so deviously fictive, that patients began claiming they had multiple personalities, split-off selves they said were the result of their severe traumas. The acme of this cultural and therapeutic frenzy was the construction of a whole new diagnostic category: multiple personality disorder, a diagnosis that, in the 1980s, was fairly easy to obtain if you came to see your therapist with complaints of forgetfulness or strange feelings of detachment, both of which were supposed signs of other personalities lurking around the patient like invisible ghosts.

Eventually the fad died down, in part because psychologist Elizabeth Loftus definitively showed that it was eerily, easily possible to induce false memories in a substantial number of people by simple suggestion. Her work, perhaps more than anything else, signalled the end of the trauma party that had left its thumbprints all over the excessive 1980s. Now multiple personality disorder does not even exist as a diagnostic category any more. It has been replaced by a diagnosis called dissociative identity disorder, which shares some features with its precursor but is rarely used. While we can be thankful for that fact, this history also reveals how uncomfortably unstable and suggestible psychiatry's diagnoses really are, how they sometimes arise in large part out of cultural constructions and committee consensus and not out of what we would most want them to stem from: blood, bile, torn tissue or altered neurotransmitter levels.

Diazepam, the vaunted tranquilliser for the relief of anxiety and tension, was another instigator of diagnostic drift. By 1969, six years after it was approved and marketed under the brand name Valium, diazepam had become the top-selling pharmaceutical in the US, a status it retained for the next fourteen years, peaking in 1978, with more than 2 billion tablets sold. Once that drug came on to the market, suddenly hundreds of thousands, and then millions of women were suffering from a bad case of nerves. It's not that anxiety didn't exist before diazepam but rather that diazepam, once it was born, gave vast numbers of people who were tense by nature a chance to turn their character trait into an illness. Once that trait had been named a sickness, and the person with that trait a patient, the new medication became necessary.

But for all the popularity of diazepam and the other benzodiazepines, the birth of fluoxetine caused a cultural shift in the US more seismic than anything in psychiatry that had preceded it. Yes, chlorpromazine forever changed the face and fate of madness, but its relevance was restricted only to those with a truly rare disorder, pushed to the sidelines of society. The drug never became a household word. Likewise, the tricyclics and the MAOIs never penetrated deeply into popular culture. For the most part, these drugs were reserved for the severe mental pain that accompanies the rare event of a major depressive episode. More common is a condition called dysthymia, a milder form of depression, the equivalent of a persistent low-grade fever. Individuals with dysthymia, glass-half-empty characters, usually function fine but possess little capacity for joy.

When fluoxetine came on to the market, in early 1988, people experiencing dysthymia were ultimately the ones who made the drug a runaway success. It was as though everyone with any kind of depressive streak came forward with palm held out. Researchers began to discover, serendipitously, that the drug was not tied tightly to major depression after all. In fact, much like chlorprom-azine and its off-label uses a generation earlier, fluoxetine could successfully treat not only a nation of dysthymics but also those with conditions not even in the *DSM*. *Time* reported, for instance, on a patient named Susan, a self-described workaholic who got irritable around her periods and who had once thrown her wed-ding ring at her husband. On fluoxetine, the jagged edges of her personality were planed into something smooth, and functioning was so much easier that life became a joy. Eventually the concept of depression ballooned to embrace the irritable Susans, the work-aholics, the pessimists, the panicky and the malcontents, to the point where the diagnosis included personality types as much as any specific psychiatric syndrome. Practitioners in the field now prescribe fluoxetine for a wide range of conditions from panic attacks to cataplexy, suggesting that perhaps all of these disorders share a common neural substrate with depression.

Of course, these developments were all to the benefit of Eli Lilly, and the drug company promoted the diagnostic drift, encouraging GPs and psychiatrists to treat even mild complaints with their new concoction. Lilly instituted a 'Depression Awareness Day', when anybody could call an 800 number to see whether he or she was depressed, punching in numbers on the phone's keypad to answer yes or no on a ten-item 'exam' featuring statements such as 'I get tired for no reason'.

The publication of influential psychiatrist Peter Kramer's *Listening to Prozac*, a bestseller that by and large painted a glowing picture of a drug able to remove the thorns in anyone's character, did nothing to dispel the building enthusiasm. The book not only helped raise the popularity of the drug but also caused the definition of depression to dilate. After all, if fluoxetine was an antidepressant, then daily disappointments and quotidian diffi-culties – misfortunes big and small – had to be subsumed within the concept of depression in order to justify the large numbers of people taking the medicine. University of Toronto historian Edward Shorter, in his *History of Psychiatry*, considered by many the standard text in the field, draws a distinction between the solid science involved in the discovery of fluoxetine and the mere scientism beneath its promotion to the masses. 'Good science lay behind the discovery of fluoxetine as a much safer and quicker second-generation antidepressant than imipramine and the other tricyclics,' he wrote. In contrast, 'scientism lay behind converting a whole host of human difficulties into the depression scale, and making all treatable with a wonder drug. This conversion was possible only because clinical psychiatry had enmeshed itself so massively in the corporate culture of the drug industry. The result was that a scientific discipline such as psychiatry nurtured a popular culture of pharmacological hedonism, as millions of people who otherwise did not have a psychiatric disorder craved the new compound because it lightened the burden of self-consciousness.'

It is a serious problem to which psychiatry seems to be particularly vulnerable. There is not, for instance, an epidemic of pulmonary specialists touting drugs for profit. One naturally wonders what it is about the profession of psychiatry that makes it so susceptible to compromise, both financially and diagnostically. Psychiatrists themselves are responsible for the oil spill of depression diagnoses, and contrary to what Robert Whitaker has written, it may be that this diagnostic proliferation is all the explanation we need for why depression is on the rise. In truth, one *hopes* that diagnostic drift is the answer to the mysterious increase in depression, since, while it is a troubling phenomenon, it is reversible, at least in theory, which makes it less troubling than the thought of brain-damaged patients gobbling their psychotropics because they really have no other choice, their neurons so perturbed that their descent into depression happens faster and faster, with shorter intervals of time in between, until relapse is inevitable and addiction all but guaranteed.

All-Purpose Fluoxetine

Fluoxetine and other serotonin boosters were heralded as psychiatry's second big pharmacological breakthrough in the treatment of depression. The drugs were supposedly more advanced, more effective and above all cleaner than the tricyclics and the MAOIs discovered in the 1950s. On closer examination, however, the SSRIs, while in some ways an improvement on the previous class of antidepressants, were not quite the breakthrough the field claims. Because the serotonin system is so widespread, the drugs cannot, by definition, be clean, meaning they cannot actually target a specific site in the brain. The problem when it comes to truly understanding depression, then, is not just the particular negative side effects, such as sexual dysfunction, that SSRIs cause by disabling disparate neural systems. It's also, oddly enough, their 'positive' effects. When serotonin boosters are given to non-depressed subjects, for instance, the subjects become peppier, chattier, more social and in general more upbeat. 'What's wrong with that?' you might ask. Nothing in general, except that although this outcome might seem desirable on the one hand, it's also, on the other, an obvious indication that these purportedly superior drugs are essentially blanketing the entire brain, much like ibuprofen for a headache. But while fluoxetine might act as a buffer to reduce pain, it does not treat the *cause* of depression, which remains unknown, and therefore the drug has little to teach us about the origins of the disease.

Similarly, studies with animals have shown that when fluoxetine is given to baby rats removed from their mother, it reduces the frequency of their ultrasonic cries, again suggesting that the drug is more like morphine or cocaine. It is able to assuage general distress, in other words, but unable to tell us as much about depression as the earlier drugs like imipramine did. The tricyclics, in sharp contrast, do nothing for already non-depressed subjects except give them nasty side effects. But because tricyclics work only on depressed subjects and relieve only depression, they may be a superior torchlight into the mechanisms of pathological despair.

The final time I talked with her, Ann Bolo, having recently celebrated her daughter's first birthday, was finally off fluoxetine, unable to tolerate any longer its sexual side effects. While the drug is touted as non-addictive, Bolo found that to be utterly untrue. 'Getting off Prozac was one of the hardest things I ever had to do,' she claimed, and described enduring withdrawal effects that stunned her: electrical zapping sensations in her head, dizzying migraines, all-consuming nausea and a deep despair that she rode out with exceptional strength and commitment. 'There were so many times in those first weeks,' Bolo said, 'when I was like, *All right, I give up, put me back on the drug.* But my marriage was at stake, and prior to having the baby I hadn't been depressed, so I hung on to the belief that I'd get my old self back.' And she did. Others, however, are not so lucky. Many, many patients are sustained on SSRIs for years, for decades, and when they try to go off, they cannot tolerate the withdrawal. Others, as Whitaker has written, have relapses while on the drugs, causing them to increase their doses and only further perturb a brain already tilted by the onslaught of synthetic chemicals.

Still, psychiatry continues to tout the SSRIs as one of its biggest innovations to date, and takes it one step further by claiming that at long last it is practising medicine in truly scientific ways. Jeffrey A. Lieberman has gone so far as to assert that in the first decade of the 21st century, 'the once stagnant field of psychiatry showed all the signs of a profession undergoing intellectual rejuvenation.' It's an opinion that stands in direct opposition to what Cornell University psychiatrist Richard Friedman, director of the Psychopharmacology Clinic at New York–Presbyterian Hospital, has bluntly stated, 'It is hard to think of a single truly novel psychotropic drug that has emerged in the last thirty years.'

Rising Doses

I'd like to think psychiatrists such as Lieberman are correct. After all, I have a vested interest in a vibrant and intellectually honest psychiatry, seeing as I daily swallow a number of its drugs. On the one hand, I have been on a serotonin booster since I was twenty-five years old, and on a tricyclic for six years before that; I am currently fifty-four. For thirty-five years, then, I have been trying to soothe my brain with psychiatry's medicines, but I cannot confidently claim that I am better because of it. The picture is mixed. Prior to the SSRIs, I swallowed imipramine. I did not get well and seemed to have no real future prospects of getting well. On SSRIs, however, I have been able to stay out of mental hospitals, to write nine books, to bear two babies who are now adolescents with their own keen interests and proclivities, to manage a marriage and then a divorce, and, just as importantly, to nurture a circle of friends. If that isn't an advertisement for psychiatry, then I don't know what is.

On the other hand (and there is always another hand when it comes to the slippery subject of psychopharmacology), the 10 milligrams of fluoxetine I first took twenty-nine years ago, and which so magically removed the dead-weight symptoms so that my whole world became a gorgeous glimmer, worked for only a little while, and it wasn't too long before I needed 20, then 30, then 60, then 80, then 100 milligrams of fluoxetine in order to get the relief that the initial tiny 10 milligrams had provided. What the rising doses and the relapses that preceded them suggested, of course, was that my brain was adapting to the drug and that my illness, far from being quelled, was raging right along beneath the blanket fluoxetine provided.

Yet even though I was terrified of having to raise the dose continually, fluoxetine had exerted such a powerful effect against my obsessive-compulsive behaviour, and my bipolar depressions, that I became completely dependent on it psychologically and perhaps physically. The idea that one day it might not work for me any more horrified me, and I spent more than my fair share of nights fretting about a future that would turn into a rerun of my past, which had been full of the window grills set into the mortar of the mental hospitals that housed me. The thought of backsliding petrified me. More than anything else, I needed my medication to work, but the signs increasingly suggested that I could not count on fluoxetine, that it was at best a temporary fix and that eventually I'd have to dose myself so severely that I'd do real damage to my liver, which metabolises the drug, or to my kidneys or, God knows, to my brain.

But 100 milligrams of fluoxetine is a whopper of a dose, and when I relapsed even on that, sometime in 2005, I finally switched to another serotonin (and noradrenaline) booster, venlafaxine. This I did with real regret and fear, and when that still didn't work, my psychopharmacologist upped the drug's punch with the atypical antipsychotic olanzapine, which also increases the availability of serotonin at the synapse. For a short time, as I recounted earlier, I replaced the olanzapine with lithium, but ultimately the lithium did not keep my depression away, as I'd so hoped it would. Thus I went back on olanzapine. The combo has worked wonders for my mental state, but the venlafaxine gave me high blood pressure, necessitating that I take another drug called lisinopril to bring my blood pressure back to normal.

As I've indicated, the problem with the olanzapine, both before and after lithium, was that it so intensified my appetite that I was beyond satiation, such that the mere mention of food caused my mouth to water. I would eat marshmallow fluff straight from the jar and wolf down multiple Mexican enchiladas filled with rotund beans and covered in mole sauce. Yes, I was warned about weight gain in connection with olanzapine, but I had no way of truly comprehending how much my body would balloon and how badly the accumulation of internal fat would damage my organs and put me at real risk for a stroke or a heart attack. A single warning from a single doctor when I was in the depths of despair could not adequately convey the message that by swallowing this new drug I was effectively agreeing to deeply damage the body upon which I rely to survive. As the olanzapine toyed first with my metabolism and then with my body, my weight went up, up, up, with the end result that I am now an overweight diabetic. High blood sugar is destroying my eyesight, so that without glasses everything looks fuzzy, with ever-stronger lenses necessary for me to get a clear view. At the back of my mind is the fear I will go blind. When I see the doctor, he checks my feet very carefully because diabetics often get festering sores from poor circulation and in the long run risk amputation. My high sugar has also caused my kidneys to malfunction, so that my mouth is always thick with thirst. My urine, far too infrequent, is thick with sediment. And my blood lipids, dangerously high as a result of olanzapine, put me at risk for pancreatitis and coronary heart disease.

To put it bluntly, I am not ageing well. I am unhealthy, and this is largely due to psychiatry's drugs. And yet I cannot live without these drugs. After more than thirty years of a steadily rising dose and an increasing number of drugs, I am quite certain my brain has been permanently altered and that my neural systems would not be able to function without these daily doses. At times, scared of dying before getting to see my children have children, I have tried to go off my drug buffet, but the withdrawal has been physically horrible and mentally dangerous. The depression has been so deep that I once bought a gun, and another time wrote suicide letters to my children, which I later sealed, undelivered, in a zip-locked bag. Eventually I gave up the chase and went back on my medications, which have returned to me my mind while wiping out my body and, in so doing, have all but proved René Descartes's claim about the mind–body split. I often wonder what would have happened to me had I never begun taking imipramine, or fluoxetine after that. Would it have been possible for me to move out of the depression on my own? There is of course no way to know. But given my experience, given the fact that I am dying as I live, dying more quickly than I would be were I not sustained on these drugs, I cannot give them an unqualified round of applause.

The Brain Bank

The Harvard Brain Tissue Resource Center at McLean in Massachusetts, known colloquially as the Brain Bank, collects people's brains upon their death and studies them, searching for the flaw that is schizophrenia, for the telltale tangles of Alzheimer's, for the beautiful, rich dendritic connections that mark a healthy cortex.

One day I found myself calling them, and when someone on the other end answered and said, 'Brain Bank', in a crisp voice, I was suddenly unsure of what to say. I stammered out a hello, followed by silence, and in the silence the static popping on the line was the only thing connecting us.

'Brain Bank,' the person said again, as though I had not heard.

'Yes,' I said. 'I know.'

'Can I help you?' the person said, and I realised I could not tell if the voice was male or female and suddenly I feared I was talking to a computer when what I needed was a human who could help me through whatever it was I had to say, to give.

'I am calling because I'd like to . . . to . . . donate my brain,' I said, the last three words spilling together in a rush.

The person on the other end did not respond and again I stood there listening to the crackle on the line, looking out my large window at the apple tree, where clusters of reddening fruit studded its beautiful branches.

'Donate. My. Brain,' I repeated, articulating each word, suddenly, strangely, emboldened.

'Okay,' the disembodied voice said. 'You can make the donation online.' And then the voice gave me the Web address and, poof, was gone.

I stood there stunned, holding the phone, which after some seconds started to beep frenetically. I hung up and went online and once at the site filled out the forms that will allow McLean, at the time of my death, to cut a wide hole in the top of my head and remove my brain, after which they will stuff my empty skull with cotton and sew up the incision so that no one at my open-casket funeral will know. Meanwhile, back at their laboratory, my brain will be halved, each hemisphere preserved in formaldehyde until a scientist is ready to cut the delicate slices of neural tissue that might give some clues as to what these drugs really do after decades of use. This is my contribution to the psychopharmacological snarl we are in, the only way I can think to really and truly help. In the meantime I will find some way to live with my rising sugar, my failing eyesight, my fading memory and the occasional motor tics that cause me to jerk in weird and unsettling ways.

Etchings

Now that I am divorced, I live part-time with my two children and full-time with my new domestic partner and our four horses in Fitchburg, Massachusetts, on 32 hectares (80 acres) of field and forest, where apple trees line the sides of the driveway and orchards spread as far as the eye can see, growing up and down hills alongside stately barns painted a bright red and crisp white, with picturesque horses burnished to a rich gleam. In effect, we have no neighbours here, making the evening darkness that much deeper. The nearest house is probably 3 hectares (8 acres) away. At night the tiny tangerine squares of its windows glow with a distant warmth. It's hard to meet people in the country, but our house, just recently raised and built, has the feel of the many human hands that helped to put our abode together.

If you go out back, make a left, walk through our pasture where the rudbeckias swing in the wind, trudge up the hill where rocks maybe millions of years old protrude, pass through the forest where your footsteps on the golden pine needles may be the only sound, you will eventually come to a small cemetery, surrounded by a black iron fence and a filigreed gate that looks like dark lace but is tough to the touch, and cold. Open the gate and the hinges squeal in protest, but you can step into the sacred space where the gravestones are worn by wind and weather. Each one is inscribed with something different but all profess love. *Here Lies Our Dearest Mother. May Abner Find His Way on Wings to Heaven's Pearly Gates.* All of these graves are from the eighteenth and nineteenth centuries. My children and I have walked among the stones and trapped the designs on their surfaces – poems, angels, clocks – by taping tracing paper to a grave and rubbing sideways with a shorn pencil. The etchings give off a ghostly feel. They flutter in the wind, a reminder that even in tiny country towns, thousands have come before us in this ancient world whose first light was struck, like flint against steel, in a blue beam billions of years ago. At home, I would look at our etchings and wonder about the people who lay beneath the gravestones. What had they done when their eyes failed them and there was no such thing as corrective lenses? What happened when the tooth cavity gave way to rot and the nerves pulsed in pain?

I know that depression, which has been recorded ever since the written word came into existence, has been treated in all kinds of ways that are bizarre to our modern minds. In the time of Philotimus, a notable Greek doctor several centuries BCE, sufferers complaining of a light head were instructed to wear a lead helmet in hopes of a cure. Chrysippus of Cnidus, a contemporary, believed that people with depression should eat more cauliflower while carefully avoiding basil because it could incite someone to insanity.

Depression's treatments have morphed over time, as has the disease itself, reminding us that suffering is never stagnant, that even discrete illnesses take the shape of the culture's currents. In the 1st century CE those afflicted by depression often felt it as a severe sort of body dysmorphism. Rufus of Ephesus, another Greek doctor, ministered at different times to all of the following confused souls: a man who believed himself to be headless, a patient who thought he was a piece of pottery and a third who believed he had sloughed his skin like a snake and it was peeling from his body. There were patients who seemed possessed by psychotic delusions, as in the baker who believed he was made of butter and would melt away in the sun, or other patients who believed that they were made of glass and thus were incredibly careful not to sit down, convinced that they would crack or break apart. Treatment consisted of herbs and bloodletting and occasionally of sexual stimulation of the genitals, whose 'rotting unreleased sexual fluids', it was believed, could give off 'noxious fumes' that would disturb the brain. A millennium later, with the rise of Christianity, from the Middle Ages onwards depression was seen as a sin and was treated with exorcisms or worse. Some demon, the thinking went, had inhabited the body of the depressive and he could be cured only through religious ritual or punishment.

The prior treatments for depression seem quaint, almost poetic. There was Rufus's 'sacred remedy' for instance, a liquid concoction of 'colocynth, yellow bugle, germander, cassia, agaric, asafoetida, wild parsley, aristolochia, white pepper, cinnamon, spikenard, saffron and myrrh', all mashed together and sweetened with honey and 'given in four-dram doses in hydromel and saltwater.' If medicines such as these worked, they did so because patients believed they would work. We know now that a menagerie of spices and herbs mixed with honey cannot possibly combat the deep despair that depression is. And yet for a time it did. There may well come a day when people look back at the cures of our own age and see them as deeply delusional, evidence of primitivism. Potions that started as a simple string of numbers in the chemist's workroom? There may come a time when we can so directly manipulate gene expression that depression becomes a button we can simply turn off, or when neural interventions such as deep brain stimulation or trans-cranial magnetic stimulation will wipe away depression as if it were a stray mark on the blackboard of the brain. Who's to say what will happen, and when and how?

In the meantime, we have our less-than-perfect tablets and our choices, which are as limited as the medicines themselves. One can choose to wait depression out and hope that in the process one's brain won't be irreparably scarred from the pell-mell of stress chemicals spilling inside the head, or one can submit to pharmacological intervention and hope to remain unharmed in the process. Is there not a third way, another option, an exit? Therapy? Church? Yes, these are also possible avenues, but maybe not for deep depressions, the kind that comes in the full glare of the summer sun and clutches your throat and takes you down in daylight.

I touch the gravestone etching my children and I have done. The paper is so thin, so insubstantial, every bit as vulnerable as that scrap with its cry for *HELP* that I came across beneath the pillow in room 332 at the abandoned asylum. I don't believe in heaven and I don't believe in hell of the sort that Christianity describes. I do believe it is possible, though, to lose your mind and I also believe that there is no suffering worse than this. Because of that, when one emerges from a deep depression, the whole world looks brand new. You touch everything tenderly, and with wonder. The streets gleam. The cars shine like lollipops. The trees shoot upwards and lose themselves in lace.

This feeling is not due to fluoxetine, or to imipramine, or to any other chemical concoction you might be taking. It happens because depression, when it departs, leaves gratitude in its place. Your life becomes a new bud, a leaf. No drug can match this high, and it is here where you are your best, your most human, your healthiest self. Celebrate softly. Go ahead and sing. I do, even when I know I am withering away. It's another day down, another day done, in gratefulness.

5

Placebos

The Dancing Disease

Placebos are extraordinary drugs. They seem to have some effect on almost every symptom known to mankind, and work in at least a third of patients (usually) and sometimes in up to 60 per cent. They have no serious side effects and cannot be given in overdose. In short, they hold the prize for the most adaptable, protean, effective, safe and cheap drugs in the world's pharmacopoeia. Not only that, but they've been around for centuries, so even their pedigree is impeccable.

– Dr Robert Buckman and Karl Sabbagh (1993)

Mr Wright

In 1957 psychologist Bruno Klopfer reported on the amazing case of a man he called Mr Wright. Mr Wright was suffering from advanced cancer of the lymph nodes. Tumours the size of oranges studded his skeleton and wound throughout his organs. He was so near death that he was more malignancy than man, his face pale on the pillow, an IV plunged into one of his stringy veins.

Some people, as they near the end of a long battle with cancer, their hair gone and their teeth loose in their sockets, are ready to exit, exhausted by the demanding treatments, by the burn of radiation and the poison of chemotherapy. But Mr Wright, because he had a severe anaemic condition, was not eligible for the treatments of the day, which were radiotherapy and nitrogen mustard. He had wasted away all on his own, without the help of cures that also kill. But his will to live, his desire to see the day, was strong, and the shadow of death that fell across his hospital bed, a dark hole into which he would soon dwindle and disappear, terrified him.

Then one day Mr Wright – 'febrile, gasping for air, completely bedridden', according to his doctor – overheard people talking about a new cancer cure called Krebiozen, a horse serum available in the United States, which was being tested at the very hospital he was in. Hope sprang up like a stalk inside him. He begged his doctor for a dose, and his doctor, although doubting the drug would help at this late stage, nevertheless loaded his syringe and took his patient's wasted arm.

Three days passed as Mr Wright lay quietly in his hospital bed. On the third morning after the shot of Krebiozen had been administered, his doctor returned to examine him, and an incredible thing had happened. Before the doctor arrived, Mr Wright had swung his feet over his hospital bed and for the first time in months stood up straight on the floor, strong enough to support himself, to walk, even to stride, which he did, out of his room and down the ward to the station around which the nurses flurried. The doctor found this man who had been at death's door now joking, flirting, cavorting. X-rays showed that the tumours had shrunk from the size of oranges to golf balls – having melted 'like snowballs on a hot stove'.

No one could quite believe it, but no one could deny it either, because here was the man, once washed out but now ruddy with health and hope. Within ten days Mr Wright was discharged from the hospital, cancer-free, and he went home to pick up where he had left off before cancer came to claim him, stepping back into his life as if slipping into a perfectly fitted suit. He returned to work. Perhaps he went out to dinners, eating red slabs of steak and whipped potatoes with slabs of butter melting at their crests and salads with frilled lettuce and crimson tomatoes sliced into wheels arrayed on a plate of crystal. Perhaps he drank fine wines and champagnes where the bubbles rushed to the top when the cork was pulled out with a satisfying pop. He was here. He was alive and loving it.

Days passed, weeks passed and Mr Wright remained free of malignancies. Within two months, however, reports came out in the news saying that the Krebiozen trial had concluded and the drug was worthless. Soon after that Mr Wright's tumours returned and he was back in the hospital, once more staring at the drain hole of death, at the shadow falling across his bed.

His doctor then did something that doctors today would never be permitted to do. He told Mr Wright a story, a lie. The news reports, the doctor said, were wrong. Krebiozen was in fact a potent anti-cancer drug. Why, then, Mr Wright wondered, had he relapsed, and so badly? Because, his doctor said, Mr Wright had unfortunately been given an injection of the stuff from a weak batch, but the hospital was expecting a new shipment and it was guaranteed to be two times stronger than even the most potent Krebiozen to date. Mr Wright's doctor delayed administering anything to his patient so that his anticipation would build. After several days had passed, the doctor rolled up Mr Wright's sleeve, Mr Wright offered his arm and the doctor gave his patient a new injection – of pure water.

Again hope made an entrance. Mr Wright let all his tumours go. Once again they shrank and disappeared until no trace of them could be found in his body, and once again he left the hospital. It's not hard to picture him dancing his way through his days. A second remission! Mr Wright lived for a further two months without symptoms and then, unfortunately for him, came another news report. The American Medical Association, after numerous tests on patients, issued its final verdict on Krebiozen, confidently declaring the drug to be useless. Mr Wright's tumours reappeared, and this time, within two days after his readmission to the hospital, he was dead.

Ancient Placebos

Remember that two-thirds of patients on an SSRI would likely have improved on a placebo alone. This may go some way towards explaining why ancient medicine, as unscientific as it was, could be so effective; it consisted almost entirely of placebos. For instance, Huang Ti, the Yellow Emperor, who ruled almost five millennia ago, lists over two thousand drugs and sixteen thousand prescriptions that were used largely unchanged in China for thousands of years. Likewise there are 265 drugs in the Sumerian-Babylonian-Assyrian annals, and more than six hundred touted in ancient India. The practice of using these various potions and concoctions persisted across time. According to psychiatrists and researchers Arthur and Elaine Shapiro, the London *Pharmacopoeia*, first published in the seventeenth century, includes all of the following so-called remedies:

> Usnea (moss from the skull of victims of violent death); Vigo's plaster (viper's flesh, live frogs and worms), Gascoyne's powder (bezoar, amber, pearls, crabs' eyes, coral and black tops of crabs' claws); triangular Wormian bone from the juncture of the sagittal and lambdoid sutures of the skull of an executed criminal, theriac, mattioli, mithridate, bile, blood, bee glue, bones, bone marrow, claws, cuttlefish, cock's comb, cast-off snake skin, fox lung, fat, fur, feathers, hair, horns, hooves, isinglass, lozenges of dried viper, oil of brick, ants and wolves, powder of precious stones, seasilk, sponge, scorpions, swallows' nest, spider webs, raw silk, teeth, viscera, worms, wood lice, human placenta and perspiration, saliva of a fasting man, sexual organs and excreta of all sorts.

Theriac, used to treat poison and buried there in that list, was an especially popular placebo. It had anywhere from thirty-three to a hundred different ingredients, the main one being viper's flesh, with sometimes a dash of opium. Unicorn horn was one of the most expensive remedies, costing about four-hundred-thousand pounds in today's money. Bezoar stone, which healers claimed was a crystallised tear from the eye of a deer bitten by a poisonous snake, was in fact gallstones, or deposits of gunk found in the stomachs of livestock. The Chinese sometimes used what they claimed were ground dragon bones to treat convulsions, and liver for blood diseases and night blindness. While almost all, if not all, of today's medical men and women would claim that every cure just listed is bunk, the fact is that many people in prior centuries got sick and then got well on dried dung or crystallised tears or the flesh of vipers. How could this be?

The answer is simple: placebo.

The Pharmaceutical Factory in Our Heads

In the 1970s came the discovery of endorphins, which are opiate-like chemicals the body manufactures all on its own and which play a key role in the placebo effect, especially in cases of pain. The discovery led scientists to uncover a rich supply of nerves linking the brain to the immune system, which in turn resulted in the rise of a new branch of medicine called psychoneuroimmunology. Studies in this new medicine suggested that placebos may work to decrease pain – something they are especially good at doing – by increasing endorphins in the brain.

At the University of California, San Francisco, for example, in a 1978 double-blind experiment with young people who had recently had their wisdom teeth removed, most patients were given a placebo and reported significantly less pain. Then some of the subjects were given naloxone, a drug that is typically administered in A&E departments in cases when a patient has overdosed on heroin or morphine. Naloxone works by blocking the opiate, thereby immediately reversing the effect of the deadly ingestion. In this study with the wisdom teeth patients, once they were given naloxone, the pain relief they had experienced as a result of the placebo suddenly vanished. Once again the young people were in pain. This outcome provided researchers with a strong suggestion as to how placebos might work. It must indeed be that they released the brain's natural opiates – endorphins – and that as long as this release wasn't blocked by naloxone, or by some other organic means, then these endorphins would allow us to find real relief.

Blue and Pink Tablets

The *form* of the placebo has implications for its function. For instance, when it comes to tablets, scientists have discovered that blue placebos tend to make people drowsy, whereas red or pink placebos induce alertness. In the 1970s several professors at the University of Cincinnati took fifty-seven second-year medical students and divided them into four groups. Two groups received pink tablets and two groups blue tablets, and of the two groups receiving the same colour, one group received one tablet and the other group two tablets. All of the tablets were inert. The students then listened to a one-hour lecture and after that went back to the laboratory to fill out forms rating their moods.

The results? The students who had received two tablets reported more intense responses than the students who had taken only one tablet. And of the students who had taken the blue tablets, 66 per cent felt less alert after the lecture compared to only 26 per cent of students who had taken the pink tablets. Medical anthropologist Daniel Moerman believes that the colour of a capsule or a tablet has a strong significance to the imbiber. Blues and greens are cool colours while reds and pinks are hot colours. A study in Texas showed that red and black capsules were ranked as strongest while white ones were weakest. 'Colours are meaningful,' Moerman wrote, 'and these meanings can affect the outcome of medical treatment.' Blue tablets make us drowsy while carmines perk us up. And large tablets have more power over us than medium-sized ones, especially if they are multicoloured.

The research on the size and colour of tablets makes one wonder if we might also be more strongly affected by tablets embossed or engraved with a name: *Tagamet (brand name for cimetidine), venlafaxine, olanzapine, Abilify (brand name for aripiprazole), Concerta (brand name for methylphenidate)*. Are drug companies not hoping that if they carefully and suggestively label their medicines, we will give their tablets extra credence? Clearly the name matters. It is always multisyllabic and often suggests technological prowess. You cannot call a placebo *Tim*, for instance. The name should bring to mind test tubes and Bunsen burners with their petal-shaped flames. The name should also connote, somewhere in its utterance, the pure peace of good health, the abilities with which *Abilify* will endow you, the consonance of *Concerta*, when all the world makes solid sense.

Even more persuasive than tablets, at least in the treatment of headaches, are placebo injections. A meta-analysis of a drug called sumatriptan – which, when first introduced, was available only as an injection and then later as a capsule or a nasal spray – looked at thirty-five trials treating migraine sufferers with sumatriptan versus placebo and found that, of those patients taking a placebo tablet, only 25.7 per cent reported that their headache was mild or gone, compared to 32.4 per cent of those treated with a placebo injection reporting relief. This may seem like a small difference, but it is statistically significant and could be expected to happen by chance only twice if the experiment were repeated a thousand times. Over and over, research has revealed that when patients are injected with an inert substance they report more pain relief than those who have simply swallowed a tablet. Perhaps there is something about the needle, the press of the plunger as the supposed miracle liquid seeps below the skin and into the muscle, finding its way into the circulatory system, and at last to the wet red charm that sits within its curved cage. While a tablet can be quiet, simple, its magic subtler and singular, there is drama in a shot.

But if placebos can be especially effective for pain relief, they decidedly do not work on people who have Alzheimer's disease. Evolutionary biologist and sociobiologist Robert Trivers, in tracing the historical necessity of deceit, has found that what the brain expects to happen in the near future affects its physiological condition. This goes part of the way towards explaining why people in pain who receive a placebo they are told is a powerful pain reliever feel better after taking the inert substance. In fact, they feel better even *before* taking it. Our brains are anticipators. They prepare for the known future, and in the case of pain, that means they release endorphins. People with Alzheimer's, however, have lost the ability to see into the future and thus to prepare their brain and the associated neurotransmitters for the treatment.

Hope

Of course, none of this so far answers the question of exactly *how* endorphins get released in the first place. It seems to have something to do with belief, with hope, with faith. Even the smallest spark of it helps our heads to secrete chemicals so soothing that their analogues are illegal around the world. People who think they are drinking alcohol, but in fact are not, will nevertheless get tipsy. The opposite of hope is also very telling. Where it is absent, or unknown, medication sometimes fails to work. Diazepam, for instance, has been shown to affect a person only if he knows he is taking it.

But while there have been many studies done to predict the personality type of placebo responders, they have proven inconclusive. If only we knew! Then we would have a clear class of people to whom we could confidently feed inert substances and who could be assured of getting real relief. No such study, however, has been able to find a personality type, or rather, it would be more accurate to say that all of the studies conflict with one another. Some claim that people who respond to placebos have neurotic personality types; others claim that introverts are more likely to be fooled by placebos; while research from the UK has found that extroverts are the group most susceptible to placebos. Scientists have claimed at different times that placebo responders are both quiet and ebullient, that they have poor ego formation and super-egos the size of a city, that they are judgemental as well as easily swayed, that they are trusting and sceptical. The net sum suggests that there is no definitive profile of a person likely to respond to a placebo. Everyone is a responder – maybe not all of the time but some of the time, in some situations, in great pain or fear, perhaps, or with wants so large that they outstrip the self who holds them. We do not know. The only thing we can say for sure is that 30 to 60 per cent of the population can be fooled by a trick, by a sugar tablet, by water, by an injection of saline or a bright pink sphere glittering in the palm.

Sham Surgery

Still more powerful than tablets with even the most alluring of names and injections with even the keenest of needles is some-thing called sham surgery, which has been performed not once, not twice, but many times, and to very good effect. There are of course ethical snarls involved, but despite these obstacles, sham surgeries do happen. In the late 1950s and early 60s two different surgical teams, one in Kansas City and one in Seattle, did double-blind trials of a ligation procedure – the closing of a duct or tube using a clip – for very ill patients suffering from severe angina, a condition in which pain radiates from the chest to the outer extremities as a result of poor blood supply to the heart. The sur-geons were not told until they arrived in the operating theatre which patients were to receive a real ligation and which were not.

All of the patients, whether or not they were getting the procedure, had their chest cracked open and their heart lifted out. But only half of the patients actually had their arteries rerouted so that their blood could more efficiently bathe its pump. Each patient was sutured up in the exact same manner and was followed up by a cardiologist who did not know whether the patient had received the sham surgery or the real surgery.

The outcomes? Sixty-seven per cent of those who'd had an actual arterial coronary ligation reported subjective improvement – less pain and more energy – whereas fully 87 per cent of the sham surgery subjects felt better. The need for nitroglycerine uniformly decreased, dropping 34 per cent in the surgical patients and 42 per cent in the sham surgery patients. Both groups were able to exercise longer. All in all, the patients who'd undergone the sham surgery did even better than those who'd had the real thing. As one sham surgery patient put it: 'Practically immediately I felt better. I felt I could take a deep breath.' He estimated that he was 95 per cent better, and went from taking five doses of nitroglycerine a day before surgery to only twelve doses total in the first five weeks following the surgery.

For perhaps even better effect, sham surgery can be done in conjunction with a high-tech laser rather than a scalpel. There is a procedure called transmyocardial laser revascularisation (TMR), 'the latest whistle in the surgical approach to angina'. In TMR an incision is made in the side of the chest between two ribs. The outer layer of the heart is removed so that the heart muscle itself is exposed. A laser beam is then fired directly into the muscle, with the goal of carving a channel through which blood can flow, thereby unblocking a clogged pump and allowing oxygen-rich blood to saturate the heart. Afterwards, the outer layer of the heart is put back in place and the patient is stitched up.

In one US study, published in 2000, three hundred very sick patients were enrolled in a placebo-controlled trial of a TMR-related procedure. Of these, 90 per cent had previously had bypass surgeries and 65 per cent had had heart attacks. The patients were divided into three groups. The group undergoing the mock procedure received only simulated laser treatment, while the low-dose group received fifteen laser shots and the high-dose group twenty-five laser shots. In the six months following these surgeries, all three groups had surprisingly similar results. Every patient, regardless of the group he or she was in, displayed striking improvement, with patients who'd received the mock procedure showing gains at a rate 8 per cent higher than for those who'd received the high dose. Exercise tolerance increased all around. Angina attacks went on the wane. 'Electrical machines', wrote one scientist, 'have great appeal to patients, and recently anything with the word "laser" attached to it has caught the imagination.'

Sham surgeries have successfully been performed on hearts, on herniated discs, on sciatic nerves, on mangled knees and on the inner ears of patients with Ménière's disease, which causes vertigo, tinnitus and hearing loss. In patients suffering from Parkinson's, a disease caused by dopamine deficiency, sham surgeries are so powerfully persuasive that researchers have even discovered an increase in the patients' dopamine levels afterwards. This terrible clenched condition can be ameliorated by the combination of a scalpel and a tall tale about how you, a Parkinson's patient, suffering a partly paralysed body, have undergone a serious medical procedure designed to restore movement to your wayward limbs. Upon seeing the surgical scars, upon hearing how high-tech your procedure was, you can become fluid again, mobile again, for some period of time. As with the release of endorphins, it appears that the hope, the belief in the surgery, sparks an increase of dopamine production in the substantia nigra, a part of the brain that controls when we waltz, run, walk or fall.

Clearly, placebo cures are subject to style and perception. But if patients are made drowsy by blue tablets and alert by red ones, and if they project more power on to a large tablet than they do on to a medium-sized one, why is psychopharmacology not taking all this rich information into account in its research and development? Why are not all antidepressants some beautiful shade of vermillion that brings to mind sunsets in Venice or Floridian warmth? And why are there not more sham surgeries being performed on patients, like Mr Wright, who are at the end of the road, those treatment-resistant souls who cannot be helped by any tablet no matter its size or shape? The field could be doing sham lobotomies and sham deep brain stimulations.

Perhaps even more appealing would be the instituting of sham trans-cranial magnetic stimulation (TMS), as high-tech a procedure as one could ask for, which involves passing across the patient's head magnets whose current collides with the brain's own magnetic field and may cause a rerouting of the nerve cells, such that their stuckness, the sign of so much mental illness, finally loosens and floats away, taking with it the debris of depression, the confetti of mania, restoring the sufferer to sanity. While TMS and vagus nerve stimulation (VNS) – in which a battery pack is placed under the skin and connected by wire to one of the body's vagus nerves, delivering constant current to the brain – mostly seem to help people achieve remission if their depression is mild, these treatments do have the flair, the fluorescence, that is perfect for the placebo. Both could turn out to be stupendously powerful interventions.

Pharmaceutical research often focuses on how to make medications so strong that they will trump the placebo in trials. For decades, in fact, psychiatry has bemoaned the placebo as the behemoth of its studies, as sugar tablets equalled or outperformed capsules of fluoxetine and sertraline and venlafaxine more than half the time in double-blind studies, and even in successful trials the advantage of drugs over the placebo, you'll remember, was minimal. But viewed another way, placebos can be embraced as treatment methods in their own right rather than disdained as something with which psychiatry must contend or compete. Why, for instance, is no one asking the obvious question about how to strengthen the performance of the placebo so that it more regularly – and more spectacularly – beats the drug? A related issue is that even when the psychiatric drug does beat the placebo, researchers are failing to take into consideration the possibility that those patients on the drug may be having, at least in part, a placebo response of their own – that old adage of 'working with the drug'.

Talking Therapy

Some say that psychotherapy is the purest form of placebo we have. People make this claim because patients who enter psychotherapy seem to improve: their morale goes up, their ability to care for themselves increases, they report feeling more hope and less loss. But these improvements are not due to any particular kind of cure, or indeed, as we shall see, any special expertise on the part of the doctor. So what, exactly, *is* happening to patients to cause their improvement? The answer: not much, or nothing medical anyway. It appears that people get better in psychotherapy because they endow the process with meaning, projecting on to it their hopes and their healing, just as they do with a sugar tablet, a shot in the biceps, or a sham surgery.

Placebos are usually defined as inert substances, but in fact there's nothing inert about a placebo. As soon as the patient puts the tablet in her hand or rolls up her sleeve for a shot or looks at the round face of the doctor, wearing wire-rimmed glasses, magic begins to happen. That inert sugar tablet becomes like the mezuzah that graces the doorway of believing Jews. That needle shimmers with luxuriant light. The face of that doctor has about it a gravitas, such that even the cleft in his chin is a sign of profound wisdom. All of this meaning – all of these symbols and the sense they make to the person in pain – comes directly from some portal within. The placebo is a key that unlocks our endogenous opiates, part of our complex immune system which shakes itself out and gets down to work, finally. The placebo is the push we need to step over some threshold, dragging our body behind us, and once we're on the other side, healing begins.

Psychotherapy, of course, is not a sugar tablet, a needle, a scalpel or a laser. It cannot be contained like a tonic in a bottle. But who says placebos must be actual objects, with weights and measures? Cannot the face of a handsome therapist with the golden seal of his diploma hanging authoritatively on the wall reassure the patient? Cannot a glance between therapist and patient be a salve in its own right? It can, and it often is.

Psychotherapy comes in many different styles; in the United States they have more than four hundred different kinds of treatment, leaving out entirely the shamans and exorcists on the other side of the seas. There are also numerous therapy options in the UK. There is psychodynamic therapy, where you explore the way your past pollutes your present. There is Gestalt psychotherapy, where you speak to your loved ones through role-playing you do with your doctor. There is cognitive behavioural psychotherapy, where you learn to restructure your negative thoughts. There is dialectical behavioural therapy, philosophical therapy, Freudian therapy, Adlerian therapy, so many different schools and such a splatter of approaches that one wonders how to choose.

Given the almost absurd plethora of treatment options, it may come as some relief to know that studies have more or less definitively shown that you can pick any school of psychotherapy that you like, whether on the NHS or available privately, because all the different kinds of treatments yield pretty much the same result. Yes, that's right. Research demonstrates that not only do *all* schools of psychotherapy seem to work but also that they all work equally well when it comes time to tally the points. No matter the school, those who receive psychotherapy of some kind are on average more psychologically well than 75 per cent of people who don't, an outcome that suggests, if you don't want to wait for a referral and if you happen to have extra cash to spare, a private psychotherapist might not be a bad investment.

In fact, research shows that even the slackers who come only a few times still make some gains from having given therapy a go. That's because the very act of disclosure appears to have a profound effect on health and well-being. In the 1980s researcher James Pennebaker, a psychologist at Southern Methodist University in Texas who would one day be tapped by the FBI to study al-Qaeda communications, organised a series of disclosure experiments with university students. Of the two groups he studied, the first was assigned to write about ordinary everyday events, to describe, for instance, the laboratory where they were writing, or the act of washing and drying their dishes. The other group was told to compose a story about a traumatic event in their lives. Participants in this second group became deeply invested in their stories, the prose powerful and compelling, and many cried as they were scribing. The stories they told had a hold on the reader because they were so genuinely felt. This was not the most striking outcome, however. Pennebaker followed up with the two groups of students after the experiment had concluded, checking to see how often they visited the university health services in the months following the writing assignments. The students who had written about a trauma, it turned out, went to the clinic less frequently than did the students who had written about mundane details.

When this experiment has been repeated with different subjects and in different countries – from New Zealand to the Netherlands and from Belgium to Mexico – the results are always the same. Disclosure itself has a protective effect on health and well-being. This is likely why psychotherapy of any and every kind helps the majority of people. It has nothing to do with the techniques of the clinician and everything to do with the stories the patient chooses to tell. That's partly because merely pondering the events of our lives doesn't provide meaning or psychological growth or health. It's when we use 'causal words' – such as 'because', 'cause' and 'effect' – that we get to the root of things and show improved health as a result. Our own words are the potent tablets. Our own words strengthen our immune system, tamp down inflammatory cells and release endorphins in our brain, thereby allowing us to live well.

Here, in fact, is how little the particular clinician performing the treatment matters. Research demonstrates pretty convincingly that you really don't need a psychotherapist at all to get the benefit of the talking cure. This is probably hard to hear if you spent, say, seven years on your doctorate, plugging along so that you would have the right to grace your last name with those three esteemed letters, the capital *P* and the lowercase *h* followed by the capital *D*. But one study showed conclusively that the correlation of the effect between the experience of the therapist and the therapeutic outcome was 0.01. Other studies have also had similar results. In other words, effectively zero. No relationship whatsoever – a result that has been confirmed many times. Your next-door neighbour Bill or your Aunt Jo would likely be just as effective a therapist as that Sigmund Freud lookalike you've been making appointments with.

How can this be? Another 1979 study done with university students – this time a group of disturbed individuals – illuminates the conundrum. In this study, researchers sent half of the students to highly skilled therapists (with twenty-three years of experience on average) and the other half to kindly university professors of English, philosophy, history or mathematics. The professors were chosen for their radiant warmth, their wit, their engaging personality styles and their seeming willingness not only to draw a person out but also to listen empathically. The researchers also had two control groups, one of which received no treatment at all, while the other received only minimal treatment. Not surprisingly, the students who received up to twenty-five hours of discussion with a therapist or a professor did significantly better than the control groups, but there were no significant differences in outcome between the group who saw the premier therapists and the group who saw the kindly professors. The researchers attributed the positive change in the students to 'the healing effects of a benign human relationship'.

It's something about warmth. About connection. Something about the process of making meaning and myth with another person who cares. This can salve the suppurating wound of panic, can warm the chill of dysthymia. We live in an age when it would be an understatement to say that medication is in style, what with one in every eleven British adults popping antidepressants for syndromes we can't quite call diseases because we have no affiliated diseased tissue to show for our psychiatric state. But while the pathophysiology of mental misery is far from being understood, no one doubts it is real.

Almost four centuries ago, René Descartes hypothesised that the soul was located in the brain's pineal gland, a tiny structure in the shape of a pine cone lodged deep in crenellated paste. By separating the soul into its own space, Descartes gave birth to the mind–body problem. But no one really thinks any more that there are two separate entities known as mind and body. We know – do we not? – that we are all body and that being all body is an astounding, miraculous, never-ending curiosity and weight. We know that all our tangles of emotions, whether arising from seeing a sunset or contemplating suicide, are neurochemical phenomena. It's all about synapses and liquids coursing through our heads. And yet these very real, very visceral human hurts can be healed by a gentle hand on top of our own, by a maths professor who likes to listen. Something about the telling of stories can make our miseries bearable, and is this not in essence what a placebo response is? 'Placebo' comes from the Latin for 'I will please' and when our maths professor puts down his chalk and sits in his rumpled suit and listens with his head cocked slightly to one side, the person on the other side is pleased. He is placeboed. And he is helped.

A placebo is not just a sugar tablet or a bunch of sham sutures. A placebo can be an event as well as a thing. Anytime a person endows something with meaning, whether it's a relationship or an occurrence, he is held in a warm embrace; he is helped by something that does not exist except as dream or hope or expectation. Much of the power of the placebo comes from the one who is hurting, which means we can start to see the sheer energy in states of sickness – what we are capable of doing when down and supposedly out, how strong we really are, even in our weakest moments, with our brain always ready to find us some faith.

Nocebo

It makes sense that if the power to heal comes from within the walls of our own bodies, then so too does the power to hurt. Consider the strange story of a 26-year-old man enrolled in a double-blind clinical drug trial aimed at testing a novel antidepressant. The subject did not know whether he was receiving the inert capsules or the real thing, although events suggest he believed he was taking the actual antidepressant because one day he overdosed on his capsules, taking twenty-nine of them, after which he became quite ill and his blood pressure fell so steeply that at the hospital he required intravenous fluids. Once the man understood, however, that he had overdosed on the dummy capsules and not the real thing, his adverse symptoms immediately reversed and he was fine.

This is not a singular sort of story. There are numerous accounts of voodoo death in indigenous cultures. For instance, in William Brown's 1845 ethnography of New Zealand aborigines, there is the tale of a Maori woman who ate fruit she was later told had been taken from a tabooed place. The woman then believed that she had somehow sullied the holiness of the chief and that she would die as a result. Sure enough, within a day of eating the fruit, the woman was dead. In another account, in North Queensland in Australia, a well-known witch doctor in the area pointed a bone at one of his fellow natives who had become a convert at the local mission. The young man, now serving as the principal helper of the missionary, subsequently became weak and then actually ill and in anguish. When a doctor was called to examine him, he found no fever, indeed no signs or symptoms of any disease, and yet the young man was in great distress and was clearly wasting away. Once the doctor learned that the witch doctor had pointed a bone at the young man, he sought out the witch doctor and threatened to cut off his food supply unless he reversed the spell. The witch doctor immediately agreed to go see the young man and, upon visiting his sickbed, assured him that no harm would come to him, that it was all 'a mistake, a mere joke', whereupon the young man instantly recovered.

Voodoo death is a form of what is called nocebo, a phenomenon that shares many similarities with the placebo; in fact it *is* the placebo, only turned totally around. Like 'placebo', the name comes from Latin, and means 'I will *cause harm*', although that would be putting it lightly, given that the nocebo phenomenon can kill you just as surely as a bullet to the brain. Nocebos show once again the power of human thought to completely affect our somatic systems. Researchers believe that nocebos precipitate a slew of toxic hormones in our brains and bodies such as the stress hormone cortisol, which can kill in excess, and adrenaline, which shares some similarities with forms of speed and can also kill in overdose. The mixture of these harmful hormones creates a cocktail that can cut the lifeline short. Nocebos and placebos, it turns out, reveal a lot about not only the role of expectation, faith, fear and belief, but also the extent to which our bodies are themselves pharmaceutical factories producing psychoactive drugs in considerable quantities.

Nocebos are about the incredible power that lies within the borders of our bodies, the power to heal and the power to kill. This power is also, however, social in nature; it belongs to each of us individually, but it is activated by interaction with others and illuminates the significance of contact and connection. Our lives cannot be lived in isolation, or at least not fully. All primates are social creatures. In fact almost all animals of every kind are social creatures, but *Homo sapiens* may be the most social of all. Consider this: when a newspaper releases a story about a suicide, the suicide rate can suddenly rise. Marilyn Monroe committed suicide in August 1962. The suicide rate spiked by 12 per cent in the month following her death. Similarly, when a fatal car accident is reported in a widely circulated newspaper, the number of car crashes increases in its immediate wake.

Perhaps the most dramatic example of this odd kind of human contagion occurred during the deadly dancing plague of 1518, in the Alsatian city of Strasbourg, which had been suffering from famines, a series of them rising out of bitterly cold winters and scorching summers, the sun pounding in a sky white with heat. Before the deadly dancing plague began, the city was in distress of biblical proportions, with sudden hailstorms pelting its citizens from clouds cracked open as if by the grasp of God himself. It's easy to imagine the citizens of Strasbourg as frayed, in extremis. And then, one July during this duress, a woman named Frau Troffea suddenly began to dance fervently in the street. She danced for four to six days straight and then was taken away to a shrine. At that point, others began to dance, putting down their satchels of baguettes and apples, the detritus of their lives, dancing by both daylight and moonlight. At the end of the week, thirty-four people had joined in and were dancing up and down the street. From there the contagion grew. Within the month, more than four hundred dancers filled the city, moving as if struck by a spell. Some died from heatstroke, others from heart attacks or exhaustion. Still the dancers twirled around the fallen bodies, unable or unwilling to stop even as more fell and more joined the ranks of the dead.

As the plague worsened, concerned nobles brought in esteemed doctors. At first they blamed astrological or supernatural causes, then ruled those out and attributed the deadly dancing plague to 'hot blood'. Perhaps because it would have been impossible to bleed hundreds of people in perpetual motion, the village authorities decided on a quite different treatment. They would instead encourage the dancing, bring it to its apex in the hope that, once it crested, it would dissipate and recede, like a wave crashing and washing out. The grain halls were emptied to make room for more dancers and a stage was constructed to hold them. Musicians were hired to urge the dancers on. The dancing grew more and more frenetic, with the afflicted townspeople going at it day and night until, as the village authorities had predicted, the plague ran its crazed course and at last the flailing citizens stopped. But not, however, before dozens had died. Died of dancing, yes, but really of the social contagion that had transmitted the dancing from person to person.

Caring Clinicians

As has already been discussed, the rates of depression are climbing despite the fact that we supposedly have superior medications such as SSRIs to treat the syndrome. More and more people are getting sick. And as we have seen, sickness is often a social act – almost always contagious. Could the high rates of depression be due to the nocebo effect? And if this is the case, do we not have the answer, a way to stem the tide? A hand held forth? A saline solution administered by a doctor who cares? It's possible that these may very well turn out to be the best cure of all.

Studies of the placebo effect by Ted Kaptchuk, a Harvard University researcher, definitively show that the more care you lavish on a person, the more symptomatic relief that person will get. One of Kaptchuk's studies of patients with irritable bowel syndrome examined the effects of sham acupuncture. The catch here is that *both* groups of patients received the sham version of the acupuncture. The difference is that in one group the sham acupuncture was administered by a clinician who was cold and curt, whereas in the other group the sham acupuncture was administered by a clinician who was warm, who took the time to sit with the patient before beginning the 'treatment'. The caring clinician was instructed to have a 'warm friendly manner', to sympathise with how difficult the condition must be for the patient and to stare thoughtfully into space for about twenty seconds. The curt clinician, by contrast, was instructed to say as little as possible to the patient during the 'procedure'. The results? The patients who received treatment from the caring clinician had a huge decrease in pain and in irritable bowel symptoms in the weeks that followed, while the patients who had been with the curt clinician got far fewer benefits. Placebos require that we be kind, in other words, and they prove that kindness and compassion have potent biological consequences.

Medicine, however, may not be at a place where it can embrace these findings. That's true especially of psychiatry, a profession that has long fought for the status of a science. It's almost inconceivable that it would willingly backtrack into something as soft and fuzzy and even, yes, schmaltzy as *caring*. What about the PETs, the fMRIs, the studies suggesting the genetic underpinnings of psychiatric syndromes like schizophrenia and bipolar depression? But this is a false dichotomy. Science need not be tossed out the window in order for psychiatry to embrace the placebo. After all, the placebo is a biological phenomenon worthy of scientific study. Furthermore, even with successful placebos, we still need medicine. The placebo is not a cure-all; it doesn't work on dementia, and it's hard to imagine it working for the hallucinations and delusions of psychosis.

But the placebo can still be a significant part of the armamentarium with which we fight potent pain of all kinds. Psychiatry must take a step back from its neurological love affair and recall its roots, which were bio-psycho-social in origin. It is a profession that, from the beginning, intended to treat the whole human, not just his neurons. So much has been lost in the craze to medicate, most especially the magic that happens whenever two people talk or touch.

Stung

Just outside the window of the study I used back before my divorce grows a large apple tree. It had never produced any fruit until two autumns ago, when the tree was flush with its first apples. In the haze of its leaves, red globes bent the branches with their weight. When the wind blew, a handful of the apples would release their grip and smash on the ground, cracking open on impact, their interiors a satiny sheen of dense white. As the autumn passed, the fallen apples sweetly rotted, fermenting in the strong sunlight of the Indian summer days and perfuming the air with the smell of spiked cider. Bees and wasps, woozy with hunger, alighted on the gore of smashed fruit and suckled on the sweetness. Their heady humming filled the air. From my study window I could see as many as twenty wasps with their stingers pushed into the plushness, their bodies vibrating as they worked the nectar and juice.

One day, wanting a solid apple before the frosts came, I climbed a rickety ladder and thrust my hand up into the tree's criss-crossed boughs. As my hand curved around a smooth globe, it was immediately attacked by unseen wasps – *sting sting sting.* I leapt off the ladder and hurled the apple into the air, pursued as I raced towards the house, hunched and batting at my hair, swatting every which way at the seemingly omnipresent wasps. Once I was inside, with the door slammed shut behind me, the wasps hung in the air on the other side of the glass as if suspended from string, then finally flew away.

My hand had been stung I don't know how many times, so swollen it was more mitten than hand. The pain was pure fire. I thrust it under a flow of cold water but it continued to grow in a grotesque way. The already taut skin stretched over my hand tighter still, with numerous welts the colour of vexed crimson. Oh how it hurt! I turned the water on full force and as cold as it would go but it was no match for the deep and persistent burn of the welts. And then, standing there by the sink, alone in my home with no one to help me, I thought I felt a funny tingle in my lips. The tingle danced its way down my tongue, which I was sure was swelling now too, and came to rest in my throat, which I touched with my other hand in an effort to assess if it too was going to swell, scared now because I'd heard stories of people who died when their throats closed up from anaphylactic shock. I'd never been stung by a wasp before, not to mention an angry phalanx of them, so perhaps I was allergic and was finding out, as they say, the hard way. Should I go to the hospital? Should I call my husband at work? I was panicked, which made it hard to think, never mind move. I just stood by the sink with my hand still under the running water, trying to trace the tingle. It felt like my lips were growing into two huge scarlet crescents on my face. I pressed on their puffiness with my fingers, thinking, *No air, no air, no air.*

In the midst of all this the doorbell rang. A delivery man had arrived with a parcel. Through the plate glass doors, on which a wasp was climbing, I could see his van rumbling in our driveway. I wobbled my way to the front door and opened it. The delivery man wore a uniform, which I found somehow comforting, the officialness of it. The parcel he was holding, an enormous cube wrapped in cardboard with a plastic sleeve, was labelled with my name. If I repeated my name to myself, I wondered, would that help pinion me in place?

The delivery man held out his electronic signature pad but then, seeing my face, took it back and asked if I was okay.

I told him I'd just been stung by a horde of wasps. 'I'm swelling up,' I said, but I couldn't complete my sentence, not for lack of air but because tears now burned at the back of my throat.

'Let me see,' the delivery man said softly, and he put down the parcel and his signature pad. I held out my hand, and he examined my pocked palm and knuckles. 'I was an EMT for years,' he explained, referring to a previous job as an emergency medical technician.

'Why'd you quit?' I asked.

'Ten dollars an hour,' he said.

'Do you ever miss it?'

'Yes,' he said, and then nothing more. With his forefinger he traced my raised red welts.

'I think it's in my throat too,' I said. 'I'm afraid my throat is swelling up.'

He palpated my neck, then leaned in close and looked at my lips, all while he stood on one side of the threshold and I on the other. 'You're fine,' he announced.

'I am?' I said, and the relief was real, a weight wafting away.

'Put some cortisone cream on the welts,' he said. 'But you're not having an allergic reaction.'

I asked him how he knew.

He looked at his watch. 'We've been standing here for four minutes,' he said. 'Anaphylactic shock happens very quickly. You're steady and stable.'

'Oh,' I said, and I thanked him.

'Not a problem,' he said.

'I really mean it,' I said. 'Thank you so much. I thought I might be dying.'

'Not today,' he said, and laughed. He held out his electronic pad again. 'Sign here,' he said, and I picked up the probe and swept my signature across the electrified surface, watching the magic of my name appearing solid and sure.

Then the delivery man left. The parcel he'd brought was huge. It was a tuba, meant for my husband. But I was so relieved not to be dying, so comforted and elated to have been healed by the arrival of the delivery man, that I slit open the parcel right there on the kitchen floor and lifted the massive brass instrument into the light. The tuba was complexly shaped, flaring into something like a trumpet flower at the place where the music escaped its pipes and curves to rise into the air and meld with the music of other players in a symphony somewhere. I could almost hear it.

I slung the tuba over my shoulder, filled my lungs with all the air they could hold and blew into the cold round mouthpiece, blew and blew until the instrument finally answered with a solid sound as low as a foghorn, no tremble, a sound that only someone healthy and whole would be able to make. I was that healthy person, standing in a kitchen one autumn day as evening approached. The air smelled like apples and the wasps were on the other side of the window and the sun was descending, casting its late afternoon rays over the grass and turning it a deeper shade of green, backlighting the pine trees and fringing the clouds with fire. Mysteriously, I wasn't hurting any more. The stings were gone, each one like a bubble burst, and my hand and the veins at the rim of my wrist had returned to their normal colour, the welts erased by the simple touch of a stranger.

6

Psilocybin (Magic Mushrooms)

God's Flesh

A Strange Swelling

In February 2008, 53-year-old Carol Vincent found a strange swelling on her body. Having just recovered from a bout of illness, she dismissed it as the last flutterings of the flu. Her fiancé persuaded her to consult her doctor, which she did, almost breezily, assuming he would tell her that the enlarged knuckle-like node was of no real concern. Instead, as her doctor pressed and palpated, a shadow passed over his face and fear took hold in Vincent. The next thing she knew she was being X-rayed and biopsied. Later, dressed and seated in her doctor's well-appointed surgery, Vincent was informed that she had lymphoma, a kind of cancer for which there is no cure and no consistently effective treatment either. As days and weeks went by, the strange swelling migrated and multiplied, appearing in her armpit and the cradle of her collarbone.

Vincent, a writer and an entrepreneur who owned an advertising agency in Victoria, British Columbia, had a full life, a life she loved, a life that included a home, a fiancé, a grown son and meaningful work. A born fighter, she wasn't ready to give up on any of it. As she waited to find out whether the cancer would progress to the point where it would require radiation and chemotherapy, she decided to do everything in her power to conquer her disease. She gave up sugar, caffeine and flour; she cleansed and juiced, drinking puréed wheatgrass so thick it coated the sides of the cup and left a mark above her mouth. She logged on to the Internet for hours each day, searching for studies, experiments and medications. Information gleaned from Google informed Vincent that she had seven years to live, ten at the absolute outer limit. 'Emotionally it was very stressful,' she said. 'An anvil over my head. Every single decision was tricky. Should I drink super-clean wheatgrass juice or just eat chocolate chip cookies because life is short? Do I pay off my mortgage or rack up my credit cards?' Before long, when the strange swellings abated, Vincent began to believe that her diet might be healing her. High on hope, she was shattered when the hard nodes returned, in new places on her body. A certain paranoia, or heightened awareness, overtook her. Was an excrescence emerging on her ankle? What was that bump behind her ear? Her body became a bomb, detonating slowly, over days, then weeks, then months, so that even though the end was some unknown number of years away, Vincent began to lose hope.

An Epidural for Death?

Eventually, however, when she was nearing the point of surrendering hope entirely, it would return in the form of Roland Griffiths, a psychopharmacologist and professor of behavioural biology at Johns Hopkins University in Maryland. Griffiths was in the midst of an experiment that involved giving psilocybin, the active ingredient in so-called magic mushrooms, to fifty-one end-stage cancer patients in an effort to alleviate their fear of death. Psilocybin, along with LSD, a similar hallucinogenic, is in a class of drugs known as psychedelics. As opposed to psychotropic drugs such as chlorpromazine, lithium, the tricyclics, the MAOIs and the SSRIs, whose primary function is to alter the mood or function of the brain, the main action of psychedelics is to change actual perception or cognition, bringing the brain somewhere beyond ordinary consciousness.

Trained as a strict scientist and known for his meticulous research methodologies, Griffiths also continues to maintain a rigorous practice of meditation that he began about two decades ago. He is passionate about meditation, maintaining that it 'opened up a spiritual window for me and made me very curious about the nature of mystical experience and spiritual transformation', prompting 'an existential question for me about the meaningfulness of my own research programme in drug-abuse pharmacology.' His meditation eventually caused a swerve in his thinking, and this stern scientist began to meander and to muse. He started to wonder about wonder itself. And from that wondering grew his interest in psilocybin and its effects on the human psyche. Shifting his laboratory focus away from animals and drugs of abuse, Griffiths homed in on psychedelics. In 2006 he published his landmark study of the drug, straightforwardly titled 'Psilocybin Can Occasion Mystical-Type Experiences Having Substantial and Sustained Personal Meaning and Spiritual Significance'.

The idea and the experiment were not new, of course. The novelist Aldous Huxley first tried psychedelics in the early 1950s and famously continued ingesting them to the very end. In 1963, expiring of laryngeal cancer and unable to speak, he made a written request of his wife to inject him with LSD on his deathbed so that he could leave this world in a psychedelic swirl of stars. What Huxley wanted, and what the work of Griffiths could realise, is for death to be less of a physiological process and more of a spiritual one.

Around the time of Huxley's death, unrelated to the author's personal experimentation, an anaesthesiologist at the Chicago Medical School named Eric Kast, finding normal analgesics insufficient for managing the most intense pain of his dying patients, decided to explore whether LSD might be an effective alternative. In a study published in 1964, he compared the analgesic properties of pethidine and hydromorphone to those of LSD. The subjects of the study were fifty people suffering from various severe cancers, gangrene of the feet and legs, and a single case of shingles. Kast's statistical analysis showed that LSD proved superior to the more common analgesics. On LSD, not only did the patients develop 'a peculiar disregard' for their suffering and for the seriousness of their situations, but also they discussed their death more freely and with considerably less fear.

Building on the success of these findings, Kast went on to study 128 cancer patients to whom he gave 100 micrograms of LSD, this time looking not only at the drug's potential to alleviate pain but also at its ability to alter attitudes towards illness and death. In this experiment, after the initial administration of the LSD, patients experienced dramatic pain relief in two to three hours, and their fear of death was reduced for ten days following the psychedelic session. Emboldened by these results, Kast did yet another LSD study, this time with eighty people whose malignant and terminal diseases gave them a life expectancy of just weeks or months. All eighty of Kast's subjects knew about their diagnoses and were fully aware of the limits on their lives. In this group, 100 micrograms of LSD not only offered powerful relief from pain but also brought about 'happy oceanic feelings', along with enhanced communications between patients and an increase in morale and self-regard that made the physiological and spiritual aspects of dying easier to bear.

The Original Magic Mushrooms

Kast and Huxley were among the earliest psychedelic pioneers, but they were not the ones to bring into popular use the drug that would eventually help Carol Vincent and so many others.

That honour belongs to R. Gordon Wasson, a public relations executive for J. P. Morgan & Co. and an amateur ethnomycologist – someone who studies the historical uses and sociological impact of mushrooms. As a businessman who wore a pressed suit to work every day, he was hardly a likely candidate for the job of mushroom messenger. In fact, up until his honeymoon Wasson had hated mushrooms, calling them toadstools or 'excrescences'. His Russian-born wife, however, convinced him of their majesty and beauty.

Wasson, converted by his wife into a 'mycophile', had heard stories of magic mushroom ceremonies in Mexico that supposedly occurred only under the cover of darkness and were led by a sacred shaman. Research revealed to Wasson and his wife that when Cortés overtook Mexico, he discovered that the Aztecs were using different kinds of mushrooms in their religious rites, calling them *teonanacatl*, meaning 'God's flesh'. That may be because some of the Indians believed the mushroom grew only where droplets of Christ's blood or saliva had graced the ground. The Mexican mushrooms fascinated Wasson and his wife. Were they real? What made them so special? Were they purely a plant of the past or did they still exist? With these questions uppermost in his mind, on 29 June 1955, Wasson and his friend Allan Richardson travelled to a remote Mexican village in Oaxaca, in the Mixteca region, in search of *teonanacatl*. It was a trip about which Wasson would write a *Life* magazine story two years later.

The village was small and dusty and sunstruck, its streets eerily empty. At an altitude of about 1,675 metres (5,500 feet), it was so remote, and the past so well preserved, that even the unique language – Mixtec – was intact. In the town hall Wasson found a young Indian man, a *síndico*, the official in charge, sitting in a large empty room. Wasson leaned down and asked the *síndico* if he could help him 'learn the secrets of the divine mushroom'. Nothing could be easier, the *síndico* replied, instructing Wasson and Richardson to come to his house at siesta time. The two men did so and encountered there, in a ravine, hundreds of moist mushrooms. Wasson and Richardson knelt in the grove and gathered their goods, hearing the wet snap of the stalks as they picked, heaping their finds into a box, and then trudging uphill, high above the *síndico's* house, to meet María Sabina and her daughter, the two *curanderas*, or healers, about whom the *síndico* had told them. 'We showed our mushrooms', wrote Wasson, and 'they cried out in rapture over the firmness, the fresh beauty and abundance of our young specimens. Through an interpreter we asked if they would serve us that night. They said yes.'

Thus Wasson and Richardson found themselves, that evening, as the first known white men ever to partake in an ancient Indian mushroom ceremony. The ceremony took place in the lower chamber of the *síndico's* house after eight o'clock. At about ten thirty, the *curanderas* began to prepare the fungi, washing each individual mushroom and praying over the entire lot. The room was filled with Indians sitting on mats, waiting to be served. Children were also present, although they did not partake, and as the evening progressed, they slipped quietly into sleep. Before midnight the mother and daughter shamans passed out the mushrooms, giving each adult a portion and keeping most for themselves. María Sabina snapped a flower from the bouquet on a table to snuff out the candles' flames and all light was lost. Richardson had promised his wife he would not ingest any mushrooms, the price of her agreeing to his undertaking the expedition in the first place, but he found himself swept into the ceremony, as was Wasson, for whom this was the culminating moment in a long pursuit. Both men bit into the fresh fungi and chewed them slowly.

After ingesting the mushrooms, they lay on their mats in dense darkness, in a world, in a culture radically removed from anything they knew. After half an hour had passed, spectacular visions began appearing to Wasson – a steady stream of gorgeous geometrics, then palaces of pearl, arcades, gardens, chariots pulled by mythological beasts. Each image was perfectly etched, clearer than clear, so that Wasson felt that for the first time he was really seeing reality. Then he suddenly broke away from the body on the mat and floated free. The walls of the home dissolved, and his spirit whirled in space, looking down on caravans of camels passing through ancient archways, a balmy blue lake and tier upon tier of mountains rising all the way to the horizon.

Throughout the ceremony the shamans sang, chanted and occasionally danced. Sabina, hands clasped together in prayer, cried out: 'Am I not good? I am a creator woman, a star woman, a moon woman, a cross woman, a woman of heaven. I am a cloud person, a dew-on-the-grass person.' Sometimes her voice changed, and this was because God was speaking through her, giving her the answer to whatever question had prompted the mushroom ritual in the first place.

For the Mixtecos this night was an exception, brought on by their American guests. They did not typically use *teonanacatl* as a drug of recreation. The mushrooms were utterly sacred to them and were meant as a means of consultation when problems arose. The problem might be concrete, such as determining who had stolen one's donkey or how one's son was faring if he had left the village. The mushrooms, singing through the shaman, could let the distressed parent know whether his son was alive or dead, prospering or in prison. Sometimes the question had to do with health – would the suffering villager recover or perish? – and if the shamans received word that the person would perish, then this was what happened, often within days.

Wasson and Richardson were utterly awed by their experience. On successive trips they brought along the world-renowned mushroom expert Roger Heim in an effort to identify all the types of hallucinogenic mushrooms and to procure enough of a supply that it could be used for laboratory study. Eventually mushrooms were sent to Albert Hofmann, the first man to synthesise LSD, at the laboratory of the pharmaceutical firm Sandoz, in Basel, Switzerland. Hofmann ate a few and recorded his experience – 'everything took on a Mexican character' – and later discovered their active ingredient, psilocybin.

Back in Boston, Timothy Leary, a psychologist and professor at Harvard University who would become famous for the admonition to 'turn on, tune in and drop out', learned about the magic mush-rooms and then ate them in Cuernavaca, leading him to conceive of and implement the Harvard Psilocybin Project, whose goal was to study the effects of hallucinogens on a wide range of subjects: prisoners, parishioners, divinity students, the dying.

Psychedelic Psychotherapy

Despite Wasson's 1957 *Life* magazine story, however, the earliest experiments with psychedelics continued to be with LSD rather than psilocybin. The Czech psychiatrist Stanislav Grof, for instance, a founder of transpersonal psychology, did what he termed 'psyche-delic psychotherapy' with patients in Prague in the early 1960s. 'When psychotherapy was combined with administration of psych-edelics,' he wrote, 'all our patients, irrespective of their diagnostic categories, sooner or later transcended the realm of postnatal biog-raphy and of the individual unconscious.' Grof describes patients on LSD undergoing profound spiritual and symbolic deaths and rebirths as their psyches stretched well beyond the concepts described by Freud. Psychedelics, it appeared, could radically alter an individual long after the drug was taken, allowing those who were cramped and caged by severe psychiatric diagnoses to feel, for weeks or even months after their sessions, a freedom and a kind of 'cosmic con-sciousness' that had before been completely unavailable to them. Over and over again Grof witnessed in these patients what he termed symbolic death and rebirth, so that 'fear of their own physiological demise diminished, they became open to the possibility of con-sciousness exiting after clinical death, and they tended to view the process of dying as an adventure in consciousness rather than the ultimate biological disaster and personal defeat.'

Grof emigrated to the United States in 1967 and became part of the treatment team at Baltimore's Spring Grove State Hospital, where there was among the clinicians a great interest in the promise of LSD for dying patients. Some testing had begun as early as 1963, and it accelerated two years later when a member of the team, a woman in her early forties named Gloria, developed metastatic breast cancer. Her severe pain and emotional distress gripped the rest of the team. All of them wanted to help their colleague in some way and decided to try an LSD session, for which Gloria was prepped over a period of one week with daily psychotherapy focusing on her interpersonal relationships and life history. Two weeks after this psychedelic session, Gloria wrote a lengthy description of her experience under the influence, concluding:

> As I began to emerge I was taken to a fresh windswept world. Members of the department welcomed me, and I felt joy not only for myself, but for having been able to use the experience these people who cared for me wanted me to have. I felt very close to a large group of people. Later, as members of my family came, there was a closeness that seemed new. That night, at home, my parents came too. All noticed a change in me. I was radiant, and I seemed at peace, they said. I felt that way too. What has changed me? I am living now and being. I can take it as it comes. Some of my physical symptoms are gone – the excessive fatigue, some of the pains. I still get irritated occasionally and yell. I am still me, but more at peace. My family senses this and we are closer. All who know me will say that this has been a good experience.

Five weeks later, Gloria died peacefully, leaving behind a Spring Grove staff now dedicated to exploring the role of LSD in terminal cancer patients. The surgeons and oncologists at Baltimore's Sinai Hospital, unusually open-minded doctors, agreed to refer their patients to Grof and the other staff members for guided LSD sessions.

In 1967, the same year Grof arrived, Spring Grove hired the equally youthful Walter Pahnke (both were born in 1931), a dynamic researcher and psychiatrist who had been a student of Timothy Leary's, to helm its LSD project. Two years later the team moved into the Maryland Psychiatric Research Center, where there was a sensory deprivation tank, two treatment suites that could be monitored with cameras, sleep study laboratories and a sensory overload department. In the late 1960s and early 1970s, more than a hundred terminal cancer patients underwent LSD therapy at the centre. The typical patient was one with a very poor prognosis, and on whom all other available treatments had been tried and had failed.

Pahnke had a background in philosophy and divinity as well as a medical degree. He was also known as something of a dare-devil; he was an avid motorcyclist, and pursued a host of hobbies that contributed to his eclectic energy and joie de vivre. In the summer of 1971, he added scuba diving to his list of avocations. Unfortunately, his life was cut short in tragic fashion when he died in a scuba diving accident off the coast of Maine, where he and his wife and children were on holiday. He had slipped into the sea with second-hand equipment bought from a friend, and with no real knowledge of how to dive. His body disappeared into the Atlantic, and despite an extensive search by the coast guard and the work of several psychics, he was never found. Pahnke's early and mysterious death put a brief dent in psychedelic research, leaving the Spring Grove team without a leader until Grof, who had worked closely with Pahnke before his death, was appointed to take over the position.

Grof's self-professed objective was 'to formulate a theoretical framework that would account for some of the dramatic changes occurring as a result of LSD therapy.' He looked for patients who exhibited anxiety, depression, emotional tension and social with-drawal, and for whom the available analgesics were not working. Patients also needed to have a life expectancy of at least three months, since Grof and his team were interested not only in the immediate results of psychedelic therapy but also in its longer-term impact.

Grof designed the therapy to consist of three stages: (1) the initial preparatory period, (2) the psychedelic session itself and (3) a post-session period during which the patient processed the material that had emerged under the influence. The preparation stage usually lasted two to three weeks and consisted of Grof and the treatment team exploring with the patient his or her history and present situation. Unresolved conflicts were given special attention. The goal was not only to flush to the surface the issues that might arise during a psychedelic session but also to build trust between the patient and the staff. Grof and the team believed that trust was an essential aspect of a positive psychedelic experience, especially because dramatic and frightening material might emerge and the patient needed to know that he or she was in good hands. 'We did all we could', Grof wrote, 'to create an opportunity for the patient and their relatives to discuss their feelings about each other, about the disease and about the seriousness of the situation, including the imminence of death.' During his work with patients in Prague and again in Baltimore, Grof had witnessed psychedelic sessions during which the patient experienced death and rebirth, or memories of birth and prenatal experiences that Grof believed were not simply artefacts of the drug but rather real and valid memories that the psychedelic made accessible. As part of the final preparatory stage, then, Grof and his colleagues explained to patients that their psychedelic journey might take them to realms far beyond those described by traditional psychiatry.

The treatment room and its set-up were of vital importance. Patients wore headphones for most of their session, using music as a means of both transportation and transformation. Black eye masks blocked out the physical world and encouraged patients to travel inwards, to the depths where, Grof believed, resided ancient archetypes and symbols with the potential to bring about a new relationship with one's remaining life and imminent death. The room was filled with the fragrance of flowers and burning incense, decorated with flowing drapes and other props designed to facilitate comfort and ease.

Grof gave his patients between 200 and 600 micrograms of LSD, a considerable dose that takes only about twenty to forty minutes to make its effects felt. During the initial phase patients sat quietly with the staff, looking at the family photographs they had been encouraged to bring with them. Once the drug 'hit', the patient lay back wearing the eye mask and listening to the headphones piping in a selection of music compiled by a music therapist. Grof took the music choices very seriously, because he believed that music helps bring primitive emotions to the surface of the mind while simultaneously urging patients to 'let go of their psychological defences and provid[ing] a dynamic carrier wave, which takes the patients through difficult experiential impasses.' The music was usually a combination of classical pieces and ethnic rhythms and chants from spiritual practices around the world. If the music became too intense for the patients, they could take off their headphones and remove their eye masks. When this happened, the treatment team would reassure the patients and encourage them to 'return into their inner world as soon as possible.'

Among the hundreds of terminal cancer patients whom Grof treated during his time as the leader of Spring Grove was Matthew, a brilliant doctor and an atheist. As his cancer closed in around him, he became weak, anxious and despairing. He experienced considerable nausea, and as the disease progressed, the weight dropped off him, leaving behind a frail man. Given that his mental and physical health had always been perfect, Matthew was devastated by his new condition. When the disease struck, he had been right in the middle of a stunningly successful life, with a beautiful wife, three children and an exciting, fast-paced career. Having never pursued religion or anything even remotely spiritual, he felt utterly unprepared for the rigours of disease and death.

Matthew received 200 micrograms of LSD intramuscularly. For the first hour it appeared that nothing was happening. Then, suddenly, he became ecstatic about the music pouring in through his headphones. 'The music sounded divine to him', Grof wrote, 'and he was losing his boundaries and merging with its flow.' He felt an intense need for physical proximity and reached out to one of his guides, Joan Halifax, who for a time had been Grof's wife and was one of his research collaborators. She held Matthew for four full hours while he tossed and turned on his mat, a wasted man, muttering mystical phrases such as 'one world and one universe', 'all is one', 'nothing and everything' and 'it is either the real thing or it is not', before concluding with the declaration 'So I am immortal . . . it is true!'

Matthew's wife, who periodically came to the door of the room during the session to check on him, was shocked when she heard these words coming from his mouth and also when her husband, normally distant and stiff, wanted to embrace her, to feel himself 'melting into her'. Over the remaining days of his life, his physical condition deteriorated rapidly, but husband and wife, previously emotionally estranged, developed a deep connection that was, both independently said, the most powerful part of their marriage. Knowing that death was near, Matthew, who had been unable to deal with the thought of his demise, told the treatment team that he was okay, and that when it was time to go he was ready. He died shortly thereafter, in peace and without the pain that had racked him throughout his fight with cancer. 'The changes that we observed in cancer patients following psychedelic therapy were extremely varied, complex and multidimensional,' Grof maintained. There was an 'attenuation or even elimination of fear of death and radical changes in basic life philosophy and strategy, in spiritual orientation, and in hierarchy of values'.

At the other end of the spectrum of belief was 45-year-old Jesse, another cancer patient whom Grof treated. Jesse, a committed Catholic, was one of sixteen children, and had been orphaned as a young boy when his parents died in a car wreck. Thirteen years earlier he'd had a squamous cell carcinoma in his upper lip, and now he was back with a similar cancer that was spreading with ferocious speed throughout his entire body. Ulcers and leaking tumours had sprouted all over his skin. Wrapped in bandages that were soaked in the fluid of his cancer and emanated a repulsive odour, Jesse saw himself as an outcast and a terrible burden on his girlfriend, Betty, and her sister, the women who dutifully cared for him in their small flat.

During preparation for his psychedelic session, Jesse expressed a strong and overwhelming fear of death, which he saw in two ways: first, as the ultimate end of his physical and mental self, a step into utter darkness, and secondly, as a possible continuation of his consciousness that would be judged by the Catholic God he believed in. Jesse assumed that the judgement against him would be severe because of the various sins he felt he'd committed, and he therefore sensed that he would be consigned to the fires of hell. Given his two views of death, he was clinging to what little life he had left with all his strength.

Jesse's case history demonstrates how psychedelics reflect confirmed religious belief even as they provide the opportunity to go beyond the dogma often associated with such belief. During Jesse's psychedelic session he saw countless images and scenes pass before his eyes: scrapyards where emaciated corpses writhed in agony, the spiking fires of hell, rotting offal and then, suddenly, a huge orange ball of fire – appearing as if from nowhere – into which all the mess and stink were poured to be cleansed in the high heat of the flames. Jesse envisioned himself being consumed in the fire and yet his soul survived and appeared before God on the final Judgement Day. At the judgement, scenes from Jesse's childhood streamed before him, and at last he experienced God not as a physical being but as a palpable presence of pure divinity and love. God was judging him favourably now, deciding that his good deeds far outweighed his bad. Then Jesse received a powerful message that came to him without words: when he died, his soul would survive; he would come back to Earth in a form not yet revealed. Thus this confirmed Catholic came to believe in the Eastern concept of reincarnation. 'The perspective of another incarnation', Grof and Halifax wrote, 'freed him from clinging to his body.' Five days after the session he died at peace.

Researchers acknowledge that it's not clear how psilocybin reduces a person's anxiety about mortality, not simply during the trip but for weeks and months following. 'It's a bit of a mystery,' admits Charles Grob, the lead investigator in the ongoing end-of-life psilocybin study at the Harbor-UCLA Medical Center in California. 'I don't really have altogether a definitive answer as to why the drug eases the fear of death, but we do know that from time immemorial individuals who have transformative spiritual experiences come to a very different view of themselves and the world around them and thus are able to handle their own deaths differently.' John Halpern, former director of the Laboratory for Integrative Psychiatry at McLean Hospital in Massachusetts, holds a similar view: 'On psychedelics you have an experience in which you feel there is something you are a part of, something else is out there that's bigger than you, that there is a dazzling unity you belong to, that love is possible, and all these realisations are imbued with deep meaning. I'm telling you that you're not going to forget that six months from now. The experience gives you, just when you're on the edge of death, hope for something more.'

Psychedelics and Spirituality

The Good Friday experiment is perhaps the most famous study of the role of psilocybin in spirituality. Conducted in 1962 by Walter Pahnke, who would go on to run the LSD project at Spring Grove, the experiment gathered twenty Protestant Harvard Divinity School students outside the Marsh Chapel at Boston University to receive a capsule of white powder right before a Good Friday service. Ten of the capsules contained psilocybin and ten contained nicotinic acid, an active placebo that causes flushing in the face. Of the ten students who received the psilocybin, eight said they had a mystical experience, wandering around Marsh Chapel while saying things like 'God is everywhere' or 'Oh the glory.' Their behaviour convinced Pahnke that a psilocybin high shared many aspects with a full-fledged mystical experience of the sort described by the philosopher William James.

Persuasive as it is, however, recent scholars such as Rick Doblin, the founder and executive director of the Multidisciplinary Association for Psychedelic Studies (MAPS), located in Santa Cruz, California, have found methodological flaws in Pahnke's study. Doblin, from 1986 to 1989, did a follow-up of the Good Friday experiment, identifying all but one of the divinity students who had taken part in the original, and interviewing the sixteen who agreed to participate, including seven of the ten who had taken psilocybin. All seven of these subjects told Doblin that 'the experience had shaped their lives and work in profound and enduring ways.' Doblin found, however, that the study had failed to mention that some of the students had struggled with fear during the experiment. One of them even charged from the chapel and raced down the street, filled with the conviction that he was meant to announce the next Messiah, after which he ultimately needed to be restrained and administered a tranquillising shot of chlorpromazine to bring him back inside the chapel.

Critics of psilocybin and other psychedelics claim that a mystical experience inspired by these agents is a dishonest shortcut to nirvana. They call the phenomenon 'chemical mysticism' – not of equal value to an enlightened state achieved, say, through days of fasting or hours of meditation and prayer. The idea that one can pop a tablet and touch God was and is distasteful to people who believe that true mysticism is achieved only by a lifetime of pious behaviour and service to the divine. Those who adopt this viewpoint are also wary of scientists deciding what is or isn't a mystical experience, a determination that they claim should be made by theologians, ministers, rabbis or priests.

But the counterargument points out that psychedelic plants have been used for centuries to facilitate communication with worlds beyond our own and are themselves part of a sacred circle which is not a shortcut but rather an aperture we go through with careful, meaningful preparation and a sense of awe. From this perspective, taking the psychedelic is itself a sacrament that allows users to touch the numinous, the transcendent, the very face and body of the divine. In fact, some scholars have even argued that psychedelic plants may be at the root of all religions, may be the very reason why they exist in the first place. Imagine primitive *Homo sapiens* ingesting psychedelic plants, something they in all likelihood did, and seeing visions for which they had no explanation except that there must be a world beyond our world, a sacred spot that demanded our respect. Perhaps from these experiences they deemed necessary a life of prayer and piousness alongside a palpable belief in divinity.

Timothy Leary was among the scholars who believed that psilocybin and other psychedelics gave rise to valid mystical experiences that could radically revise mind and body, belief and behaviour. While carrying out research at Harvard University from 1961 to 1963, he tested psilocybin on thirty-two prisoners in the nearby Concord State Penitentiary who had volunteered for the experiment. Leary's goal was to see whether the drug would reduce rates of recidivism once inmates were released. In this experiment the drug was given to the inmates in group therapy sessions over a period of months, so that each prisoner had several psychedelic experiences. Leary and his colleagues, in an attempt to disassemble the rigid hierarchy that defines prison life, took the psilocybin along with the prisoners and conducted the sessions while under the influence. The result was that prisoners who received psychedelic group psychotherapy did indeed have markedly lower rates of recidivism than their non-drugged counterparts.

There was, for instance, the case of S., a 48-year-old man whom Leary described as a hardened criminal, having spent a total of fourteen years behind bars, a hulking man who had devoted years to larceny, fraud, drunkenness and an assortment of other petty misdemeanours and felonies. Under the influence of psilocybin, however, S. experienced waves of sadness washing over him, and he seemed to soften. For the first time he turned almost tender, seeing his life as it was – wasted, with so much time lost to being locked up. 'Out of the shell of a hardened criminal', wrote Leary, 'emerged a sensitive lonely child-like human being.' When S. was released from prison some weeks later, he found himself disoriented but nevertheless managed to get a job on a construction crew and was later promoted to foreman. Eventually, S. opened an auto body shop. At the time of Leary's writing, it had been two years, and S. had not gone back to prison.

It must be noted that Doblin found flaws in Leary's study similar to the ones he pursued in Pahnke's Good Friday experiment. Still, Leary's psilocybin study is undoubtedly the inspiration for a current study taking place in a Brazilian rainforest where prisoners – men who have committed murder, rape, child molestation – are brought to participate in a ceremony that involves drinking ayahuasca tea. Ayahuasca is a hallucinogen, a mind-bending, mind-blowing chemical that researchers are hoping will transform hardened criminals into reflective, responsible citizens. 'I'm finally realising I was on the wrong path in this life,' one prisoner told a reporter in 2015. 'Each experience helps me communicate with my victim to beg for forgiveness.'

Of all the intellectuals who investigated the psychedelics, Huston Smith, the renowned scholar of religious studies who chaired the Massachusetts Institute of Technology's philosophy department during the turbulent 1960s, is the one who perhaps best found the middle ground between critics of chemical mysticism and supporters of psychedelic journeys. Smith himself had many psychedelic-inspired mystical experiences and did not doubt their authenticity, but he stressed that set and setting were critical to the outcome. There is a huge difference, he pointed out, between someone who has prepped deeply for a session, who goes into it with intention and the true desire to quest, who has questions to be posed to the drug, and the person who imbibes LSD tossed into the punchbowl at a party. In many ways it was Smith who laid the groundwork for Doblin and Griffiths and the other researchers who would return to the psychedelics a generation later.

The Drug War, Finally Fading

Though researchers are bringing psychedelics back into their various fields of study these days, it is difficult for us to imagine, given the paucity of psychedelics in a fight-against-drugs world, how freely available they were in the 1950s, '60s and '70s, so freely available, in fact, that they eventually leached out of the laboratories and into the streets of a culture undergoing seismic shifts. The drugs became part of protests and alternative lifestyles, eventually causing the Nixon administration, in October 1970, to sign the Controlled Substances Act, making all psychedelics illegal. Likewise, the Misuse of Drugs Act was passed in the UK in 1971. In both countries drugs such as LSD and magic mushrooms were put into the highest-risk drugs categories with the most severe penalties attached, effectively erasing these substances not only from the culture but also from science. Indeed Richard Nixon once famously called Timothy Leary 'the most dangerous man in America'. There were exceptions, and for a short time researchers like Grof were still able to obtain funding for psychedelic studies, but it was with such increasing difficulty that by the mid-1970s all research had come to a halt, and the fecund body of knowledge gleaned from the psychedelic work done by Grof, Pahnke, Leary, Kast and others got buried and eventually all but lost to memory.

It is only in recent years, with the fight against drugs finally fading, that a new group of scientists are lifting the lid and peering at past work to draw inspiration and design from those pioneers. Almost five decades after governments put the kibosh on psychedelic studies, there is something of a rebirth going on both in the United States and abroad. Research is taking place at several universities, among them Johns Hopkins University in Maryland, New York University, University of California, Los Angeles (UCLA), Imperial College London and University of Zurich, but permission remains hard to obtain because psychedelics are stained by the excesses of the 1960s, a fact that makes both the scientists and their respective governments extremely cautious. Charles Grob of UCLA, along with Roland Griffiths of Johns Hopkins, John Halpern of McLean Hospital in Massachusetts, and Stephen Ross of New York University, make up a group of researchers unearthing the studies of yesteryear, dusting them off and putting them back into practice, returning to buried roots where the results are intact and ready to be built on. 'It feels a little bit like Rip Van Winkle,' Grob has said, referring to a folklore of a man who falls asleep for twenty years, and indeed it seems so, as reams of studies rife with tantalising suggestions that have been locked away are finally beginning to be reopened. 'It is enormously exciting to find what is, in essence, a treasure trove of information from the past,' Grob continued. 'At the same time we want to be very careful. We don't want to be associated with flower power. We want to be seen as serious scientists.'

The goal of these recent end-of-life psilocybin experiments is to determine whether it is possible to reduce or even remove the fear of dying in end-stage cancer patients and perhaps, in future years, in healthy subjects as well. Grob, who calls psilocybin 'existential medicine', envisions treatment centres where the dying could go to get psilocybin administered safely and therapeutically. Rick Doblin, however, finds that use of the drug too limiting. 'Why confine this to just the dying?' he asks. 'This powerful intervention could be used with young adults who could then reap the benefits of it much earlier.' He's referring to the fact that subjects who have undergone psilocybin treatment report an increased appreciation for the time they have left, a deeper awareness of their roles in the cycle of life and an increased motivation to invest their days with meaning. 'Imagine allowing young adults, who have their whole lives in front of them, access to this kind of therapy,' Doblin said. 'Imagine the kind of lives they could then create.'

A Complete Mystical Experience

As for Griffiths, he was undoubtedly influenced by Pahnke's Good Friday experiment; in some ways his first psilocybin experiment is a continuation of Pahnke's work. In a 2006 study, Griffiths recruited thirty-six healthy adult volunteers, none of whom had ever taken a psychedelic before. All of the volunteers did two sessions; they got psilocybin in one session and a placebo in the other. In an attempt to correct for the failure of Pahnke's double-blind design, Griffiths opted for an active placebo that contained methylphenidate, better known by the brand name Ritalin, a strong stimulant usually used to treat attention deficit disorder. Sixty-one per cent of Griffiths's subjects had a 'complete mystical experience' during the psilocybin session, compared with only 11 per cent during the placebo session. Furthermore, on a questionnaire completed two months after the experiment, many of these volunteers ranked the psilocybin experience as among the most meaningful in their lives, with fully two-thirds of them including it in the top five most spiritually significant events in their life, and about 15 per cent rating the encounter at an absolute peak, the most meaningful thing they had ever experienced.

At a fourteen-month follow-up these rankings shifted only slightly, and Griffiths also found sustained positive changes in personality. This is especially notable, as many psychologists believe that the basics of personality are firmly set by early adulthood and unamenable to change. Some people are risk-averse, others have an openness to new experiences, and the general belief has been that these tendencies, being hard to overcome, lead people to live their lives within the boundaries of their basic traits. These experiments with psilocybin throw this assumption into question, however. Fourteen months after ingesting the drug, those who had had profound mystical encounters had also undergone significant increases in their openness, which is one of the five personality domains that researchers believe are unchangeable but, according to Griffiths's work, it actually isn't.

Apparently, then, psychedelics can loosen the bonds that hold us in place. Psychedelics can stretch and even snap our tightest tethers. Becoming more open has profound implications for a person. It permits him to take more meaningful risks. It widens the circle of possible relationships, allows for creativity, increases empathy and makes 'the other' less of a foreigner and more of a friend. Thus it is fair to say that Griffiths's healthy psilocybin subjects were changed in lasting, profound and positive ways. Griffiths, who has unabashedly said he can't think of anything more important to be studying, considers the implications far-reaching:

> The core feature of the mystical experience is this strong sense of the interconnectedness of all things, where there's a rising sense not only of self-confidence and clarity, but of communal responsibility, of altruism and social justice, a felt sense of the golden rule: Do unto others as you would have them do unto you. And those kinds of sensibilities are at the core of all the world's religious, ethical and spiritual traditions. Understanding the nature of these effects, and their consequences, may be the key to the survival of our species.

So if psilocybin can reliably induce these life-altering experiences, why have the hundreds of thousands of people who have taken magic mushrooms recreationally not had this profound experience?

Grob explains that in addition to the carefully controlled setting of these studies and the opportunity to process the experience with the researchers, the subjects are primed for transcendence before they even take the drug. 'Unlike the recreational user, we process the experience ahead of time,' Grob said. 'We make it very clear up front that the hoped-for outcome is therapeutic, that they'll have less anxiety, less depression and a greater acceptance of death.' Subjects, in other words, intend to have a transformative experience.

For all the convincing eloquence of these explanations, however, something feels fuzzy about a phenomenon in which a cancer-ridden patient takes a tablet and overcomes her fear of death not just for the moment but for all the weeks and months that follow. A recent British study can help us understand what might be happening here. In this study, David J. Nutt, director of the neuropsychopharmacology unit at Imperial College London, and others on his team used an MRI to scan the brains of healthy volunteers dosed on psilocybin in order to 'capture the transition from normal waking consciousness to the psychedelic state'. The researchers found that the states of unrestrained consciousness that accompany the ingestion of psilocybin are associated with a deactivation of regions of the brain that integrate our senses and our perception of self. In depressed people, Nutt explains, one of those regions, the anterior cingulate cortex, is overactive, and psilocybin may work to shut it down. In 2016 Nutt and associated researchers dosed twelve treatment-resistant depressives with psilocybin. Each subject had been depressed for about eighteen years on average and had failed to respond to standard interventions like SSRIs and electroconvulsive therapy. Within a week after taking the psilocybin, every single patient had experienced substantial improvements in his or her depressive symptoms, and after three months, five of the twelve subjects had enjoyed a complete remission.

Perhaps the patients in these various studies are able to capture

enduring benefits from psilocybin precisely because they are processing their drug experiences again and again with research staff
and, in doing so, changing the way their brain encodes positive
memories. The phenomenon might be similar to how other memories work: when we remember something sweet-smelling, the
olfactory neurons in our brain start to stir; when we remember
running, our motor cortex begins to buzz. If this is the case with
psilocybin as well, then merely recalling the trip could resurrect its
neural correlates, allowing the person to re-experience the insight,
the awareness, the hope.

Griffiths is unearthing and continuing the pioneering work
of the 1960s and '70s, having completed a study using psilocybin with cancer patients who have a life-threatening diagnosis.
Additional studies have been done at New York University, where,
according to lead investigator Stephen Ross, cancer patients
receiving just a single dose of psilocybin experienced immediate
and dramatic relief from their fear of death, lasting for at least six
months. Likewise, Grob found in his psilocybin study of terminal
cancer patients at UCLA that all subjects achieved a sense of serenity regarding their death that had not been present prior to their
taking the psychedelic. Subjects filling out post-session question-
naires in Griffiths's study made claims including 'all things were
alive' or 'all things seemed to be conscious' or 'all things seemed
to be unified into a single whole'. These consistent responses led
Griffiths to the conclusion that psilocybin is able to reduce or even
remove the fear of death because the patient experiences 'an intuition that consciousness is alive and pervades everything'. Once the
person grasps that, he said, 'from there it is not a great stretch to
contemplate the possibility of the continuity of consciousness – or,
more traditionally, immortal soul.' In the end, then, it's really the
'perceptual shift' the drug accomplishes, the ability to relinquish
the limiting view that we are reduced to our bodies, that brings
about the reduction in the fear of death that we see in patients
taking psilocybin.

The Crab

None of the drug's history was known to Carol Vincent, who learned of Griffiths's cancer patient study when her adult son read about it online. Here was something she could do, Vincent thought. She sent in her name on a long shot and was pleasantly surprised when the Johns Hopkins team got in touch with her to conduct intensive phone screening, after which she flew to Baltimore to meet Griffiths and his colleagues and to undergo still more psychological and physical testing. By this point, fast approaching the life limit she had been given for the disease six years earlier, Vincent had become definitively depressed. She had tried almost every natural cure available and still her nodes continued to swell, a constant reminder of her foreshortened future. 'I thought a lot about death and dying,' she said. 'It was so relentless. I remember crossing at an intersection. A car came towards me. Instinctively I jumped out of the way but afterwards I wondered if maybe I should have just stood there.'

Now fifty-nine, Vincent was accepted into Griffiths's double-blind study. She would receive two doses of psilocybin on two separate occasions five weeks apart. One dose would be high and one would be either high or low. No one would know which was which. In April 2014 Vincent stepped into a Johns Hopkins treatment room researchers had stripped of its medical veneer and made to look like a comfortable living room. In doing this, they were adhering to the idea, first put forth by Huston Smith, that set and setting are paramount for those ingesting psychedelic drugs. Vincent had two guides who would accompany her for the duration of her trip. She was not frightened. Her guides, Griffiths's colleagues, asked her what her intentions were. 'This is not about just having a good time,' she said. 'My intent is to find ways to deal with my diagnosis and to recover my normal state of mind as much as possible.'

In asking each subject to create a clear intention that informs and shapes her psilocybin experience, researchers are separating recreational drug use from therapeutic drug discovery. They are also linking their clinical investigations to history, mirroring the way psychedelics were used by Grof and others in the 1960s and 70s, and, going back still further, the way they were and are used by ancient and indigenous Indian tribes, evoking seriousness and sacredness. In some sense, then, the 'new' work with psychedelics is actually very old, springing not just from studies done forty or fifty years ago but from rituals that date back to 500 CE. It's as if the mushrooms play the part of an oracle that will reveal some sort of truth to those who seek its secrets.

In order to emphasise the noetic quality of the quest, Griffiths gives his subjects their psilocybin in a goblet, which he believes further connects the use of the drug to its ancient roots. Vincent clasped the goblet coolly. In it lay a fat capsule of psilocybin. Her guides, Mary and Taylor, sat by her side. She had been instructed to bring some meaningful mementos from home, pictures of loved ones and trinkets. After she swallowed the drug, she and Mary and Taylor looked at the objects together while Vincent explained what each one meant. During this time Vincent was hyper-aware of her mind, waiting and waiting for the drug to hit. Her photographs assumed a grainy appearance and began to disassemble into dots, and then came a dizziness. Vincent felt faint. Mary suggested that she lie on the sofa. Mary then put headphones and an eye mask on her. Through the headphones poured the most exquisite music Vincent had ever heard – concertos and chanting, the music physical, palpable, lifting her up on crystal crescendos and then dropping her back into dark depths that frightened Vincent at first. Then colours came and the feeling of space, deep space, as Vincent faced a massive and monolithic structure that was dark, impersonal and cold. She saw a gold shield, a huge black vault and then motifs so drenched in stunning colour that Vincent wept for their beauty. *Where's the God?* Vincent asked. *Where's the human? Where's the connection?* She posed her questions to an endless expanse of space and at first got no answers.

What she did get, however, was a collage of images – a fish, a rabbit, a huge pirate ship, a castle – and then a massive dark force coming closer and closer. In a moment of pure courage, Vincent reached out to touch the monstrosity, only to have it turn soft as fog. As she experienced this, a superhero in a red cape blew by and, from time to time, a white cartoon crab made an appearance, clacking away.

At one point Vincent believed the drug had worn off. She sat up, took off her eye mask, and went to the lavatory. When she returned she looked again at the pictures she had brought with her. Then the eye mask went back on and more music poured through her, at first just the plucking of a guitar, followed by rhythms of greater and greater depth. 'The music became heavier and heavier and loaded with global pain,' Vincent said. She felt the agony of everyone in the world and she saw that her pain was but a fleck in a huge and complex network of suffering. The crab came back, and Vincent would later come to understand that this was her cancer, this silly little thing that did not have nearly the resonance, the meaning, of the dazzling deep space, of the gorgeous tapestry of swirling colours, of the hugeness of history and the accumulation of tears. Consciousness, it seemed, had a continuity to it that could well extend beyond her death. But this realisation is not what truly comforted Vincent. The crab was what did it for her. Through the crab, with the crab, Vincent saw that her illness and death were not nearly the big deal that she had made them out to be. 'I was told to lighten up a little,' she said. 'To lighten up a lot. I was told to have a sense of humour; after all, the crab was a cartoon.'

When her trip was over, six hours after it had begun, Vincent was changed. Though personally an atheist, she had felt connected to something larger than herself, 'some kind of communal energy'. She could understand that the world wouldn't come to an end just because she did. Her mandate was to laugh about it. 'You die and you say, "I'm here. I'm home. I'm back".' Through psilocybin, Vincent found a quilt in a corner of the universe, a safe space she believed she would go to when her time came.

The Ultimate Existential Medicine

Vincent was the last subject in Griffiths's study of terminal cancer patients, but Griffiths is in no way finished with his inquiries into psychedelics and how they might help, or even heal, the human brain. He is now exploring the role of psilocybin in smoking addiction, giving it to people hooked on cigarettes to see if it might help them stop. So far he's found that it does. Out of fifteen nicotine-addicted subjects, 80 per cent have kicked their habit for six months or more. William, one of Griffiths's subjects in the cigarette study, puts it this way: 'Psilocybin reveals to you how pointless your addiction is. You see the majesty of the world, and polluting it and yourself comes to seem like sin.'

Vincent and William both used the drug as a lens through which they peered into worlds that gave new perspective to their conundrums. As with the Indians whom Gordon Wasson observed, if you pose to psilocybin a problem, any problem, it reflects back to you visions, voices, entryways and exits. Your whole mind swirls in a glittering test tube; all your fixed notions melt in the high heat of a trip, cleansed so that you can suddenly see around corners and down slopes previously too steep to navigate. The problem Carol Vincent posed to psilocybin had to do with fear of death. The response was a deep knowledge of universal unity which revealed to her that her own infinitesimal speck was a part of the warp and weft that would change shape upon her passing, but would also endure forever. What William got when he posed to psilocybin the problem of his nicotine addiction was a sense of the sacredness of his life and all life, to which, he saw, he was deeply connected. In filling the lobes of his lungs with tar, he was in some ineffable sense charring the very chain of life to which he was irretrievably linked.

It would seem that psilocybin could be used for almost any struggle. As an illuminator, it is, as Grob has said, 'the ultimate existential medicine'. And while at present it is limited to the laboratory and cannot be obtained legally by the ordinary citizen looking for a quest, there may well come a time when it is more widely available as an indispensable aid to people with a broad range of conflicts. Indeed it is Rick Doblin's mission to legalise psychedelics for 'things that are not diseases, like personal growth, spirituality, couples counselling.' Given that the drug seems to reveal to people the sacred interconnectedness of all life forms, psilocybin might indeed prove useful in everything from the treatment of violence and antisocial behaviour to chronic pain and clinical depression or agoraphobia and generalised anxiety disorder.

How can a single drug have so many potential applications? The answer to this lies partly in the nature of most mental illness, which is characterised by mental rigidity and stereotypical thought patterns, the monotonous 'I hate myself' of depression or the repetitive fears of contamination in OCD. 'Psilocybin can be of benefit for these types of troubles,' Doblin said. 'The drug breaks down neurotic defences and allows people trapped in bad psychiatric states to think flexibly, to think openly, to be open to novel experience.'

Although he believes there will come a time when psilocybin will be legally available to clinicians and patients who might best benefit from it, Doblin acknowledges that this is a way off. The excesses of the 1960s are fading but still with us. Griffiths hopes for a time when spiritually minded people can use the psychedelic to enhance and deepen their journeys. Charles Grob wants to see centres for the dying where the drug can be safely administered to those seeking serenity on their way out. These ideas are not new so much as they are a return to questions and quests from the past. All of these visions and views spring both from ancient shamanic traditions and from the more recent work done in the 1950s, '60s and '70s, before psychedelics were made illegal.

Griffiths has said that understanding the effects of drugs like psilocybin, indeed understanding the effects of all psychedelics, may be the key to the survival of our species. His comment goes well beyond the idea of psilocybin for the psychiatric patient or for the dying or for the seeker of spiritual truths, and places psilocybin at the very centre of our troubled world, as *the* potential answer to what ails us all. But could a psychedelic really save our place in a shredded planet, a world so saturated with CO_2 that the glaciers are slipping into the sea as thousands of animals go extinct, a world where civilians are shot down in the streets, where radicals put bombs on planes and take down towers in the name of religion? We live in a time of rampant corruption and continuous violence, of profound poverty and obscene wealth, spinning, it sometimes seems, into an abyss. What role could psychedelics possibly play for us in such a world?

Perhaps, actually, a profound one. The early psychedelic pioneers like Grof and Pahnke, along with newcomers like Griffiths and Grob, have accumulated literally hundreds, maybe thousands, of case studies in which subjects ingest either LSD or psilocybin. And one after the other the subjects almost invariably experience the sacred quality of consciousness and come to see how it seeps beyond the circle of our own skulls to infuse all living things, thereby promoting a deep sense of interconnectedness along with a belief in the divine. No one who has taken these drugs under these researchers' supervision has come away from the experience thinking he is grand and big. In fact the result is just the opposite. People tend to experience themselves as small, as a mote absorbed into some larger and sacred framework. They consistently report feelings of deep empathy for others. Carol Vincent, listening to black spirituals while on a psychedelic, claimed to feel the pain of all the slaves we had stolen and forced to work, and wept for what had happened; others have reported feeling a newfound empathy for friends, spouses, children. It appears that the drug imparts beneficence, brings out the best in the humans who use it, eradicates the hubris at the heart of so many of our troubles and leaves in its place an open humility from which love and kindness easily flow.

Imagine, then, and just for kicks, our politicians taking psilocybin, not at a London bash but in a place where set and setting have been carefully constructed; imagine the United Nations doing the same. Imagine even terrorists taking a substance that showed them how small they were in a world where everyone is intimately connected. What kind of priming would be necessary to bring about such revelations in our leaders? And even with proper priming, would the drug reveal such truths to a scar-hardened warrior? Or might the opposite happen? Does the drug conform to the psyche of the person who takes it, so that fighters would experience the valour of violence while cancer patients, already laid low by their diagnoses, experience their diminutiveness? Or does the drug really lead us to a Platonic destination where an ineffable yet solid truth resides, a truth of the sacredness of consciousness and the utter significance of love? If this is true, then perhaps Griffiths is right and psilocybin really could change the world, by changing consciousness – one mind at a time.

7

MDMA (Ecstasy)

The Marriage Medicine

Sanctuary

Their marriage was coming apart. They were fighting over this and that, pointing, pacing, shouting, slamming and then the silence, which was maybe worst of all, how it just continued on and on, minutes stretching out into an hour and then a whole day, as the rain dripped down or the sun perversely shone, laying bars of light along the maple floor.

Their names: Kelly and Thomas Shuge. Their stats: forty-four and fifty-three, respectively. Their marriage: twenty-three years, going on gold (or was it silver?) – worth saving, that much they knew. But the fights cast a pall they couldn't seem to stop, and had forced their love into some cramped corner, where it dwindled down even as Kelly's terminal cancer grew and grew, throwing a suffocating blanket over the life they'd built together for so many years.

Kelly was a talker. She always had been. She talked with friends on the phone. She talked over glasses of wine and on a stool at the kitchen worktop with her legs crossed. She'd talk about her day or her darkness with equal ease, something Thomas had never been able to do. He kept quiet and let pain blow over. Like wind or weather, it always eventually went away. Why bother with all that digging? The world was going to do what the world was going to do, and you'd best save your energy for the grind. Thomas had broad hands and worked with wood. He could take a piece of raw pine and shape it into a ship, or a table, or a bed with a half-moon headboard. Kelly loved to watch him work. She loved the way he dipped a rag in fragrant stain and wiped it over the piece, his hand slowly circling as the hue deepened to bronze or chestnut brown.

Kelly had been diagnosed with cancer five years earlier; it wasn't news, but still she wanted to talk about it. She wanted to talk about her fears, her hope, her highs and lows, about the chemo treatment and the different types of tumours, whether there was something in the water that could have caused this; she had a lot to say, and she kept saying it and saying it until Thomas thought his head would explode and he sought solace elsewhere.

'Where are you going?' Kelly would cry after him, but he never answered because he didn't know. Where was he going? Without her, what would he do? Sometimes he'd wake up in the middle of the night and see her sleeping next to him, her body shawled in shadow as if she'd already left, as if he could put his hand right through her and come out empty on the other side, and the ache in his throat was so severe he had trouble breathing. *Sanctuary.* That was a word that came to him often these days. He'd picture a place in the forest, a cleared spot ringed by trees, a place to put his head. Her head. Somewhere they could go, together.

Things got bad enough between them that, despite her illness, Kelly thought about divorce. They saw a couples counsellor but didn't get anywhere. It was all tit for tat, both of them skating on the surface of things, stuck in their *if only*s. And then one day, Kelly's oncologist told her about therapists who were using a drug called MDMA (illegally under current law in both the United States and the UK) to help couples communicate more effectively while also mediating the anxiety and trauma of an end-stage diagnosis.

MDMA, known in the mainstream as ecstasy or simply E, is not your average anti-anxiety medication. It shares not a single molecule with our old standbys like lorazepam, diazepam, alprazolam or clonazepam. MDMA amplifies the sensual world, so that music sounds richer, a touch tingles more intensely and ordinary thoughts drop away in favour of keener insights and understanding. While MDMA shares similarities with psilocybin (both are used to ease end-of-life anxiety in patients with cancer diagnoses), the drugs also differ in important ways. Psilocybin is a hallucinogen, which means that it causes its imbiber to see and hear things that are not really there: rays of light, figures from your past, dark matter, fluorescent swirls and geometric patterns, silvered plateaus and melting meadows that appear to go on for miles. On MDMA you will not experience any of this because, while it is a psychedelic, it is not a hallucinogen. MDMA bathes the brain in oxytocin, which is why users feel so much affinity for those around them, and also why it is so effective at treating trauma. Traumatised patients on MDMA are able to recall their horror in an atmosphere of total trust. Psilocybin, by contrast, would probably not be suggested for a trauma victim because it dissolves the ego, the border between you and the external world, which a trauma victim might find deeply frightening.

In the Beginning

The German pharmaceutical company Merck synthesised MDMA in 1912. After it was patented, however, the drug was all but forgotten. The goal of the researchers had been to come up with a good vasoconstrictor to reduce bleeding, something that MDMA does not do. Therefore, much like lithium, it was shelved for years, unused. No one knows who the first human to take MDMA was. It was used briefly in a classified study sponsored by the US military in the 1950s, but only on animals, ranging from mice to monkeys. The first documented appearance on the street was in Chicago, in 1970, when tablets containing MDMA were confiscated, and the drug began to seep into the culture at large in the early to mid-1970s. Alexander Shulgin, a Californian chemist who would come to be known as the 'godfather of psychedelics', concocted his own batch of MDMA and took it in ever higher doses. In his laboratory notes from September 1976, Shulgin wrote: 'I feel absolutely clean inside, and there is nothing but pure euphoria. I have never felt so great or believed this to be possible. The cleanliness, clarity and marvellous feeling of solid inner strength continued throughout the rest of the day and evening. I am overcome by the profundity of the experience.'

He wasn't the only one. Therapists caught on to the drug as well, and because the US government had not yet criminalised it, a small but significant subset of them began to use it as a therapeutic aid with their patients. Some, like psychologist and psychotherapist Leo Zeff, another pioneer in the field of psychedelics, took careful and copious notes that give us a remarkably clear picture of how MDMA affected patients in psychotherapy. On MDMA, patients were able to easily retrieve otherwise inaccessible memories, some of them traumatic, and to explore these frightening recollections in a state of absolute serenity. Previously self-hating patients enjoyed total self-acceptance and got to see the world without the lacerating edge of cynicism that so often accompanies neurotic suffering.

Ann Shulgin, Alexander's wife and a practising therapist, also began using MDMA in couples therapy, finding that MDMA had the power to restore vibrancy and energy to worn-out pair bonds, not only during the actual high but also after the drug had worn off, with her patients often able to integrate the psychedelic point of view into their quotidian lives. As of yet there are no quantitative data to tell us how many couples have taken MDMA, and for what particular problems, or, most significantly, what the outcomes have been. All we have are qualitative accounts that describe how previously polarised couples were able to trust each other again deeply, perhaps in part because MDMA improves one's ability to listen empathically, enabling couples to verbalise their root issues. MDMA appears to unclog the plumbing between two individuals so that positive feelings flow freely.

Banned

Psychedelics have been imbibed for centuries by people seeking spiritual enlightenment, but thanks in part to Timothy Leary, who welded them to the 1960s counterculture – when drugs like psilocybin and LSD were taken by the palmful – they were fast made illegal and relegated to the fringe, associated in most Americans' minds with tie-dye and Deadheads (a term coined for the fans of the rock group Grateful Dead), their favourite guitarist Jerry Garcia strumming stoned on a stage. At MAPS, the Multidisciplinary Association for Psychedelic Studies in California, Rick Doblin, in addition to re-examining past experiments with psilocybin, is trying hard to change these associations. Unaffiliated with a university, MAPS is a non-profit organisation that develops and funds clinical trials to investigate a range of psychedelics in treating physical and psychological conditions that have proven resistant to more traditional pharmacological approaches. According to Doblin, 'Leary didn't do psychedelics any favour when he made them agents of rebellion. There was a sort of arrogance to his stance. He was telling people to sever themselves from society, to go form communes, to go back to the land. It was a rejection of the dominant culture in the extreme.'

If Doblin is correct and Leary's goal was to cut psychedelics off from the dominant culture, he was supremely successful. According to the US National Household Survey on Drug Abuse (NHSDA), by 1972, despite the exhortation to 'tune in and turn on', only 5 per cent of Americans, most of them under the age of eighteen, had used psychedelics. Nor did use of hallucinogens become part of the mainstream, with still only 14 per cent of the population reporting lifetime usage a quarter of a century later, in the mid-1990s. Most of us know people who smoke weed, but how many of us are friends with people who regularly imbibe psychedelics? 'There's been this sense', Doblin said, 'that these drugs are dirty, dangerous and that those who use them are somehow irreparably irresponsible, perpetually spaced out and not the kind we'd like to keep company with.'

MDMA as Medicine

While the dominant culture may continue to conflate Leary and LSD, or Deadheads and psychedelics, and cast a less than favourable light on this admittedly mysterious class of drugs, the medical community is undergoing its own revolution. Fifty-odd years after Leary, researchers around the world are newly and seriously interested in investigating psychedelics for their potential capacity to ease everything from death-related anxiety to cluster headaches, and to aid in the treatment of addiction, post-traumatic stress disorder (PTSD) and autism.

Charles Grob, in addition to conducting his end-of-life psilocybin study at the Harbor-UCLA Medical Center in California, has worked with transpersonal psychotherapist Alicia Danforth to publish a phase-one study in which adults with dual diagnoses of autism and social anxiety are given MDMA to see if the drug might help them more effectively relate to others. Danforth and Grob have reason to believe that MDMA could be crucial in breaking down the barriers autistic people face, especially their extreme difficulty in connecting to the 'neurotypical' world. There are ample accounts from those with autism who have taken MDMA independently, without medical guidance, stating that the drug makes it possible for them to function – not only while they're on the drug, but for weeks and sometimes months afterwards. In Danforth's own study of how autistic adults experience the subjective effects of MDMA, she found that 91 per cent of respondents reported an increase in feelings of connectedness on MDMA, while 86 per cent of them said that communication became easier.

Though this study is a profound breakthrough in the treatment of autism, the use of psychedelics for this purpose isn't an entirely new idea. In fact, as Grob and Danforth found in their research, throughout the 1960s more than a hundred minors with autism or the now obsolete diagnosis of 'juvenile schizophrenia' participated in trials in which they ingested psychedelics, and in at least six of these studies LSD was administered to children as young as five. Lest our only reaction be shock, however, it's worth noting that while the autistic children were under the influence of these drugs, researchers observed that they displayed an increase in vocabulary and emotional responsiveness to others, mood enhancement, more eye-to-eye contact and a decrease in compulsive behaviours. LSD was also given to mute catatonic schizophrenics, who finally spoke, a result that spurred still more studies on treating non-communicative autistic people with psychedelics. But as we saw with psilocybin, despite the promise of psychedelics in the treatment of autism and catatonic states, government bans in the early 1970s decisively discouraged all investigations with psychedelic compounds.

John Halpern, of McLean Hospital in Massachusetts, is, like Danforth, investigating MDMA's effects on high-functioning autistic patients who want help connecting to the neurotypical world. Halpern has surveyed autistic adults who self-medicate with MDMA. 'We don't want to put the cart before the horse,' he said on the day I spoke to him. 'We need good medical research that validates what we're seeing, which is that MDMA is a game changer.' Halpern went on to describe how one of the autistic people he'd been observing had insisted that on MDMA he could appreciate and respect other people's feelings and that once the MDMA wore off he was still able to remember the behaviours he'd learned while under its influence. Halpern paused, touched a smooth stone on his desk, a flat rock the colour of caramel with visible white veins branching through its body, of the sort that I might see on the shelves of my own rock-collecting doctor. His hope, he said, was that they would get the necessary funding to conduct high-quality medical research that would confirm what has already been suggested anecdotally. 'Some psychedelics, and MDMA in particular,' he said, 'are powerful empathogens that could be made into medicines to treat a whole range of conditions, from distinct diseases to shadow syndromes, like extreme shyness.'

An empathogen is the name given to a psychoactive drug, like MDMA, that brings about emotional communion or openness – in other words, empathy. Halpern pointed out the range of human problems that, in one way or another, involve connection and its impairment. '*Delic*', he said, typing the suffix into his computer and staring at the screen, 'means "to make aware, to reveal". That's what these drugs do. They reveal people to each other; they increase one's awareness of the signals others are sending. And because they're pro-social, they give people who are stymied by, say, shyness a chance to interact with others.' Halpern, like Ann Shulgin before him, has evidence from those who use psychedelics like MDMA illegitimately that these empathogens have therapeutic potential not only for the treatment of social phobias and autism but also for couples counselling.

For Trauma

Psilocybin and its close cousin LSD also have empathogenic properties, but of all the empathogenic psychedelics, MDMA may be the most potent. Along with psilocybin, it is experiencing a second life. No longer the 'hug drug' of the 1980s and '90s clubbing culture, it appears now in pristine clinical settings, one of which is run by Michael Mithoefer, a psychiatrist in private practice in Charleston, South Carolina. Mithoefer completed a US-government approved trial of MDMA for the treatment of severe post-traumatic stress disorder, with stunning results. In 2011, with the support of MAPS, he and his team created a double-blind design in which twelve severely traumatised patients were given MDMA and psychotherapy, and eight patients were given an active placebo and psychotherapy. The researchers used the Clinician Administered PTSD Scale (CAPS) as a means of measuring symptom reduction after intervention. In the placebo group, only two out of eight subjects had a significantly lowered CAPS score post-intervention, whereas in the MDMA group, ten out of the twelve subjects had significantly lowered CAPS scores and were able to maintain those scores at a two-month follow-up. Furthermore, in the MDMA group, ten of the twelve patients were so improved that they no longer met the *DSM* criteria for post-traumatic stress disorder. The second phase of the study allowed seven subjects who had previously taken the placebo (six of whom had failed to respond to the placebo and one of whom had relapsed after the placebo) to now try MDMA. They found a clinical response rate of 100 per cent, and the three people who had previously said they weren't able to perform their jobs on account of their post-traumatic stress disorder were now able to work once again.

The drug appears to act by allowing traumatised victims to recall their terror in an utterly peaceful frame of mind, thereby forging new neuronal associations in the brain. According to Halpern, 'it is because empathogens give people the ego strength to tolerate frightening images or thoughts that they are so useful for people who have had traumatic experiences.' Under the influence of MDMA, victims of violent crime and veterans of war have both the mental stamina and the serenity to talk about what happened without fear. The drug creates a state in which the subject is calm and feels deep trust in his or her therapist, which allows for a more profound processing of the trauma. On MDMA patients are able, perhaps for the first time, to explore their trauma, rendering it with words rather than reacting with mute terror. Part of how post-traumatic stress disorder afflicts those who suffer from it is by increasing blood flow to the amygdala, the part of the brain responsible for feelings of fear, and decreasing blood flow to the cortex, where reasoning takes place and narrative is built, thereby making it much harder for people to reframe and revise painful life events. The thinking is that MDMA may reverse this phenomenon, allowing trauma victims, who sometimes blame themselves, to feel instead a deep sense of compassion, not only for others but also for themselves.

The Love Hormone

Kelly Shuge turned out to be one of the people MDMA could help. Her experience paints a remarkable picture of how certain psychedelics can improve and intensify relationships. Prior to MDMA, Kelly and Thomas were polarised, their different coping skills fracturing their marriage and keeping them apart emotionally and physically. Kelly agreed to try MDMA – during six guided therapeutic counselling sessions – with the hope that she would learn to deal with the anxiety her cancer was causing her in a way that was less noxious to Thomas. That's not what happened, though. The drug helped her, but in a different way than she'd imagined it would. Under the influence of MDMA, Kelly had 'a powerfully empathic experience of what it was going to be like for her husband to lose her' her therapist explained to me. 'That empathic experience was so strong that it just cut through the bickering and the strain. Kelly was able to see the suffering in her husband's heart and to communicate that understanding to him, and it just drastically improved the time they had to spend together.' Four months after her MDMA sessions, Kelly died in her husband's arms.

One theory about how MDMA achieves its special pair-bonding effect has to do with the rising levels of oxytocin it promotes. In a 2004 study in the Netherlands, researchers measured the concentration of oxytocin in fifteen MDMA users' blood, operating from the hypothesis that as 'pro-social' feelings increased, so too would levels of oxytocin, known informally as 'the hormone of love', so named because of its capacity to forge human bonding. That the researchers guessed correctly is no surprise given that ample studies of animals had already shown that, under the influence of MDMA, the brain is 'just flooded' with oxytocin, according to Doblin. Oxytocin, an extremely powerful hormone that has the capacity to alter human and animal behaviour, has been researched extensively in prairie voles, an animal known for its monogamous sexual habits. The prairie vole is one of the few mammals on this planet to stick with a partner for life. If you inject a female vole with an oxytocin antagonist, however, she will show a complete receptivity to a new mate. Cease the oxytocin antagonist and the rodents immediately return to their first-picked partner and happily resume their loyal lives.

Like prairie voles, humans also manufacture oxytocin, and have the capacity to do so in large amounts. Without oxytocin we would likely have trouble loving our offspring, especially right after birth, when they've ripped us up and lie there screaming, looking less like a human than some sort of surrealist depiction of an alien life form. Yet love these little creatures we usually do, often immediately, and probably because the oxytocin that causes the spasms of labour to begin with also sticks around after the birth and is triggered once again in huge amounts by breast-feeding, not to mention in lesser but still significant amounts whenever we touch or are touched. Without oxytocin, chances are good we'd be reduced to robots.

Raves

Oxytocin is a chemical you can easily procure. In fact it is sold in mail-order catalogues as an aphrodisiac. MDMA, at the present time, is harder to get hold of. If we were living in the late 1970s or early 1980s, however, we would be able to obtain it without a lot of trouble, but there'd be no guarantee that what we were buying was pure. Back then, before the government got wind of this empathogen, you could find it in a nightclub and even charge it on your credit card. The tablets sometimes came in a brown bottle labelled 'Sassyfras'. (MDMA is in part derived from the sassafras plant.) Before the drug achieved widespread recreational use in the United States, batches were cooked up primarily by a group of therapeutically minded chemists around Boston called the 'Boston Group'. But as the drug became more profitable, large laboratories dedicated to making and distributing empathogens sprang up all across the country. Like any good thing, MDMA, or 'Adam' (a reference to the Eden-like state it induced), became a topic of gossip. It entered the mainstream enough to be written about everywhere from *Newsweek* to the 'Doonesbury' cartoon strip. People began to abuse it, taking dose after dose during all-night raves – MDMA dance parties, Dionysian in the extreme.

For the chemical chefs behind MDMA, business was good, even great, to the extent that their main concern was what to call the stuff, how to find a name that best reflected its amazing properties. The name is not the sole reason ecstasy finally caught the attention of police officers, legislators and distressed doctors who were seeing people post-rave, dehydrated and depressed from dancing and drugging all night, but it has something to do with it. 'Ecstasy', so christened in 1981 by an early distributor who thought it would sell better – '"Empathy" might be more appropriate,' he said, 'but how many people know what it means?' – has a sort of sliding sound, and because Americans supersize everything from their cars to their sweets, some of them slid down the slide of ecstasy, using it to excess and causing a ruckus as they went along. When the biggest distributor for the Boston Group in the Southwest opened his own laboratory, in Texas, production went into overdrive, and by 1985, at the height, almost a quarter-million doses a month were being produced by the new 'Texas Group' alone. According to Jerome Beck, of the Institute for Scientific Analysis in Berkeley, and Marsha Rosenbaum, the director of the US Center for Drug

Studies, 'the quiet use of Adam in limited therapeutic circles had been transformed into a phenomenon. Ecstasy was now the "drug of choice" among Texas yuppies.'

Senator Lloyd Bentsen of Texas, soon to be the Democratic nominee for vice president, grew concerned about the proliferation of the drug and the accompanying raves, especially in the Austin and Dallas–Fort Worth areas – his whole huge state, it must have seemed, had gone bananas – and he sought to put a stop to it. In 1985 he brought ecstasy to the attention of the US Drug Enforcement Administration (DEA), with a request for a temporary emergency ban, at the same time that neurology researcher George Ricaurte, at Johns Hopkins University in Maryland, published a study which showed that MDMA caused neurotoxicity in rats. The tactic proved to be successful, and on 31 May of that year, the DEA did indeed issue a one-year ban. 'We saw it coming,' Doblin said. 'We saw that this incredibly valuable substance was going to be criminalised, and so we organised, and did whatever we could to stop it.'

After the DEA criminalised the drug, Doblin sued, a move that forced the issue into court, where an administrative law judge looked closely at the evidence for and against MDMA. Doblin and his group argued that Ricaurte had given his rodents doses so huge they would burn through even a bionic brain, while simultaneously pointing out the fact that there were to date no deaths associated with MDMA and no evidence that it caused any kind of brain damage whatsoever in human users. Doblin's goal, and the goal of MAPS, was not to keep MDMA on the street, where it could continue to be used in excess, but instead to have it formally and legally scheduled in such a way that researchers and doctors would still have access to it for clinical purposes. Despite the fact that Doblin won his lawsuit and the judge recommended to the DEA that it put MDMA in the same category as other highly controlled but clinically useful drugs, the DEA overrode the judge's recommendation and put MDMA permanently in its highest drug-risk category, which includes dangerous drugs such as heroin and Quaaludes (the popular US name for the depressant methaqua-lone, known as Mandrax in the UK) – in other words, drugs the DEA has deemed to have no clinical or research relevance. MDMA was made illegal in the UK by 1977 but researchers could carry out experiments if they got a licence from the Home Office.

The Spurious Study

'If I thought about goals', Doblin told me, 'I'd get depressed. For me the work has to be not about what we've achieved but about the meaning in the struggle.' And struggle he has. Doblin has fought the DEA every step of the way, almost his entire professional life, about getting MDMA and its allied empathogens made available for limited legal use as prescription medicine.

Those of Ricaurte's persuasion do not make Doblin's life any easier. In 2002, almost two decades after his study on the putative neurotoxicity of MDMA when given to rats, Ricaurte published a still more alarming paper claiming he'd fed MDMA to primates and that a few had died as a result, and there was evidence of neurotox-icity in all. This study threw a serious spanner in the works into the MDMA debate. Doblin, along with Mithoefer, was on the cusp of getting institutional review board approval for his study using MDMA to treat severe post-traumatic stress disorder, but as soon as Ricaurte released his new MDMA results, Doblin said, 'They shut us right down.' Of course, who could argue with that? If our closest genetic cousins are dropping dead from the love drug, well then, you'd better stop loving the drug. Along with his published paper, Ricaurte released images of primate brains post-MDMA exposure. The images are ghostly, haunting black-and-white brains with huge ragged holes ripped in them, the damage so severe and worrisome that Oprah Winfrey did a segment on MDMA and the supposedly severe side effects it caused, along with the obvious message to just please, now, once and for all and forever, say no to drugs.

Others, meanwhile, continued to disagree. 'We've seen thousands of people safely use MDMA, sometimes as many as forty times or more,' said Julie Holland, who for a time ran the psychiatric A&E department at Bellevue Hospital in New York, and has seen hundreds of drug-related emergencies. 'There was nothing about the Ricaurte study that seemed plausible to me, and I can tell you, based on everything I've seen, based on the published data and my clinical experience, MDMA is just not a significant cause of psychiatric crisis.' Doblin, too, was left scratching his bald spot. But it didn't take long before someone started to poke around in Ricaurte's study and a grave error was uncovered. Ricaurte, it turned out, had *not* given MDMA to his orangutans and bonobos. He'd given them an entirely different drug – methamphetamine, a known toxin – dosing his subjects with large amounts, watching as their brains sizzled, and then saying the damage had been done by MDMA.

How could this have happened? Ricaurte reported that his supplier mislabelled the bottles, while his supplier counterclaims that it has never mislabelled its bottles. Ricaurte was forced to issue a retraction, but in a way it didn't matter; the damage was already done. Millions of Oprah's viewers had seen the images, while very few of them saw the published retraction. 'The Ricaurte study has definitely added to the stigma and misinformation around MDMA,' Doblin said. 'It has become part of our uphill battle.'

After Ricaurte published his retraction, the DEA gave the go-ahead to Doblin and Mithoefer for their research. That 2011 study has given rise to four others, including one in Boulder, Colorado, where the results have been promising. Of the twenty-eight subjects who were enrolled, three-quarters of those who received an active dose as opposed to a placebo achieved remission; they no longer met the diagnostic criteria for post-traumatic stress disorder. This, combined with a study of Mithoefer's in which subjects were followed for as long as forty months and were still holding strong, suggests that while MDMA might be a quick high, it's also no quickly fading cure. The positive press the post-traumatic stress disorder–MDMA experiments have generated has gone a way towards undoing some of the damage caused by Ricaurte's megaphone. Doblin now wants to focus all his efforts on getting the DEA and the FDA to legalise MDMA for the treatment of post-traumatic stress disorder and, prior to that, getting permission to conduct more studies replicating the findings of the first few.

Seeking MDMA

Doblin was quick to acknowledge that MDMA has many applications beyond the treatment of post-traumatic stress disorder. But despite the breadth and depth of MDMA's potential, he said he and his researchers would not be pursuing most of these paths right now and, with the exception of MDMA for life-threatening illnesses and the treatment of social shyness in autistic adults, probably not anytime soon either.

This disappointed me, and for a very personal reason. When I first spoke to Doblin, the marriage to my husband that has now ended was in its denouement. But I wasn't ready for our story to be over. After everything I had read, I was ready to try a tablet or two of MDMA with my husband. It was cheaper and faster, I reasoned, than taking the two-month holiday we would otherwise have needed to find our way back to the long-lost but not completely forgotten love we once had. Yes, I thought, we were perfect candidates for a blind date with an empathogen. But as it turned out, I probably wasn't about to be making these discoveries, at least not through a MAPS-funded study, and right now that's the only option there is in this country, at least of the legal variety. Of course my husband and I could have tried 'scoring' some of this stuff on our own, but I didn't want what comes off the street.

'Where *is* the MDMA anyway?' I asked Doblin. 'When the DEA gives you permission to do a study, where do you get the drug if it's illegal?'

The answer? Purdue University, where it was made in 1985 with a DEA licence by David Nichols, the former chair of pharmacology at Purdue. 'MDMA', Doblin explained, 'is an extremely stable compound', which means there's a big glass bottle full of the substance that's been sitting on a shelf in a chemist's locked safe in an institution of higher learning for years. Impervious to heat, cold, light and darkness, the chemical doesn't break down. In this sense it's unlike most other medications, which come in bottles with use-by dates stamped on their sides. I find it ironic that 'ecstasy', a state known more for its passing than its actual emotion, is, in its molecular form, something so very solid.

There was an awkward pause in my conversation with Doblin and I felt my face beginning to burn and at first I wasn't sure why, but then the question formed. 'Would you consider getting some for my husband and me to try?' I couldn't believe I was asking him this. Think about drugs too much, I guess, and you start to act like you're on them.

Doblin and I were sitting on the roof deck of his home in Belmont, Massachusetts. It was one of those gorgeous days on the cusp of autumn, before any of the trees have begun to turn, the air cooled, the greenery lush and verdant. Somewhere a dog was barking, and music came from the house next door.

Before he could answer I said, 'I'm on other medications, like Effexor [venlafaxine], for depression,' to which Doblin replied, 'You can't take MDMA with an SSRI.'

He explained why but I wasn't listening. Or rather I was, but to something else. I was listening to the neighbour's radio and to the staccato barks of the dog, and pondering the disappointment I felt in Doblin – that despite all its potential myriad purposes, all the various and significant ways MDMA could help people connect, he and his agency were pursuing only one. I was remembering something he had said to me moments earlier, about how post-traumatic stress victims – war veterans, survivors of violent rape – make MDMA seem like a serious, even patriotic drug, whereas couples counselling reverberates with echoes of hippiedom, which is what Doblin above all wants to avoid. 'Marriage can't be conceived of as a disease,' Doblin had said to me, 'so how could we devise a study if there's no discrete set of symptoms to increase, decrease or stabilise? Beyond that, couples counselling just doesn't carry the weight, the import, in the public's eye, and we need to think a lot about the public, and that eye.'

I could appreciate Doblin's reasoning, and the difficulty of the dual roles he needs to play here, part researcher, part PR manager, tiptoeing carefully along. 'My life's goal', he said, 'is to see the psychedelics made into prescription drugs.' He hoped to see this happen by 2021. But for now he had picked just a portion of that goal to focus on: post-traumatic stress disorder, with MDMA as the treatment. And I understood why, even as I disagreed with him about whether marriage can be quantified for the purposes of research. Surely there must be some scale somewhere out there that captures, for instance, the symptoms of a failing marriage, some way to measure the marriage pre- and post-MDMA ingestion.

'I'm going to find you a measurement device,' I told him, 'and if I can't find you one, I'll make one.' Doblin laughed.

We were at that point when the summer's end feels palpable, the smell of autumn everywhere in the air. The sun was slowly sinking as we spoke, inching down bit by bit, so slowly you couldn't even see it and wouldn't notice until, suddenly, there were shadows everywhere and it was evening – just like that. This is how many marriages devolve as well, the shine waning so subtly no one notices until one day in year twelve of your marriage you can't rinse the stale taste out of your mouth, and when you try to trace the path that got you here, all you see are seemingly festive landmarks: babies born, first day at school and so on. And then somehow it has been two decades.

I don't want to argue the case that divorce is a disease or that a failing, faded marriage is the same as a sickness, because that is a subject that goes, as the scientists say, 'beyond the scope of this paper'. But even if divorce is not an illness itself, it does leave a trail littered with symptoms and syndromes – the depression, for instance, that so often comes when a dyad dissolves, or the generalised anxiety disorder that some children experience when their parents go their separate ways. I'm rooting for a return, of sorts, to a time when MDMA was used by therapists like Shulgin and Zeff to treat marriages at their breaking point. And while Doblin may wish to steer clear of 'the soft stuff' and reserve MDMA for those decimated by a particular kind of distress, there is a part of him that understands how wide the reach of MDMA could, and perhaps should, be. I know this because he gave me the name of a practitioner who uses MDMA in her therapeutic work with couples.

I drove out to see her. I told her I was on the edge of divorce, and that the edge felt bad – shaky and sharp both. Her office was filled with flowers, trillium and irises and lilies with long golden tongues. She had a statue of a laughing Buddha and somewhere a fountain burbled and splashed. Her hair, blonde and flowing, put me in mind of a pelt. I wanted her to simply give me two tablets, one for him and one for me, but she wouldn't do that. Instead she wanted the whole sorry story of our decline, and even after I'd told it to her, over a series of weekly visits, she still wouldn't give me the goods.

'You may be too sensitive,' she said, 'and given all the medications you're on I'd have no idea how to dose you.'

'Let's start small', I said, 'and go from there', but she wouldn't do it and eventually I lost interest in trying. I've never taken an empathogen, or any other type of psychedelic for that matter, and it seems like such a loss to me. Could MDMA really have saved my marriage, or would it have been just another chemical tool added to my already considerable stash? I have no way of knowing.

In the meantime the season continued to change. The leaves were all coming down. The days were shorter and then shorter still until at last the sky was daily drained by four in the afternoon, with the tiny spot of the sun setting and the frost stiffening the grass and glazing the masses of fallen leaves. What can we do when we are lost to each other, when the temperature plummets, when the snow blinds us to even the familiar landmarks? Someday. Somewhere. Somehow. This is what I tell myself. *Delic*: to open. Maybe I don't need a drug to see the wonder of the world, but I also didn't need a drug to see the relationship dissolving, going to pieces, falling in flakes at our feet.

Divorce may not be an illness, but it sears the soul all the same. I dream that we will one day meet and that, spurred by MDMA, we will recover the love we lost, even if only for an afternoon. I'd like him to see me as he once did, and vice versa. I'd like to be twenty-four, not fifty-four. Someone once told me that she took MDMA and all she did was weep. That is a possibility. Still, I want to see through that oxytocin-soaked lens. In the meantime I'll wait. If Doblin's goal is to make MDMA a legal prescription medicine by 2021, then I really have only four years to go. By then, who knows, we both may be remarried. But there's enough love here that it deserves to be recalled, if not rekindled.

8

PKMzeta/ZIP (Memory Drugs)

The Spotless Mind

Memory Erasers

Strange things were happening to me. When friends came to visit I'd say, 'Let me show you around', and the odd way they looked at me let me know I'd already given them the grand tour of my new home months, weeks, maybe just days ago. The house felt to me like a maze, all crooked corridors and dark doors, a floor plan I couldn't seem to memorise even after we'd been here for six whole months, long enough to learn the layout of a bungalow with four bedrooms and two bathrooms ugly enough to want to forget. 'Let's redo those bathrooms,' I'd say to my husband, and then I'd launch into my design ideas and he'd ho-hum, having heard it all before. But when? My mind, it seemed, was going the way of the wood I coveted – gnarled and pitted, washed out by weather. It felt as if there were ragged holes in my brain through which both fact and fiction were swiftly falling.

In an increasingly ageing society – in England and Wales, according to the Office for National Statistics, the aged sixty-five and over population increased from 8.3 million in 2001 to 9.2 million in 2011, an increase of 11 per cent – memory is more than a hot topic of conversation. While I may be showing some form of early cognitive decline, it won't be long before my contemporaries have to acknowledge that their brains aren't as shiny as they once were either. Our collective ageing, and the huge profit potential for clinical interventions that slow or even reverse age-related forgetfulness, has researchers on the fast track to find a cure for the dreaded Alzheimer's and its companion scourge, mild cognitive impairment (MCI), a condition that frequently develops into Alzheimer's.

Memory research, however, is about much more than Alzheimer's. Scientists are using fMRIs to peer deep into our mental machinery, and studying the brains of fruit flies as well, all in an effort to better grasp not only how we remember but also how we forget. The goal is to create a drug that can be administered to addicts or trauma survivors. While MDMA can change the emotional tone of trauma so that the memory no longer sears or scares, some scientists are looking to go even further by developing a drug capable of completely erasing a frightening incident, or, for addicts, of wiping out a series of recalled ingrained associations and behaviours that they have been unable to shake.

Current memory research, then, reflects our own contradictory needs. We are, on the one hand, a society terrified of losing our past, while at the same time we seek the means to wipe our slates clean – if not the whole blackboard, then at least those nightmare scrawlings: whether it's the collective trauma of a serious terrorist attack or disaster or the personal trauma of the rape in the rain. We covet a memory scrubber so specific, so technologically savvy, that it can cleanse certain spots while leaving the rest of the plot untouched. At the moment this is just a dream, an ambition, what the scientists are stretching towards as they probe for ways of helping us navigate the minefield of memory, both when it wanes against our will and when it clings, keeping us spellbound by something we'd rather be rid of.

But just because scientists haven't yet managed to work all the magic we might wish for doesn't mean they haven't come up with some pretty amazing discoveries about memory. Alain Brunet, for example, a clinical psychologist at McGill University in Montreal, had a hunch about a common drug that he believed could be repurposed into a mental eraser. Unlike MDMA, which is illegal without a special permit and therefore impractical for scientists to obtain, Brunet's drug is readily available including in the United States and the UK. The drug is called propranolol, a commonly used beta blocker prescribed for those suffering from high blood pressure or, in other cases, performance anxiety. The drug works by blocking the action of the chemical noradrenaline, which is involved in arousing strong emotions, particularly during fight-or-flight mode. Brunet understood that traumatic memories retain their power because every time we recall the event, we reactivate our fear circuitry – the clammy hands, the rapid heartbeat, the high startle response. What would happen, Brunet wondered, if he could get traumatised subjects to recall their terrible and terrifying stories while simultaneously suppressing the fight-or-flight response that keeps the trauma potent?

Unlike MDMA, propranolol does not raise levels of oxytocin, a hormone that, as we've seen, promotes feelings of peace and love, but propranolol does inhibit adrenaline, thereby allowing trauma survivors to remember with less fear. In 2011 Brunet administered propranolol to nineteen traumatised patients, asking them first to write a detailed description of their trauma before ingesting the drug. He then waited one week and had his subjects return to his laboratory, whereupon he exposed them to their own written descriptions of the traumatic event. Subjects who had ingested a placebo appeared as traumatised as ever, but those who had taken the beta blocker seemed changed. Upon hearing their tales of trauma read out loud, they showed significantly reduced stress responses. Brunet and other scientists in the field believe that the beta blocker works to dilute traumatic memories by suppressing the fear and anxiety associated with them so that the memories no longer kick the amygdala – the fear centre in the brain – into overdrive.

While propranolol is not a 'forgetting tablet' – it doesn't destroy memory but instead alters its emotional overtones – it was a big advance and provided the platform for what came next. The following year, in 2012, when I first spoke to neuroscientist Todd Sacktor, he was busy studying the tiniest particles of chemical compounds associated with remembering and forgetting in a laboratory in Brooklyn. Sacktor's father was a biochemist who had suggested to his son, almost three decades earlier, that he should take a look at a group of molecules called protein kinase C. Sacktor listened to his father and began investigating the enzymes, taking three years first just to purify and isolate them before eventually discovering that PKMzeta, a type of protein kinase C, has a star role in making our memories work the way they do.

Fast Fading

Many people assume that memory works something like a camcorder, inscribing events on to the rumpled mass of our brain, where they either flare or fade, depending on their importance. This general conceit goes as far back as the ancient Greek philosopher Plato, who analogised memory to an impression in a wax tablet. The metaphor wended its way through the ages, tweaked and amplified as our understanding shifted, but remaining, at heart, a stable image that gave way to an enduring set of beliefs about how and why we recall what we recall. In the 1970s, memory researcher Elizabeth Loftus was one of the first to dismember the camcorder–wax stamp notion, proving that eyewitness accounts were wildly unreliable and subject to suggestibility. In one groundbreaking experiment, Loftus showed it was possible to get people to create memories of something that had never happened by proposing to them that they'd gotten lost in a shopping mall; she later listened to her unwitting subjects confidently detail the discombobulating incident that had not, in fact, occurred.

More recently, psychology professors William Hirst, of the New School for Social Research in New York, and Elizabeth Phelps, of New York University, conducted a study of flashbulb memories: intense recollections – including, for example, where you were when you learned something – associated with extreme events such as the assassination of John F. Kennedy or the explosion of the *Challenger* space shuttle. On 11 September 2001, almost every American citizen absorbed a flashbulb memory of two towers falling or of a low-flying plane against a brilliant blue sky, or of columns of smoke and ash. It was a tragedy that also provided an unprecedented opportunity to ascertain how immutable flashbulb memories really are.

Phelps and Hirst surveyed several hundred people about their 11 September recollections over a period of ten years, observing the subjects' memories deteriorate even as the subjects exhibited no clue that their deeply felt stories were morphing. All the participants whom Phelps and Hirst surveyed had formed a flashbulb memory of the 9/11 attacks. It turned out that most of the forgetting, which was manifested in errors of either omission or commission, occurred in the first year after the event. The deviations ranged from simple tweaks to wholesale revisions, and even in the case of extreme changes, the subjects were unaware that they were deconstructing and reconstructing what seemed, to them, a very stable story. Researchers believe that the act of repeating a narrative somehow contaminates it, meaning that nowhere in our brain do any permanent, unmarred memories reside, no matter how much it may feel that way. Their theory has since become a central concept in memory research. If you recall, let's say, your bat mitzvah on a day when you're feeling hungry, your memory will likely focus more on the sweet sandwiches served and less on your chanting the Haftarah, and that shift in mental weight alters the network of neurons in which the memory was encoded. Each subsequent recollection does the same. It's almost sad to learn this, to relinquish the idea that there are neural nooks where pieces of our past are stored, like a safe-deposit box to which we alone have the key. That's just not the way it works. Our memories, instead, are fragile and friable.

Brain Scrub

And so we return to Sacktor in his laboratory and his years-long inquiries into the role of PKMzeta. When we recall an event, it is because a series of linked neurons are sparking, firing, speaking to one another: the auditory portion of the memory is stored in the neurons in the auditory portion of our brains, the olfactory portion of the memory is linked to neurons in the olfactory portion of our brains, and the movement portion of the memory is tied to the neurons of our motor cortex. All these neurons connect to form the whole memory gestalt. Sacktor began to realise that PKMzeta, this enzyme, seemed always to be present in the brain, especially whenever cells were speaking to one another in the act of making memories, reaching out to one another across gaps between neurons to form the bridges that allow memory to exist, with one association cemented to another and in the process a person's past created.

In isolating and purifying PKMzeta, and in seeing its constant presence and activation in neuronal networks of memory, Sacktor sensed he was on to something. But what, exactly, was it? Was PKMzeta the golden grail of memory, *the* key chemical that allows us to retain our recollections? It seemed so, especially when a recent study in *Science* reported that adding more PKMzeta to the brains of rats strengthened their memory. Jerry Yin, a neuroscientist at the University of Wisconsin, did a related experiment with fruit flies to similar results. The higher the amount of PKMzeta in their systems, the longer they remembered. And Maria Eugenia

Velez, a physiology researcher at the University of Puerto Rico, has found that PKMzeta plays a critical role in creating and maintaining addictions, cementing the associations that lead to keen cravings and thereby embedding behaviours deep in the pliable paste of the brain.

Sacktor compares PKMzeta to a sheepdog, because the molecules do one thing in a perseverative fashion: they 'herd' AMPA receptors, which are membrane proteins crucial to receiving neural signals. Once the receptors are sandwiched between the nerve cells, it is the job of the memory molecule to make sure its AMPA receptors do not drift, thereby ensuring that memory remains cohesive during chemical cascades.

Recently, though, there have been some serious challenges thrown at Sacktor and at his PKMzeta theory of memory maintenance. Richard Huganir, director of the neuroscience department at Johns Hopkins University in Maryland, did a study in which he deleted two genes in embryonic mice, one a gene for PKMzeta and one a gene for a related protein called PKCzeta. Another researcher, Robert Messing, who runs a pharmaceutical laboratory at the University of Texas, also created mice that were missing critical memory genes. The results? The mice that had been genetically altered to produce no PKMzeta had no memory attenuation or loss at all. And Messing's mice, also missing critical memory genes, were able to recall objects and to form embedded memories for fears and for places with no trouble. The most telltale sign of a healthy memory is what scientists call 'long-term potentiation', which has to do with how strong the synapses between neurons grow. It's this characteristic that is considered the bedrock of all learning and memory development. And by this measurement as well, Huganir's mice demonstrated themselves to be at regular, standard levels.

Sacktor is not shaken by these challenges to his hypotheses. A graduate of Harvard and the Albert Einstein College of Medicine, he is supremely confident, a self-belief that likely powered him through the years prior to 2006, when only a small group of people paid attention to his work. In response to these recent studies, which have stirred questions about the crowning role of PKMzeta's relationship to memory, Sacktor argues that the results are 'not too surprising'. There may be a different gene that can explain why the mice were able to remember all that they did. In other words, memory may have a back-up system that shifts into gear when PKMzeta is compromised or lost. Specifically, Sacktor believes that the back-up system is generated by a molecule closely related to PKMzeta that is formed when PKMzeta is absent. 'It turns out that when PKMzeta is genetically eliminated in mice,' he wrote, 'another gene, called PKCiota/lambda, takes over PKMzeta's function for long-term memory storage.'

As confident as he is about his hypotheses, Sacktor is a man who continues to practise science with rigour. He said he hated school and was always the fat, shy, smart kid, the one who sought solace in books, in work. Therefore, while he believed, on the basis of his observations, that PKMzeta plays a critical role in memory formation and retention, he sought out a truly novel way to test his hypothesis. Sacktor used ZIP, zeta inhibitory peptide, which blocks PKMzeta, and then observed the results. He injected ZIP directly into the brains of one group of laboratory rats that had been trained to avoid the places in their cages where mild electrical shocks were delivered to their feet, and another group that had been trained to avoid foods they associated with nausea. The rats had quickly and thoroughly absorbed these lessons, carefully walking or trotting around their miniature minefields, the spatial memory clearly engraved in their brains.

Once ZIP went to work blocking PKMzeta in the rats' brains, however, Sacktor and his graduate students watched in awe as the memories came undone, amazed to see how the rats completely forgot about the charged places in their cages and the foods they had learned to dislike, chowing down on pellets they had learned to find disgusting and, perhaps more surprising, walking every which way and getting small shocks as a result, their memories having clearly been wiped out by ZIP, like some sort of cleanser for the brain. Unlike propranolol, which had a diffuse and subtle effect and which, most significantly, left the traumatic memories intact even as it diluted the emotional tone associated with them, ZIP completely nuked the memory, and *did so selectively*. In other words, the lab rats, which had also been trained to do a variety of tricks and to respond to an assortment of rings and dings, did not forget everything. They forgot only about the wired places in their cages and the negative associations with certain foods, suggesting that ZIP was not only a fine-tuned memory eraser but also some sort of memory editor, cutting out only certain spots in the rodents' brain. Sacktor and colleagues then went on to prove that ZIP did not cause damage, because afterwards the rats were able to relearn the lessons that ZIP had eradicated.

A rodent is a far cry from a human being, or at least it appears that way. Rats are 1/165th our size, their brains no bigger than our little finger pads. But while we look a lot different from white Wistar laboratory rats, our DNA is disturbingly similar. This means that there's a reasonable chance that a variant of ZIP could work in humans in some of the same ways and that we, thanks to Sacktor, may have in our hands the first real tablet designed for forgetting, to be used, to be used ... how?

Eventually the specific science works its way down to this vast amorphous philosophical question of how we might employ something as powerful as ZIP, as well as the ethical implications of having it at our disposal. Conceivably, the drug could be used for those with entrenched addictions, wiping out the associations of neurons that 'remind' the addict of his debilitating craving. Or it could be used after a traumatic event, allowing the survivor to bypass what could become post-traumatic stress disorder, a disorder of memory gone awry. It could be used, surprisingly, for chronic pain, which researchers have found is strongly linked to memory. ZIP could eradicate a person's memory of her own pain, thereby allowing some long-suffering souls deep and much-needed relief. Sacktor himself proposes that ZIP could be used in place of a cingulotomy, a procedure in which a small region of the brain is destroyed and along with it, or so it is hoped, the all-encompassing depression or obsession that has utterly ruined the patient's life. Instead of destroying that neural tissue, Sacktor said, 'ZIP might be injected to try to "reset" the synapses in that region.' This is something that could be attempted because ZIP spreads out only 1 to 2 millimetres from the point of injection.

And then there are the more nefarious potential uses: ZIP in the hands of governments determined to control their citizens in sinister ways. But we need not even go that far to encounter the potential problems. Post-traumatic stress disorder is devastating and can rob a person of years of productive living. But still, knowing that, would we actually want to scrub away experiences from the human brain? What would happen, for instance, if we were to edit the memories of a guilt-ridden criminal? Wouldn't he or she, finally freed from the troubling weight of a bad conscience, become more likely to repeat the crime? Might our bad memories be what tether us to good behaviour? Do our painful memories hold within them clues and cues about how to navigate our current and future circumstances, illuminating for us mistakes we don't wish to repeat? Furthermore, by completely removing even the most haunting occurrences, one is in a very real sense stripping a person of critical parts of his or her life story, and of the chance to make meaning of them, which is what humans strive for and part of what brings dignity to existence. It's possible that ZIP, in wiping out barbed memories, may take too much, or more than we can afford to lose if we humans hope to be humane.

Michael Mithoefer, the psychiatrist and researcher in South Carolina who ran trials in which MDMA was used to help trauma survivors overcome crippling post-traumatic stress disorder, is uncomfortable with the potential of a drug like ZIP. Unlike ZIP, MDMA doesn't stamp out the memory. Mithoefer's subjects took

MDMA and were infused with fond feelings and an expansive sense of well-being, and in this state talked about the trauma, thereby forging new neuronal connections around it. This seems a less problematic way of treating memory disorders: the person does not lose her experience but rather learns to rewrite its emotional overtones. With ZIP, overtones, undertones and chiaroscuro all go the way of the wind as the memory plunges down some black hole where, having disintegrated entirely, it ceases to exist. There are many who share Mithoefer's reservations. In the wake of an April 2009 *New York Times* article on Sacktor and PKMzeta, Nobel laureate and concentration camp survivor Elie Wiesel also expressed scepticism. 'I am somewhat hesitant to trust the proposed therapeutic means to use forgetting as a tool for healing,' he wrote. 'Once forgetting has begun, where and when should it stop?'

That we in all probability now possess the means to do this puts us, as human beings, in a position we've never been in before, powerful in a way we are likely not ready to be. But beyond the theoretical or philosophical questions, there are also problematic practical implications in losing your past, even just a piece. According to Daniel Schacter, a memory researcher at Harvard University in Massachusetts who feels we need the past in order to shape our future, 'a rapidly growing number of recent studies show that imagining the future depends on much of the same neural machinery that is needed for remembering the past.'

With all the potential drawbacks, one would think that a drug like ZIP would spook the average citizen. But this does not appear to be the case, at least to judge by a lot of the online comments from readers of the *New York Times* in response to an interview with Sacktor that ran on 13 April 2009, about a week after the initial piece:

I'm very interested in this. Is there a possibility it will be able to work in our lifetime? Or anytime soon? I am one of those who has gone through a tragic experience . . . I need to be able to erase my memories basically up to a year ago, or the rest of my life I will never be able to be social again . . . I want to know if this procedure could be possible anytime soon. – Zach

I will like to erase my memories. I've got a lot of anxiety problems and I suffer of depression. I tried to suicide myself like three times, I think you can help me. If you want to try that drug on human beings, I'm willing to be the first one. Please answer me quickly and thank you. – Francisco Velez

I would like to know if I can get my marriage erased. It's screwing up my life. All I think about is him and it's affecting my health. I want to forget about him. – Debra

Are you accepting human trials for this procedure? I would be willing to enter into this trial as I've had such significant trauma in my life that 25 years of therapy still can't erase. I suffer horribly from PTSD and my quality of life is practically nonexistent. – Connie Bergen

Ever been so traumatized by something that you couldn't leave your bed for weeks? couldn't speak for months? couldn't wake up in the morning without massive panic attacks, despite therapy and medication for years? . . . Makes it a bit difficult to function, never mind 'learn' from . . . I'd allow this to be tested on me in a second. No regrets. – Ciarabug

I would like to know how can I become a tester for such a thing. I truly need to erase my mem. IDC if it erases all of me so be it I just want to live anew without having traumatizing mems with me. – Lynette

I am weighed down every single day by one bad memory, I've considered suicide many times, please, if you are going to do any human trials in the future I will be more than happy to take part, it can't be worse than what I feel now. – T.

I have a son who was molested from the age of 6 to 16. The perp was found not guilty. His life is a wreck from this even with all the work he has tried, including being committed for extensive treatment that he wanted to try and move on. He wants to try this drug, what can be done so he could try to get his life back? – S. Smith

How far away are you from needing volunteers for a clinical study? I would be willing. I have a 2 year old memory I really need to erase. Just emotional, nothing criminal. – Bob T.

Please experiment on me! I want to erase my memory. – Stella

I want to volunteer for a human experiment of this memory erasing drug. I am 100% serious. I am willing to be a test subject for this product. Contact me via email. – Thomas

I would also like to be a part of the testing program for this process, if it's possible. I live in Los Angeles, but I will travel anywhere in the world for this opportunity and even pay for any expenses incurred during the process. Please contact me, thank you and God bless. – Richard

I personally believe this would be a very good thing for the general population . . . I would volunteer for a study myself. I would love to be able to be rid of some of my childhood memories that still haunt me and cause me to lose sleep and distract me from daily chores. – David M.

I am interested in your research. Please tell me if it is available and where in South Africa I can get this drug. I really need your help. – Tariro Vakisai

Memory Steroids

But now we come full circle, to where we started, with forgetfulness. So far there are still very few treatments for Alzheimer's, a disease discovered more than a century ago when Alois Alzheimer, a doctor working in a mental asylum in Germany, opened the skull of a recently deceased patient whose disorder had always eluded him. Slicing into her brain, Alzheimer found odd tangles of protein fibres and a sticky plaque called amyloid, so much that the organ was basically stuffed with a deadly jam that had been muffling her memories. In the end, the patient had been so incapacitated that she could not even swallow.

The good news is that if we may soon possess the ability to medicinally edit our histories, we also, simultaneously, may be able to do the opposite. While ZIP can nuke a memory, there's a good chance that PKMzeta can enhance it, a possibility that is only becoming more necessary. Barring a cure for Alzheimer's, by 2050 millions of people worldwide will suffer from this disease or some other age-related type of dementia. Neuroscientists are brainstorming ways to prompt cells to make more PKMzeta, the theory being that if the molecule is available to the brain in larger amounts, neuronal memory circuits might not decay. 'It's just an idea, at this stage,' Sacktor admits, but one can hear the excitement in his voice – and in the field.

The current drugs on the market for Alzheimer's just treat its symptoms rather than blocking the actual mechanism for the disease. At best they can only slow the process of memory loss for six months to a year. It's probably for this reason that the discovery of PKMzeta is so exciting. If scientists can figure out a way to make PKMzeta into a drug that causes the brain to produce more of the molecule, then we just might have, for the first time, a way of treating a devastating disease that haunts a huge population.

And scientists are doing more than searching for drugs in this expedition into memory. Recently, a technique called deep brain stimulation (DBS) has shown promise in treating people with memory disorders like Alzheimer's. Gwenn Smith, director of the geriatric psychiatry and neuropsychiatry division at Johns Hopkins, said that although the sample size of her study was only six, and it was designed mainly to establish safety, 'we don't have another treatment for [Alzheimer's] at present that shows such promising effects on brain function.'

Oddly, the idea of using DBS for memory disorders came about when scientists tried to use it to treat an obese man by implanting the electrode in the region of the brain thought to be associated with appetite suppression. The obese man did not get any thinner but, surprisingly, his memory expanded significantly, inspiring researchers to look towards electrical currents as well as chemicals in their search for dementia treatments. In a later study led by Andres M. Lozano, chair of the department of neurosurgery at the University of Toronto, an electrode was implanted in the brains of subjects suffering from Alzheimer's. The electrode emits continuous electrical impulses to the brain, and PET scans show that in patients with mild forms of Alzheimer's, there was a sustained increase in glucose metabolism. That finding was significant because a decrease in glucose metabolism accompanies Alzheimer's disease, which means that the electrodes and the current they emit are able to turn around one of the primary symptoms of this devastating syndrome.

Ours is of course not the first generation to be preoccupied with forgetting. In the sixteenth century, Jesuit missionary Matteo Ricci composed his *Treatise on Mnemonic Arts*, in which he explained the method of associating ideas with images and then locating those images in 'rooms', the result being a 'memory palace' that promised preservation of what is in fact ethereal human experience, made not of mortar but rather of gossamer. The memory palace is still used, especially by so-called memory champions, who train themselves to recall huge amounts of mostly arbitrary information (a sequence of cards, for instance) to compete in contests held around the world.

But you don't need to train for memory championships in order to help preserve your memory. Studies have shown that lesser efforts, including the much-touted crossword puzzle, can make a difference in helping us recall events. And more recent research suggests that continuing to learn new skills – playing an instrument, speaking a foreign language – into old age may be the best tonic for avoiding a misty mind. These new skills may help build new neuronal pathways in a brain that remains plastic until death. Learning keeps us curious – it's not the other way around – and curious people are more likely to have strong social networks (after all, you want to share what you've learned), which may also help ward off age-related dementia.

In the end – and of course there is an end, which we know only too well – we will succumb to the challenges of ageing, no matter how many of these advancements we make. It is this fact perhaps that drives the field of memory research, into which huge amounts of funding have lately been poured by a society that knows what lies in wait. There may very well come a time when purified molecules are made into medicines that can corral your fast-fading past and your problem-solving skills even as, on the other side of the line, 'editing' medicines can strike traumas from the mind. If or when this actually happens, we, as *Homo sapiens*, tool-building creatures for thousands of years, will have added significantly to our armamentarium. The question is whether we'll have the wisdom and savvy to know how to use these tools well. Given that, since at least the Industrial Revolution, humankind has shown it has a very hard time being responsible with its own inventions, one might say the outlook is grim, even while the science shines at its most exciting edge.

9

Deep Brain Stimulation

Who Holds the Clicker?

Prosthetics for the Brain

Mario Della Grotta was thirty-six years old when he first spoke with me, in 2005. He had a buzz cut and a tattoo of a rose on his right bicep, and wore a gold chain around a neck as thick as a thigh. He was the kind of guy you might picture in a pub in a working-class neighbourhood, a cigarette wedged in the corner of his mouth and a shot glass full of something amber. He seemed, at first appearance, like someone who swaggered his way through the world, but that wasn't true of Mario. Until four years earlier, his attempts to ward off panic meant that rituals could consume eighteen hours of every day. He couldn't stop counting and checking. Fearful of dirt, he would shower again and again. He searched for symmetries. Had he remembered to lock the car door? Had he counted things up correctly? His formal diagnosis was obsessive-compulsive disorder, which the French, with a phrase that aptly gets to the existential core of worry, call *folie du doute*, a clenched demonic doubting that overrides evidence, empiricism and plain common sense. For Mario, his entire life had been crammed into a single serrated question mark.

For fourteen years he had suffered anxiety so profound and so impervious to other treatments that finally his psychiatrists, at Butler Hospital in Providence, Rhode Island, suggested psycho-surgery, or what, in the current medical climate, has often been labelled more neutrally as neurosurgery for psychiatric disorders, to avoid the stigmatisation associated with lobotomies and, their newer version, cingulotomies. Older forms of psychosurgery have been used to treat anxiety disorders like obsessive-compulsive dis-order and its close cousin, depression, since the mid-1930s. Back then, any benefits people derived from the knife were perilously balanced against the flattening of feeling and the blanching of personality that accompanied the reduction in psychiatric ail-ments. This, however, may no longer be true. Tiny implants for the brain, originally developed in the 1990s to treat movement disorders in Parkinson's patients, are now being used on some of the most intractable but common psychiatric problems: anxiety and depression. Even two decades after they were first introduced, these neural pacemakers are still highly experimental and available only to patients who have been failed by every other treatment. Nevertheless, they suggest a time in the not-too-distant future when there may be options other than drugs available to serious sufferers of both disorders.

Unlike psychosurgeries of the past, this new procedure does not necessitate the destruction of neural tissue, the cutting of whole nerve tracts between here and there, like the taking down of phone lines. In place of that older method, surgeons are installing what amount to prosthetics for the brain: implanted electrodes. When correctly programmed, these electrodes – usually eight in total, four per hemisphere – emit a constant electrical current that, theoretically, jams pesky brain circuits, the ones that say *you're worthless, you're worthless, you're worthless* or *oh no, oh no, oh no.*

This was an idea that made sense to Mario. His experience of the illness was one terrible loop the loop. He said yes to the surgery, in part because he knew that if he didn't like the neural implants, he could simply have them switched off. And so Mario became one of the first American psychiatric patients to undergo this procedure.

Psychosurgery's Earliest Pioneers

Neural implants are not new; they are merely being revived. The first researcher to confirm that brain function, and by extension dysfunction, could be localised was the French neurologist Pierre Paul Broca, in 1861. Autopsying a patient who could say only one word – 'tan' – Broca identified organic damage to what he theorised was the speech centre. But it took seventy-five years, and a Portuguese neurologist by the name of Egas Moniz, to take Broca's theory of speech localisation and apply it to madness. Moniz, who would win a Nobel Prize for his invention of lobotomy, went through the halls of Lisbon's insane asylums looking for patients suitable for the frontal-lobe surgery, which Moniz's surgical colleagues performed, first via ether injections, with the alcohol essentially burning away the brain, and later with a leucotome, a device shaped like an ice pick, with a retractable wire to whisk out grey matter. It was a procedure for which Moniz had originally gotten the idea after a neurology conference in London, when he observed a chimpanzee that had been made docile by having its frontal lobes removed.

In 1936, shortly after the first lobotomies were performed in Lisbon, the procedure arrived in the United States, where it was adapted with all-American vigour, so much so that by the late 1950s, more than twenty thousand patients had had lobotomies and the surgery was being used to 'cure' everything from mental retardation to homosexuality to criminal insanity. Its most fervent promoter, Walter Freeman, eventually performed surgeries on multiple patients in an assembly-line fashion. Post-surgery, it was common for lobotomy recipients to be perpetually placid, carbon copies of themselves, faint and fuzzy.

Not many years after Moniz and his protégés began sawing through skulls, Robert Heath, among the first researchers to experiment with the use of implants in the treatment of psychiatric cases, was studying an alternate form of psychosurgery – deep brain stimulation, or DBS – at the Tulane University School of Medicine in Louisiana. Heath took patients culled from the back wards of the state's mental hospitals, slit open their skulls and dropped electrodes down deep inside them. He implanted more than a hundred electrodes in patients over a period of six years back in the 1950s, when psychosurgery was still an industry. With the use of a hand-held stimulator, Heath discovered that electrodes placed in the hippocampus, the thalamus or the tegmentum could produce states of rage or fear, while electrodes placed in the brain's septal area and part of the amygdala could produce feelings of pleasure. Heath 'treated' a homosexual man (identified as B-19) by firing electrodes into his pleasure centre while having him watch films of heterosexual encounters, and within seventeen days B-19 was a newly made man, proving it to Heath by sleeping with a female prostitute Heath himself had hired for this demonstration.

Whether the experiments were ethical or unethical, the motivations noble or ignoble, neural implants were significant right from the start, not only because they provided hope for the clinically distressed, but also because, by confirming Broca's theory of localisation, they began to change the way we collectively thought of the brain. Though he was misguided in some ways, Heath and researchers like him demonstrated that you could prod a tiny piece of cortical tissue and get a specific response, a taste of prune in the mouth, say, or a smear of yellow in the air. This was a major paradigm shift. In earlier centuries people had believed that thoughts and emotions were carried through the head via hollow tunnels, but now the brain became a series of discrete segments, real estate, if you will, some of it swampy, some of it stately, but all of it perhaps subject to human renovation.

Unlike lobotomies, those renovations were adjustable and did not have to be permanent. In a public demonstration at a bullring in Spain, another researcher, Yale's José Delgado, provoked an implanted bull with a matador's red cape. The enraged animal raced towards him, head down, stopping only at the very last second, when Delgado, with the push of a button, fired the implant and the bull, its aggression eradicated, loped away. The potential uses and abuses of neural implants were obvious: you could control people, and perhaps you could effectively wipe out violence.

By the late 1960s, implants appealed to those in the medical and law enforcement communities who believed that urban riots were born not of poverty or oppression but of 'violent tendencies' that could be monitored or altered. The US Law Enforcement Assistance Administration handed out large sums to researchers studying implants and other behaviour modification techniques. Under one such grant proposal, in 1972 Louis Jolyon West of University of California, Los Angeles (UCLA) was to form the Center for the Study and Reduction of Violence and conduct research at various state prisons. The plan was to take inmates, implant them and then monitor their brain activity after discharge. When a *Washington Post* reporter investigated this scheme, he discovered a precedent: in 1968 officials at California's Vacaville Prison performed electrode surgery on three inmates (including a minor) with the assistance of military doctors.

A series of Senate hearings in the mid-1970s brought these and other government forays into behaviour modification to the public's attention, and the public was more than a little perturbed at the notion of mind control as a viable solution to social injustice or crime. Meanwhile, the CIA was rumoured to be experimenting with implants to break down prisoners of war and discredit rebellious citizens (Heath admitted he'd been approached by the agency), and Michael Crichton's novel *The Terminal Man*, in which the main character receives implants to control his epilepsy and turns psychotic, became a bestseller. All this, concomitant with the rise of the antipsychiatry movement, ensured that neural implants fell into disrepute.

The Sweet Spot

Implants were resurrected, however, in 1987, when a French neuro-surgeon, Alim-Louis Benabid, operating on a Parkinson's patient, discovered that if he touched the patient's thalamus with an electrical probe, the patient's shaking stopped. A decade later, neural implants were approved by the US Food and Drug Administration (FDA) for treating tremors, dystonia and some forms of pain, and 150,000 patients worldwide have since been implanted for movement disorders.

But something else was being observed as well in those implanted Parkinson's patients. Many experienced positive mood changes, or felt their worries go away. It appeared the circuits that controlled their physical shaking were somehow connected to mental quaking as well. Remember how iproniazid, the precursor of the MAOIs, turned out to make tubercular patients happier and more energised in addition to curing their tuberculosis? 'It's how a lot of medicine happens,' neurosurgeon Jeff Arle of the Lahey Clinic in Burlington, Massachusetts, told me. 'It's by extrapolating backwards. Someone then has to have the chutzpah to say, "Gee, maybe we ought to try this for certain psychiatric problems." You believe it's worth the risk. You don't know until you try it.'

By the mid-1990s a small international group of psychia-trists, neurologists and neurosurgeons was considering using the implants for the treatment of mental illness. One of their primary questions is 'Where, precisely, in a psychiatric patient would one put the electrodes?' While Heath and Delgado had demonstrated that you can crudely trigger generalised states of affect – like terror and rage – by stimulating areas of the limbic system, no one had so far found those millimetre-sized snarls of circuitry where researchers hoped the more nuanced forms of mental health, or illness, resided. 'We want more than anything', said Helen Mayberg, a leading deep brain stimulation for depression researcher at Emory University, 'to find that sweet spot, and go there.'

If finding the exact loci of depression or obsession proves to be problematic, couldn't scientists simply override people's psychic pain by stimulating their pleasure centres? That would be too crude, neuroscientists believe, akin to getting patients high. Harold Sackheim, of the New York State Psychiatric Institute, added, 'If you can get relief without invasive surgery' – this procedure does come with a small chance of haemorrhage or infection – 'you might want to pursue that other avenue first.'

And just what is that other avenue? Tablets, of course. And we have pursued that avenue. For all our consumption, though, the risk of suicide associated with antidepressants is now considered serious enough for adolescents that the US government has mandated black box warnings on labels (like those on cigarette packets) alerting doctors and patients to the dangers. Equally compelling are data that suggests antidepressants leave a staggering number of users without any relief at all. 'We have searched and searched for the Holy Grail', said depression researcher William Burke of the University of Nebraska Medical Center, 'and we have never found it.' And that's true. In its tracking of the remission of symptoms for people suffering from depressive disorders, the US National Institute of Mental Health reports rates of 31 per cent after fourteen weeks and 65 per cent at six months. But according to John Halpern, even of the 65 per cent who are helped, only 30 per cent of those, meaning fewer than 20 per cent of patients taking the drugs, feel robust relief. The rest get some symptom relief and limp along. Doctors advise the limpers to switch or combine drugs, but between 10 and 20 per cent of patients never improve no matter what medicines they take.

Mario, who'd tried some forty different combinations of medications, knew this all too well. He wanted a shot at the ordinary, a lawn he might mow just once a week. The ability to endure the mess and touch of children. He decided the implants were well worth the risk.

The Surgery

On a Monday in early February 2001, as Mario woke up next to his pregnant wife, neurosurgeons at Butler Hospital in Rhode Island were getting ready for his operation. A week or so before, in preparation for his surgery, Mario had gone to a tattoo artist and had the Chinese sign for 'child' inked into his wrist. 'If I didn't make it, if I never got to see my daughter be born, then at least I would have this tattoo,' he told me. 'Child. With it on my skin, I knew I could go to the grave with some meaning.'

Once in the operating theatre, Mario was given a local anaesthetic. His head had been shaved, his brain targeted to millimetre precision by MRIs. Attached to his head was a stereotactic frame to provide surgeons with precise coordinates and mapping imagery. He'd undergone extensive neuropsychological testing to determine where to put the implants and to provide a pre-operative baseline of functioning. Surgeons choose the brain targets on the basis of results of past lobotomies and cingulotomies, noting which lesions brought with them relief. The problem is, all sorts of lesions have attenuated anxiety and depression in desperate patients, lesions to the left or right, up or down, here or there. Without a single sweet spot, the possibilities are disturbingly numerous. No one in his right mind would get on a ship if the captain wasn't sure where to steer. But of course that's the point. Psychiatric patients who have this surgery are no longer truly in their right mind. They get on board because this is their last lifeboat.

At Butler, where Mario's procedure was done, the doctors put the implants in the anterior limb of the internal capsule. Other neurosurgeons in the past, however, have favoured the cingulate gyrus and still others the caudate nucleus. These are parts of the brain that reside in the limbic system, which is itself folded up under the frontal lobes. Helen Mayberg's target, called Area 25, the subgenual cingulate, is in front of the anterior limb, the same target for Benjamin Greenberg, one of Mario's psychiatrists, and for Don Malone of the Cleveland Clinic in Ohio. 'We chose the anterior limb', Malone told me, 'because that's where the electrodes fit the best', a slightly unnerving comment, revealing as it does the somewhat arbitrary nature of the way these decisions sometimes get made.

Success

After surgery, a deep brain stimulation patient will be retested with core questions in mind. Have the symptoms improved, deteriorated, or stayed the same? Since these electrodes were implanted, how has cognitive functioning changed, if at all? As of 2017, about seventy people in the United States had received deep brain stimulation to treat obsessive-compulsive disorder. In a sample of twenty-six patients that Greenberg conducted with colleagues worldwide, 73 per cent had a reduction of at least 25 per cent of their score on the Yale-Brown Obsessive Compulsive Scale. Some of those experienced a complete remission of symptoms of severe anxiety. Despite the success rate, and Greenberg's efforts to reach out to clinicians and recruit patients for the clinical trial, the number of people undergoing the procedure has not grown quickly. 'In the real world', Greenberg said, 'the group of patients meeting appropriate selection criteria is truly small.'

As for depression, the story is different. There have been about four times as many patients who have undergone deep brain stimulation for treatment-resistant depression, with Helen Mayberg of Emory University in Georgia participating in many of these surgeries. Mayberg's earliest deep brain stimulation procedures, performed on six patients, took place in Toronto. Mayberg placed the electrodes in the white matter of Area 25, believing that this region played a critical role in modulating negative mood states. Supporting her hypothesis is the fact that SSRIs and other anti-depressant medications appear to work by decreasing activity in Mayberg's targeted area. All six of her patients reported 'acute effects' while in the operating theatre and under the influence of the current. Among the descriptions was a feeling of 'lightness, a disappearance of the void'. The room in which the patients lay seemed suddenly brighter to them, their vision sharper. At home, family members noticed increased energy, a renewal of interest in activities that had before seemed impossible, and the ability to plan and to initiate, both of which become dulled by depression. At the one-month follow-up, two of the six implanted patients no longer met the criteria for depression; after two months, five of the six patients had improved. At the six-month follow-up, Mayberg found that a strong antidepressant reaction continued in four of her six implanted subjects, a two-thirds response rate which suggested that deep brain stimulation could be an effective intervention for severe treatment-resistant depression as well as obsessive-compulsive disorder, an 'extremely encouraging' result, according to Mayberg.

Her study was expanded to a total of twenty patients, all of whom had treatment-resistant depression and who were followed by researchers for a one-year period. In this larger study, 60 per cent of patients responded to deep brain stimulation after a six-month period, and 55 per cent of patients were responders at one year. After three years of chronic stimulation, researchers found a 60 per cent response rate and a 50 per cent remission rate. Encouraged once more by her results, Mayberg continued to implant people with severe treatment-resistant depression. Beginning in 2008 she broadened her sample to include those suffering from bipolar II depression as well, and initially implanted thirty such patients.

Area 25

Mayberg has been studying the brain for decades, trying to find the circuit or circuits responsible for depression. She started by looking at the brains of depressed Parkinson's patients using PET scans and from there went on to people without Parkinson's but with severe depression. She has homed in on what she calls Area 25, a region in the brain that shows enhanced activity when a person is depressed, along with a decrease of activity in the frontal and limbic regions, brain areas that allow us to reason, emote, remember and learn. When Mayberg studied people whose depression improved on an antidepressant, she found that their depressed frontal-lobe activity rose while the activity in Area 25 dropped. She researched non-depressed subjects who were asked to think about sad memories while undergoing a brain scan. Her results were incredibly consistent. Non-depressed subjects ruminating on depressing thoughts had a decrease of activity in their frontal lobes and an increase of activity in that pesky little Area 25, which clearly plays a significant role in whether or not we find joy in our day-to-day existence. Mayberg believes that in treatment-resistant patients, activity in Area 25 stays high and activity in the frontal lobes stays low despite our usual array of medicines and shock. 'If we couldn't talk depression down, couldn't drug it down, couldn't shock it down,' she said, 'then I believed we could go directly to Area 25 of the brain and tune it down.' Given the fact that she is placing electrodes in a region of the brain she has been studying for decades, Mayberg does not consider herself a risk taker. She has done, so far, more than two hundred implantations, with ever-increasing precision and, therefore, a higher rate of clinical success.

Recently she has turned her attention towards precisely how deep brain stimulation achieves its outcomes. She is not a localist when it comes to thinking about the brain. She does not believe, for instance, that overactivity in Area 25 is simply and solely responsible for our down days. 'I never thought depression was just about Area 25,' she said. 'It's always been about communication between multiple brain regions.' Mayberg's sense of Area 25 is that it's like a 'junction box' for the parts of the brain that work together to mitigate the effects of negative mood and depression.

In addition to the more than two hundred implantations in which she has participated, she knows of ninety other implantations that have focused on Area 25 and roughly eighty that have focused on different brain regions. One, which Mayberg was not a part of, involved a middle-aged Dutch patient who, in 2013, had endured twenty-two years of psychiatric treatment before deciding to try deep brain stimulation for his addiction to heroin. He underwent the surgery at the University of Amsterdam, where researchers drilled holes on either side of his skull and inserted long probes with electrodes attached at their ends. The researchers positioned the electrodes in his nucleus accumbens, a region of the brain thought to be responsible for addictions and their associated cravings. After the electrodes were placed, connecting wires were run to battery packs embedded in his chest. When the electrodes were turned on, they emitted constant current, with the goal of disrupting the brain circuit that researchers hypothesise is involved in addiction. In the beginning the electrodes actually appeared to increase the patient's craving for heroin – he practically doubled his dose – but once researchers were able to adjust the electrodes and the timing of the pulses they emitted, the man experienced a real diminishment of his cravings, and his use of heroin, while it did not stop entirely, dwindled to nearly nothing.

The Dangers

In addition to the now roughly 150,000 people who have been treated with deep brain stimulation for movement disorders, as of 2017 more than five hundred people around the world had received experimental implants to treat various psychiatric disorders. On the one hand, one could argue that a mere five hundred people worldwide in the last fifteen or so years does not indicate a treatment that's very promising for being used with any frequency, especially when one considers how much people have to go through beforehand simply to be eligible for the procedure. However safe psychosurgery is, then, some may feel that it does not present a real, viable alternative to psychotropic drugs, at least not for very many people. On the other hand, we would do well to remember that fully 30 per cent of depressed patients do not respond to any antidepressant treatment whatsoever. That's an awful lot of people. That translates into not only millions of pounds in lost productivity in a society but also, at its most extreme, a tragic number of suicides. Seen in this light, deep brain stimulation for psychiatric disorders achieves a real relevancy. While it is not common right now, with more research it could become so. It offers an alternative, and with that a slice of hope, to those whose suffering continues unabated.

Unfortunately, while many times the news is good, there are also plenty of patients who have experienced adverse events: suicidal thoughts and feelings, completely unmotivated homicidal rage, or its opposite, extreme apathy, or sleep disorders, a worsening of depression, sudden panic attacks. One patient who participated in the Broaden Trial for Deep Brain Stimulation at UCLA experienced such severe side effects he nearly lost his life. Watching television one night, he suddenly got up and poured boiling water all over himself, acting as if he were an automaton. Another time he felt compelled to slash his body with a knife, laughing hysterically as the wounds dripped blood. This patient, who asked that his name not be used, had the device removed but feels that his brain has been irreparably harmed in the process. 'I wrote an email to [Emory University], saying, "You're involved in studies of DBS effects. So, study me. There are people falling off the boat and you're not circling back to rescue them. Circle back and see what's going wrong." I didn't hear back.'

Doctors are understandably anxious to separate deep brain stimulation from psychosurgeries of the past, when ice pick-like instruments were thrust up through the eye sockets, and blades swished through the brain. While the finer points of brain functionality are still hazy, the surgery itself is conducted with far more precision and technological finesse than Moniz or Heath could ever have hoped for. Yet some facts remain the same. There is a gruesome quality to any brain surgery. The drill is huge; its twisted bit grinds through bone, making two burr holes on either side of the skull.

The drilling into Mario's skull was over in a few minutes. Surgeons then took a couple of hours to get the implants in place. As is the practice with brain surgery, Mario remained awake throughout and he was repeatedly questioned: 'Are you okay? Are you alert?' His head was held in place by a steel halo that screwed into his skull bone in six places. The surgeon threaded two wires just 1.27 millimetres thick through the burr holes on which the tiny platinum-iridium electrodes were strung. Picture it as ice fishing. There is the smooth bald lake, the hole opening up, dark water brimming around the aperture and then the slow lowering of the line, the searching, searching, for where the fish live.

Mario felt none of this because the brain itself, the seat of all sensation, has no sensory nerves. Next the surgeons implanted two 5 × 7.5-centimetre (2 × 3-inch) battery packs beneath each of Mario's clavicles and ran wires from the packs (the batteries of which have to be replaced every few months) up under the skin of his neck to the implants. The packs, controlled by a remote programming device, power the electrodes when the doctor flips the switch and adjusts the current. Mario lay there, waiting.

He would have to wait a while. Psychiatrists do not turn the electrodes on right after surgery. That happens later, when the swelling in the head has gone down, when the bruised brain has had a chance to heal itself and the burr holes have been sealed with new skin. At that time Greenberg would pass a programmer over Mario's chest, and the wires would leap to life.

Poised for a Comeback

With the re-emergence of neural implants, the only malleable and reversible form of psychosurgery, and the development of high-tech imaging devices and stereotactic equipment that allow for impressive precision, psychosurgery is poised to make a comeback, to step out of the pall cast by the early lobotomisers into a circle of respectability and, more importantly, possibility. Now a patient can potentially reap the very real benefits bestowed by psychosurgery without having to undergo the dulling personality changes associated with broad frontal-lobe ablation and the irreversibility of a lesion. If this seems a far-fetched notion, it's good to remember that, at one time, so did the first open-heart surgeries and organ transplants, procedures that are now performed daily.

But psychosurgery's potential comeback, its growing social acceptance, is not due only to the new flexibility of its treatments. It's also likely rooted in our growing collective realisation of the limitations of drugs and our frank disenchantment with the companies that make them. Both in the United States and the UK, we spend a huge fortune every year on psychiatric medications, even though we now know that SSRIs come with serious warnings and offer no relief at all to 30 per cent of users. We know that the companies producing these drugs claim that their high cost to consumers is justified by the research and development that is necessary, and yet, as we've seen, few if any truly original drugs have been introduced in the past few decades. Most so-called new drugs are what the industry designates 'me too' drugs, slight variations on the successful drugs already on the market, with an eye towards adapting them into one that can become a profit centre. What's more, we've learned that drug companies sometimes selectively publish only the studies with favourable results, a serious lie by omission. We also know how drug companies court doctors at conferences by paying for posh hotel rooms and other high-end goodies. We have seen companies push their sales reps to sell medications – Pfizer's gabapentin sold under the brand name Neurontin comes to mind – for uses that are almost entirely untested. How can you trust a tablet if you can't trust its progenitor?

When psychosurgery first came into vogue in North America, Walter Freeman and his cohort performed assembly-line lobotomies, going from clinic to clinic plucking patients who kicked and screamed their way to the operating table, sometimes even renting out hotel rooms for the procedure. There were no internal review boards, no ethics committees and no solid scientific studies backing the work itself. Most importantly, there was no concern with patient consent. Rather there were simply fervent testimonials from patients like Harry Drucker, who claimed, in 1938, 'Psychosurgery cured me.' And it did cure some people, or at least tweaked their lives for the better, but the cost was sometimes huge, and the damage to human dignity could be appalling. Some psychosurgery patients were made incontinent by the procedure, or worse, they lost what Moniz called their 'vital spark'.

Contemporary psychosurgeons fervently want to sidestep the excesses of the early lobotomisers such as Freeman, and have exerted tremendous efforts to separate themselves from their shady forebears. Much as today's proponents of psychedelic drugs are aware of the importance of public perception, psychosurgeons are conscious of the need to project a polished image so as not to be viewed in a dark or suspicious light. It is true, on the one hand, that it is impossible to use animal testing to gauge whether deep brain stimulation can effectively treat depression and anxiety, which means the only guinea pigs available are people like Mario. But in order for Mario to be eligible for neural implants, he not only had to have tried and exhausted every available pharmacological option at either optimal or above-optimal doses, but also had to have undergone at least twenty hours of behaviour therapy and submitted to multiple rounds of ECT. He had to understand the risks and implications of the procedure and provide his consent.

His case was reviewed by three different review boards. The US Food and Drug Administration, which regulates medical devices, gave its blessing to this experiment. 'We don't want to repeat the mistakes of the past,' said Greenberg, who in particular seemed haunted by the circus sideshow history of lobotomies. 'We want to be sure this therapy is not only not used indiscriminately, but that it is reserved for the group of people who have failed trials of everything else.'

Why so much precaution? After all, when you take a drug, you are arguably altering your brain in ways at least as profound as, if not more than, with neural implants. And when you take combinations of drugs, as many mentally ill people do, you put yourself at risk for medication-induced Parkinson's and a raft of other serious outcomes. 'That's true,' Greenberg told me. 'Look, I agree with you.' But his agreement didn't cancel out his caution. For him, the past did not feel far away.

Getting in Tune

After three weeks, Mario went back to Greenberg's office. The men sat facing each other, Greenberg with the programmer on his lap. He snapped open the laptop-like device and, using a hand-held controller, activated the implants. Mario remembered the exact moment they went on. 'I felt a strange sadness go all through me,' he said, and recalled Greenberg's fingers tapping on the keyboard, adjusting the current, pulse duration and frequency. After a few taps, the sadness went away. 'With DBS the thing has a certain immediacy to it,' said Steven Rasmussen, Mario's other former psychiatrist. 'You can change behaviour very, very rapidly. On the flip side of it there's a danger too. This really is a kind of mind control.'

This is a rare admission. For the most part, researchers insist deep brain stimulation has nothing to do with mind control or social shaping. They are simply psychiatrists targeting symptoms, they say. These doctors have seen severe psychiatric anguish and know that its remission is always a blessing. But of course any time a psychiatrist tries to tweak a patient's mind, he or she does so in accordance with social expectations.

Tap, tap. Mario felt a surge inside him. Later, outside, he peered at the world turned on, turned up, and indeed it did look different, the grass a cheerful green, the daffodils a bright yellow. When he went home, Mario wanted to talk. He had things to do. Who needed sleep?

'You're like the Energizer bunny,' his wife said to him.

'I feel revved,' Mario agreed.

Mario is not the only person to have become a little too happy on the wire. 'That's one of the dangers,' Greenberg said. Don Malone concurred: 'We don't want hypomania. Some patients like that state. It can be pleasurable. But this is just like having a drug prescription. We decide how much, when and how.'

But it's not the same as a drug prescription. A patient can decide to take no drugs, or five drugs. A patient can split his drugs with his spouse, feed them to the dog or switch to a different psychopharmacologist. Despite prescription regulations, there is tremendous freedom in being a 'pill popper'. Not so for those with implants. True, no longer is anyone dragged to the operating table in terror. No one is cut without exquisite and careful consideration both beforehand and during the procedure. Instruments have been honed, imaging devices advanced. And yet patients do not, cannot fully understand or appreciate the degree to which they will be under their doctor's control after the surgery. Once a month deep brain stimulation patients must visit their psychiatrist for what are called adjustments. (For depression patients, however, Mayberg said the rule is 'set it and forget it'.) Adjustment decisions – altering what are commonly called the 'stimulation parameters' – reflect how the patient scores on a subjective paper-and-pencil test of symptom intensity, but ultimately control lies with the treatment provider.

At a 2004 meeting of the President's Council on Bioethics,

when Massachusetts General Hospital neurosurgeon and Harvard University professor G. Rees Cosgrove concluded his presentation on the issues surrounding deep brain stimulation, another Harvard professor asked him, 'Who holds the clicker?'

Cosgrove's answer: 'The doctor.'

Long-Term Prospects and Conundrums

Mario's good mood continued. He had obsessions and compulsions, but they were smaller, and were dominated by the grand energy that saturated his existence. For two weeks he saw Greenberg every day. Greenberg adjusted the settings, turning the frequency, current and pulse up or down. Sometimes, as a setting was changed, Mario felt that peculiar wash of sadness. Then he evened out.

Six weeks went by. Mario's daughter Kaleigh was born. She was a textbook-perfect case of a baby; she screamed, she pooed, she drooled, her entire unregulated being was a little vortex of chaos. When Mario changed her nappy and saw the golden smear, in his heart he backed up – way up. He had cleaning compulsions after all. Over the next few months, his mood started to dip. He had a terrible time feeding the baby. Sometimes it seemed it took him so long to give her breakfast that it would be time for lunch already, and he'd have to start all over again. Perfect. It had to be perfect. The baby, strapped in the high chair, screamed, with squash all over her mouth. *Wipe that up*, he thought. *Right away*. He was better, yes, but not enough.

Mario went back to see Greenberg. Over a span of a few months, with Mario reporting the waxing and waning of his symptoms, Greenberg eventually got the setting right. Mario began to pick up dirty things. It was, at last, okay.

When Mario spoke about that time in his early days of recovery, tears came to his eyes. 'It was like a miracle,' he said. 'I still have some OCD symptoms but way, way less. Drs Greenberg and Rasmussen saved my life. Sometimes they travel to conferences together on the same plane. I tell them not to do it. It makes me very nervous. Who would adjust me if the plane went down? No one else in this country knows how to do it. It's like the president and the vice president travelling together.'

The hopes of implant makers, like Minneapolis-based Medtronic, the first developer of the neural electrodes, are as big as the market they imagine. They forecast a day when neural implants will treat a wide variety of psychiatric problems, from eating disorders to substance abuse to schizophrenia. Yet as these devices proliferate, so too will the ethical twisters that swirl around them. Can a severely mentally ill patient provide informed consent? Whose head is it, after all? By directly manipulating the brain, might we turn ourselves into white appliance technicians, programming speed cycles and rinses? Could it be possible to actually control the content of another person's thinking, as opposed to merely his or her affective states? And setting aside these sci-fi concerns, should doctors wade into apparently healthy brain tissue when they have yet to precisely locate mental pathology?

It isn't just critics of the procedure who worry. Even advocates of brain implants concede that the ethical issues can be thorny. At that same 2004 meeting, Cosgrove, who believes the procedure holds great promise, acknowledged the dilemmas, such as there being no possibility of large-scale, placebo-blind trials. 'We don't understand how deep brain stimulation works,' he admitted. 'We are not clear what the optimal targets are. We don't even know what the optimal stimulation parameters are, and we don't know what the long-term effects are ... It's not as simple as we make it out to be.'

And beyond all of these questions, some critics worry that rather than curing problems antidepressants have been unable to address, the implant industry could simply duplicate the problems that have scandalised the pharmaceutical world. Despite the extremely cautious way neurosurgeons and psychiatrists are going about using the implants in the treatment of anxiety and depression, and despite their impressive results, fears continue to hover that deep brain stimulation could fall into the hands of the state, or overworked prison systems, and be used as a management device. After all, both of these things nearly did happen in the last century. 'It's easy for any good neurosurgeon to do this now,' Cosgrove himself pointed out. 'That's the dangerous part – it's easy.' And if it's easy, what will stop neurosurgeons both mercenary and curious from performing these operations on people clamouring for relief? How long until implants are used to treat milder forms of mental illness? To take this one inevitable step further, what will stop people from pursuing implants for augmentation purposes? Cosgrove described one patient, for instance, who became more creative after implantation. We've heard much of this before, in the great 'Prozac: better than well' debate, but twenty-five years after Peter Kramer's influential book, people do not seem better than well. The promise of fluoxetine has faded. Chances are that neural implants may prove to be every bit as disappointing.

For Mario Della Grotta, however, it was simple. 'I've had a hard life,' he said. 'My parents got divorced. My father died. I broke my foot. I have OCD.' He paused. 'But', he said, 'I have been helped.'

Back in 1958, Swedish surgeon Åke Senning installed the world's first implantable cardiac pacemaker, which made some people nervous. The first patient, then forty-three, went on to live a further forty years, and now, pacemakers, like open-heart surgery and organ transplants, are, if not common, at least not unusual. Perhaps there will come a time when neural prosthetics will seem just as banal, when we will view the brain and its surgical manipulations without awe and hand-wringing. And yet the scary potential exists for a surgeon to acutely and immediately make memories evaporate, dreams rise, fingers freeze, hope sputter. For while it's true that we are not entirely our kidneys, we do live entirely within the circle of our skull.

For Mario, this was all armchair philosophising, irrelevant to his situation. 'I don't care what it means,' he said. 'I care that

I'm better. I'm not all better, but I'm better.' So much better that eventually he would let the batteries to his implants run down on occasion, though whether this indicated a deep brain stimulation cure or just an obsessive-compulsive disorder remission, Greenberg said, it was far too soon to tell.

Either way, Mario was proud of his progress after the procedure. His wife had given birth to their second child in the intervening years. He carried with him pictures of his young daughter, a beautiful girl. She and Mario used to play 'tent' in the morning, climbing under the quilts, where he showed her shadow puppets. A flying bird. A crawling spider. This is the chapel, this is the steeple, open it up and here are the people. While his wife showered and water hit the walls with a sound like static and cars roared outside on the roads, under the quilted tent, so close to his daughter, Mario could hear her breathe. He was not afraid to hold her hand. Some might say that Mario, with his implants, agreed to a strange sort of bondage, but he didn't think so. He would say he had been freed enough to love.

Epilogue

Where We're Headed

It all depends on whom you ask. Jeffrey A. Lieberman touts a psychiatry that has finally become truly scientific, a psychiatry that has unfettered itself from the shackles of Freud, whose theories were rooted in pure conjecture, and is embracing high-tech tools that put the profession on par with other medical subspecialties. We're seeing a psychiatry hitched to PET scans and fMRIs, machines that allow doctors to peer beyond the bony casement of the skull, catching glimpses into memory, into speech, into fear, into love. The psychiatry of the future will use these tools, and others, to become ever more intimate with our minds, and will be practised by doctors with the ability to saw open the scalp and place tiny electrodes powered by battery packs into regions of the brain that may be responsible for our mental distress.

The brain is cunningly complex, with more neuronal connections, some say, than there are stars in the Milky Way, making it one of the most intricate pieces of architecture in the known universe. How, then, will we ever truly master it? Can the brain understand the brain, or do we need a higher intelligence to interpret our grey matter? And what would that higher intelligence be? Some sort of supercomputer with enough bandwidth and RAM and processing speed to outwit us as it interprets us, explaining, finally, the aetiology of the disorders that cause chaos in our lives, disorders about which current-day psychiatry still knows so little?

What, for instance, causes schizophrenia? How durable is the dopamine hypothesis, and what does it mean that when it comes to schizophrenics, drugs which dampen dopamine seem to diminish hallucinations and drugs that increase dopamine appear to make schizophrenic symptoms worse, even though, when researchers compare dopamine levels in so-called normal subjects with those in schizophrenic subjects, they find no correlation between high dopamine levels and psychiatric problems in the general population? Perhaps more compellingly, the low-serotonin story suffers the same fate. We have been told that depression and obsessive-compulsive disorder are the result of too little serotonin in the brain, and that this is the reason why serotonin-boosting drugs such as fluoxetine work. But some depressed people have a lot of serotonin while some well-adjusted people have less.

The psychiatry of the future would be able to address these phenomena. The psychiatry of the future, an ideal psychiatry that exists perhaps only in my mind, would finally be able to point to some lesion, some spurt, some crooked molecule or cracked neural pathway amenable to repair by tonic or surgery or even just by exercise. The cure itself matters less to me than the knowledge of the aetiology, a psychiatry in which disorders can finally become diseases attached to tissue samples, blood in a test tube, the delicate cells that live in the lining of our cheeks. Perhaps the psychiatry of the future would have a good enough handle on genes to predict with satisfying accuracy who was in for what sort of trouble on the basis of his or her DNA.

Almost a century ago, in the early 1930s, neurosurgeon Wilder Penfield opened up the skull of his epileptic patient and touched the patient's brain with a probe. Despite the fact that the patient's skull was sawed open like a pumpkin, the top cut off in a circle, the patient was awake and alert. Penfield moved the probe around to different parts of the brain. When he touched the motor cortex, his patient's toes curled up, and when he tickled the speech centre, the patient began to babble. He was able to stimulate memories of sights, sounds and smells. Imagine, under Penfield's ministrations, a patient weeping while recalling a low stone wall, or, as he moved his probe to the left, aching with anger. This was one of the first demonstrations of brain specificity, proof that this roughly 1.4-kilogram (3-pound) organ is a series of regions, each one responsible for different things, all of them linked together in a stunningly elaborate network. Laughter lives in some spot in our brain. Memory is tricky and notoriously unreliable, but it has its physical place too. Memories hide in the hippocampus and then get uploaded for long-term storage as if to a friable file cabinet corroded by rust and holes. The psychiatry of the future should fully understand these places, and know how a short-term recollection graduates to a memory so meaningful and solid that it can survive the ravages of Alzheimer's.

But right now this is all a dream. While some, like Lieberman, feel they are part of a rejuvenated profession that has sloughed off Freud and solidly stepped into science, other psychiatrists, such as Daniel Carlat, who discusses how psychiatrists can be paid to push certain psychotropics, question why psychiatrists should even go to medical school, seeing as most of what they actually do is prescribe drugs they don't understand in fifteen-minute sessions. Indeed, in the future, psychiatry might become diffuse, giving up its status consciousness, as we might be getting our drugs not only from psychopharmacologists but also from psychologists, some of whom already have prescribing privileges in several states in the United States. Besides, any honest psychopharmacologist will tell you that when he or she prescribes, it's largely a guessing game – could be escitalopram or could be citalopram; there are fluoxetine doctors and then there are those who prefer paroxetine as their first response to fear or despair. And since there are plenty of patients to go around, if prescribing drugs remains a guessing game, it seems there is no good reason not to let others in on it.

I'm a psychologist by training, but I'd rather not have prescribing privileges in the future, even though that might be good for my bank account. The fact is, if I were to get prescribing privileges, psychiatry would have failed its mission as a science and, more importantly, as a *medical* science. I'd rather see psychiatry come up with a few theories that finally pan out, theories that illuminate the pathophysiology or aetiology of depression, the structure of schizophrenia, the reason for the retreat that autism so often is. The field has a history of practitioners who have developed theories, some of them quite compelling, but they have all proved to be wrong, or misguided, or not quite enough.

There was, for instance, the monoamine theory of depression which I discussed earlier – the idea that depression is the result of a deficit of monoamines, which are neurotransmitters such as dopamine, epinephrine, noradrenaline, and serotonin. But the monoamine hypothesis did not survive as a theory for at least three reasons. First of all, drugs that raise levels of monoamines in the human brain do so immediately, and yet their effects can take six to eight weeks before becoming apparent in a patient, a discrepancy for which the hypothesis has never been able to adequately account. Beyond that, the monoamine hypothesis fails to explain why some antidepressants, such as the tricyclic iprindole, have had success despite the fact that they do not raise the levels of any of the brain's monoamines. Finally, once fluoxetine and its chemical cousins were released, the monoamine hypothesis was replaced with the somewhat simpler serotonin hypothesis, which posits that depression and obsessive-compulsive disorder are the result of low levels of this single neurotransmitter. And yet the serotonin hypothesis suffers from the same weaknesses as the monoamine hypothesis, namely, that it too cannot adequately explain why the drug raises serotonin immediately and yet it can take the patient sometimes as long as eight weeks to feel better. Nor can it explain why not all depressed people have low serotonin when the neurotransmitter is measured in cerebrospinal fluid.

Lacking blood, tissue, or cells, psychiatry has had no choice but to retreat into pure description. Because the field cannot hold up a test tube of blood and find within it, say, the virus or low levels of a neurotransmitter that cause despair or delusions, it has instead relied solely on symptoms, absent any known cause. Groups of psychiatrists are constantly working to delineate the symptoms of various mental illnesses, and their work is recorded in the *Diagnostic and Statistical Manual of Mental Disorders*. The first *DSM*, published in 1952, was full of psychoanalytic language, neurotic nail-biting patients labelled as, say, reactive depressives, in concert with the dominant view of the day. Since 1952 there have been multiple iterations of the *DSM*, about once a decade, give or take, with diagnoses appearing, disappearing and transforming. The result is a slippery sort of manual. Theodore Millon, the founding editor of the *Journal of Personality Disorders* and one of the members of the committee charged with assembling the third *DSM*, published in 1980, admitted that 'the amount of good, solid science upon which we were making our decisions was pretty modest'. It wasn't that there was no research whatsoever, but rather that it was, in Millon's words, 'a hodgepodge – scattered, inconsistent and ambiguous.'

In the early 1970s, Stanford University professor and psychologist David Rosenhan devised an ingenious experiment to illustrate the flimsy nature of the psychiatric diagnosis. He rounded up seven colleagues, plus himself, and they dispersed to various mental hospitals around the country, whereupon they presented themselves as hearing a voice that said 'thud', 'empty' and 'hollow'. This was the sole symptom that these pseudo-patients complained of; they otherwise acted completely normal. On the basis of this single 'symptom', all eight of the pseudo-patients were admitted with a diagnosis of schizophrenia, with the exception of one who was diagnosed with manic-depressive psychosis. The pseudo-patients were held on their respective wards for an average of nineteen days, during which time they acted as they always did. They took notes, which the staff tended to consider part of their pathology ('patient engaged in writing behaviour', wrote one ward nurse), and never once did any mental health specialist suspect them of faking. The actual patients, by contrast, caught on quickly to the ruse, accusing the pseudo-patients of being journalists or professors checking up on the hospital. Once all the pseudo-patients were released, Rosenhan published his results, causing quite a ruckus in the field, as he had for all intents and purposes proved that psychiatric diagnosis was entirely unreliable and scarily subjective, with almost no validity.

This got under the skin of one psychiatrist in particular, Robert Spitzer of Columbia University in New York, who made it his sole mission to overhaul the entire manual, coming out, in 1980, with the third edition of the *DSM*, which was decidedly different from the two earlier versions in that it attempted to yield a picture more akin to a statistical population census rather than relying on simple psychodynamic diagnoses. Spitzer broke human suffering into quantifiable chunks, listing, for instance, all the known symptoms of major depression, of generalised anxiety disorder, of psychotic disorders, and including instructions to clinicians as to how many symptoms the patient needed to have to qualify for any given diagnosis. Spitzer and company effectively made a diagnostic manual that had real reliability – but it didn't have any more validity, and there's the rub. The description of depression, just like every other diagnosis, was decided upon by a committee subject to whims and agendas. And still today you will not find in the *DSM* any understanding of *why*, only *how*. The manual describes all sorts of suffering but utterly fails to illuminate the roots and reasons.

For the latest iteration, the *DSM-V*, published in 2013, a group of neuroscientists, biological psychiatrists and prominent doctors petitioned the *DSM-V*'s mood disorder committee to consider a new diagnosis that they were calling by a very old name – melancholia. Melancholia has been around for a very long time, so long that Hippocrates wrote about it, attributing the phenomenon to an excess of black bile. The petitioning practitioners believed that the absence of melancholia in the *DSM-V* would be a great oversight, as it has symptoms distinctly different from other kinds of depression, like dysthymia, for example, for which low-grade dejection is the defining descriptor. In melancholia, the patient shows not only psychological symptoms, such as a guilt-ridden psyche and deep despondency, but also physical symptoms such as psychomotor retardation – a slowing of the body and the mind – and distinctly disturbed sleep patterns, along with a metabolism of the stress hormone cortisol gone into 'overdrive', decidedly different from that of non-depressed people and people suffering from other types of depression. Unlike with other symptoms of depression, there is an actual way to test a person's level of cortisol. The dexamethasone suppression test (DST), which is capable of measuring stress hormones like cortisol, may therefore be perhaps the first actual objective biological measure of a mental illness, something psychiatry has long been searching for. 'If melancholia wasn't the Holy Grail', said writer and therapist Gary Greenberg, 'it was at least a sip from the chalice of science, one disorder that could go beyond appearances.'

The mood disorder committee of the *DSM-V*, however, was not open to adding melancholia to its types and subtypes of depression, despite the fact that it would have provided the field at last with one physiological test proving that at least one mental illness is a medical disease. Committee member William Coryell wrote to the petitioning practitioners, telling them he believed they were correct but that 'the inclusion of a biological measure would be very hard to sell to the mood group.' Why? The problem, explained Coryell, was not the DST's reliability, which Coryell believed was very high, but rather that the DST would be 'the only biological test for any diagnosis being considered.' The result, wrote Greenberg, was that 'the main obstacle was exactly what you would think was melancholia's strength: the biological tests, especially the DST ... A single disorder that met the scientific demands of the day, in other words, would only make the failure to meet them in the rest of the *DSM* that much more glaring.' The committee of the *DSM-V* had the chance to step into the psychiatry of the future and turned it down, falling back on patterns of the past.

Indeed, the past may be where psychiatry is content to live for however long it lives, given that, according to psychiatrist Richard Friedman of Cornell University in New York, no novel drugs have come through the pipeline in thirty years. There were the mostly serendipitous and stunning drug discoveries that this book has endeavoured to describe, the majority of which occurred between 1949 and 1959, and then fluoxetine broke the blues in 1987. But in the long run, even that medicine turned out, despite the huge hype, not to be really any more effective than the tricyclics had been.

I personally find it difficult to believe that we have now gone decades without any true innovation in psychotropic medication. Within the cocoon of my own experience, the tricyclics were dry-mouth duds, while fluoxetine spun me around twice and then took me to the dance, where I waltzed away my thirties in a state of such supreme happiness that I was legitimately worried. And it turns out I had something to be worried about. Even setting aside the warnings of Robert Whitaker and Joseph Glenmullen about the lack of knowledge regarding the drug's long-term side effects, the problem for me was that the drug wore off – or I developed a tolerance to it, call it what you will. I needed more and more of those pretty tablets, until at last my dose was both sky-high and ineffectual.

Psychiatry's answer to the problem of tolerance is to practise polypharmacy. For me, as for so many others, this meant two things. First, I switched from an SSRI to an SNRI, venlafaxine, a drug that tickles the noradrenaline receptors as well as the serotonin receptors, and then I also went on a second drug, an antipsychotic that was meant to enhance the efficacy of the venlafaxine. I don't think, however, that psychiatry's future is in polypharmacy, in doping up patients on a little of this and a lot of that and sitting back to see what happens. But I don't totally agree with Friedman and others, either, when they say that no novel drugs have come down the pipeline in thirty years. While it may be accurate in a strictly technical sense that there has been little or no recent actual invention in the psychotropics, the truth is that there has been significant innovation. There are groups of psychiatrists doing amazing things way out on the edge, not necessarily with new drugs but with old, even ancient drugs, which they are using in undoubtedly novel ways. I think the future of psychiatry is, strangely enough, right here, in tiny tabs of acid and chalices of psychedelics such as ayahuasca, psilocybin and MDMA.

We've seen already how Alicia Danforth and Charles Grob have enabled many autistic patients at University of California, Los Angeles (UCLA) to experience, for the first time, what it is like to interact with the neurotypical world without fear. The beneficial effects of these experiences last well beyond the actual 'high'. MDMA, as we know, has already proven to be incredibly effective for those suffering from post-traumatic stress disorder, and Danforth would also like to see it utilised for borderline personality disorder (BPD), a diagnosis often given to young women who have an extreme fear of abandonment, who self-harm and who experience perpetual feelings of emptiness. It is a condition marked by self-hatred and an impaired ability to connect. In the psychiatry of the past, borderline personality disorder was a condition one either grew out of or failed to; the psychiatry of the future, however, has a potential answer to borderline personality disorder with MDMA, offering those suffering from borderline personality disorder a new world view in which their worth is protected and preserved and regard for self and others can be kept totally intact.

The intrepid practitioners out on the far fringes of psychiatry who are turning to ancient or synthesised psychedelics are finding that these drugs make a real difference for those suffering from a broad spectrum of afflictions, from autism to addiction to post-traumatic stress disorder to depression to fear of death as well.

Although there are several different psychedelics currently being tested with different populations of patients, they all seem to offer the subject the same thing: insight. The psychedelics allow patients stuck in self-destructive patterns of thought or behaviour to view themselves and their role in the universe in a radically different light. They appear to illuminate death, or the limit of life, and in so doing to underscore its preciousness. Time is both highlighted and obliterated, so that patients can truly grasp that although they live in a timeless universe, they have just a short amount of it on this Earth in which to love and to work. Psychedelics like ayahuasca, made from vines and leaves, allow patients to see the uselessness of their alcohol or drug abuse and, by increasing their empathy for others, how their behaviour may be hurting those close to them. Thus a fresh resolve is born.

The newest psychedelic that psychiatry has turned to is ketamine, known on the streets for many years as 'Special K'. It is a drug employed by anaesthesiologists during surgeries, but starting in the 1990s some researchers began to investigate whether ketamine had the ability to improve mood, and to use it when all other treatments had failed. Ketamine, which is usually delivered to the body via IV infusions in clinics that are popping up with increasing frequency around the United States, is deeply different from standard antidepressant treatments. Right now ketamine infusion therapy is reserved for only those patients who are treatment resistant, who have tried numerous other pharmacological combinations over months and years, and have undergone intermittent shock treatment, all to no effect.

Suicide is on the increase, with thousands of people living in the UK committing suicide each year, and those who kill themselves are often suffering from treatment-resistant depression. Currently, select treatment-resistant patients can go to their closest ketamine clinic in the United States, which may not be run by a psychiatrist at all but by an anaesthesiologist who has had years of practice dosing patients in the operatiang theatre. And instead of being handed a prescription, they are led to a lounge chair, where a needle is inserted into a prominent vein, and then, over the course of forty-five minutes to an hour, they are infused with the drug, experiencing perhaps some dissociation although rarely any hallucinations, perhaps a bit of dizziness or confusion but nothing so severe that they aren't fit for discharge within an hour and a half to two hours. They can't drive or operate a bulldozer directly after ketamine treatment, but this, one imagines, is a very small price to pay.

What's most remarkable about ketamine so far is the speed with which it works. Unlike traditional antidepressants, ketamine comes on right away, wiping away the sludge of despair within minutes or hours of the infusion. How long does this relief last? The answer is not clear yet. It's too new. Most patients receiving treatments at a ketamine clinic will go back for a series of four to six infusions over a twelve-week period and then return for boosters on an as-needed basis. Ketamine may well be the future for the treatment of depression in psychopharmacology. It can be taken and tolerated with many other drugs, meaning you likely won't need to detox off any other medications you may be imbibing in order to qualify as a bona fide ketamine patient.

As with all other psychiatric drugs, no one really knows why ketamine works, and especially why it works so swiftly. Some theorise that the drug is neurotrophic, meaning that it allows neurons to sprout new connections to neighbouring neurons, essentially remaking your brain, which can then, post-treatment, suddenly see life in a whole new way. Within minutes after an IV infusion of ketamine, the brain gets busy sending out its sprouts, pathways that ferry new and adaptive cognitions and images from one neuron to the next, and that express themselves as the lifting of a dark and despairing mood. These potential neurotrophic abilities of ketamine make it different from the other psychedelic drugs I have investigated here, none of which, as far as anyone knows, can actually prompt the brain to send new sprouts throughout its rumpled mass. And while there have been one or two studies of psilocybin for treatment-resistant depression, ketamine is the first psychedelic to be used specifically for this purpose, meaning it's poised to have a remarkable impact, as depression affects huge swathes of people. One study even shows that ketamine can effectively reduce or altogether eradicate suicidal thoughts. But it's a treatment so new that although there has been some research, the US Food and Drug Administration (FDA) has not yet granted approval for the drug. Legal use of ketamine is restricted in the UK, where it is mostly used as an anaesthetic but in limited cases it may be available in low doses to help relieve pain.

Rick Doblin, as we know, has said his goal is to make psychedelics – especially MDMA – legal prescription medicines by 2021. On the one hand, this is a hugely ambitious goal, and seems like a leap across too wide a barrier, given that all psychedelics are classified by the US Drug Enforcement Administration (DEA) as having 'no currently accepted medical use and a high potential for abuse'. And yet without a doubt there are subterranean shifts and stirrings. As of November 2016, the FDA is allowing MAPS to move into phase-three trials of MDMA-assisted psychotherapy for post-traumatic stress disorder. Thus it is here, in this psychedelic corner, that psychiatry is truly rejuvenating itself, not only eliminating the unhelpful dregs of psychoanalytic theory but also stepping out from under the bland blue fluoxetine sky and into a place where mysterious and mighty chemicals, illegal chemicals that carry with them the aura of the 1960s counterculture, are being resurrected with extreme caution and just a little bit of glee, so stupendous are their effects.

The psychedelics provide psychiatry with a whole new model of how drugs might work, and a whole new way to think about psychopharmacology. In our current model a patient takes a drug, or many drugs, daily, a fact that has hugely benefited pharmaceutical companies, which stand to make billions off our distress. Were psychedelics ever to become more widely adopted than SSRIs and other antidepressants, the huge money-making pharmaceutical houses would be greatly reduced, replaced with small non-profits like MAPS, which would dole out drugs with little potential for profit, because one need not take them regularly to get a beneficial effect, and because, like lithium, they are, at least some of them, naturally occurring.

The psychopharmacology of the future should be genuinely insight-oriented, and in that sense would, ironically, represent a step back into the past. One takes a chemical with the powerful and profound ability to turn the mind inside out, and then spends ten straight sessions talking about the lessons learned. Many researchers, including the Pulitzer Prize winner Siddhartha Mukherjee, an oncologist at Columbia University in New York, have noted that even in antidepressants the best results tend to come when medication is combined with talking therapy. The reason for this is not entirely clear. 'It is very unlikely that we can "talk" our brains into growing cells,' Mukherjee wrote. 'But perhaps talking alters the way that nerve death is registered by the conscious parts of the brain. Or talking could release other chemicals, opening up parallel pathways of nerve-cell growth.' But whatever the reason, it is a deeply divergent model from the one we have now, in which patients are tethered to their doctors by once-monthly visits whose purpose is simply to renew the prescriptions. Psychedelic treatment, despite its past stain and stigma, offers psychopharmacology a chance for deep dignity as its practitioners accompany patients to the furthest reaches of their minds, with the doctor recast as guide, a medical man or woman who does so much more than swiftly write out a prescription.

In the future, then, psychiatrists might be shamans or, the other way around, shamans may act as psychiatrists, counselling people during and after their trips. The lingo of the *DSM* might be replaced with phrases like 'set and setting'. Patients might be instructed to come to psychedelic sessions with photos of loved ones or meaningful mementos, any object that can facilitate a profound psychedelic journey. I doubt the *DSM* will be wiped out, or that conventional antidepressants will go the way of the wind, but there's a reasonable chance that they will become adjuncts to treatment rather than the sole focus. Such a change would be huge not only for patients accustomed to monthly medicine checks but also for psychopharmacologists, who would be remade in the role of divine guide. I have no doubt that many would reject that role, which may be why MAPS is currently training therapists in how to conduct psychedelic sessions, so that if the rejuvenation were to happen, we would be ready.

I myself would be ready. In fact, I already am ready. Despite my initial failure to procure MDMA, I decided several months ago to look into psychedelics once more and went to see a therapist who uses them in her treatment. She would give me only her first name and the address of her office, which was located in a cramped corner of the city, up a flight of stairs. As with the earlier practitioner, the walls of her treatment room were painted calming colours, and there was plenty of oriental decor and a lot of flowing fabric. After I had listed for her the drugs I'm on and told her something about my history, which includes several stays in psychiatric hospitals (although none in the past thirty years), she thought better than to give me psilocybin, the drug that I was seeking this time.

'It won't work for you,' she said. 'The medications you're on would block its effects.'

Which would leave me no choice but to detox off a cabinet full of medicines in order to touch the sky. This is something I cannot do right now. I'm not willing to risk my sanity; I fought too hard for it. Given that ketamine does not require one to go off psychiatric medications, a ketamine clinic, of which there are two already in the metropolitan Boston area, might be the next stop.

What, you might ask, am I really after here? It's hard to express. It's the fact that psychedelics, given in the right set and setting, offer the user a chance to know the universal, to step outside of time, to feel the hugeness of space and the deep interconnections among all beings. Psychedelics allow users to become more than conscious; they arrive at a whole new consciousness, their awareness as sharp as a shard of glass. I want that for myself. I'd like to really see the limits of my life, to feel my borders melt away, to swirl with space and view colours so fierce that they pulse, their hues truer than anything we normally notice. Given my particular set of circumstances, I don't think I'll have this opportunity in my lifetime, but as MAPS gets closer and closer to its goal of making psychedelics legal prescription drugs, many other people will. Who knows, there may come a day when a person with clinical depression turns to ketamine or psilocybin as a first line of treatment, with conventional antidepressants used only as a back-up. That would certainly be a paradigm shift.

The 1950s and early 1960s were considered by many to be 'the golden era of psychopharmacology'. Those decades saw the birth of chlorpromazine, which turned hurting heads inside out, all the screams and demons dumped on to the floor to be whisked away by a waiting nurse. Cade's rediscovery of lithium finally gave those afflicted with mania and bipolar disorder a chance to live a more placid life. And then along came imipramine and the MAOIs, perhaps the most significant of all the drug discoveries of that time: finally we had chemicals that could weaken the grip of even the darkest depression, a disorder that 300 million people worldwide currently suffer from. Yes, for sure, the 1950s were rife with discoveries, each one made in some serendipitous fashion, chemicals for rocket fuel repurposed into psychic energisers – who would have thought?

Once the 1950s were over, though, the discoveries dried up, with the bright exception of clozapine, a drug to treat schizophrenia, and the SSRIs, which Peter Kramer came to call cosmetic medicine, a drug that could dull the jagged edges of an irritable person, a drug not for the person but for the personality, a designer drug that could help people be bolder, more charming, more patient, nicer. Of course that's not all the SSRIs did. Although they were and perhaps still are used abundantly for all sorts of minor ills, they also gave people like me a shot at a regular life, a life lived outside of institutions. But as we've seen, when compared with the tricyclics, the SSRIs were found to be no more effective in treating anxiety and depression, and they could also cause suicidal idea- tion. Meanwhile, they continue to be used in relative ignorance, as no one seems to know what their long-term side effects are. In other words, the holy grail has not been found.

It could be, however, that psychedelics long used as sacred drugs in more shamanic cultures will bring us closer to what we are always seeking: peace of mind. These drugs are so powerful that they can actually *cause* love, as is the case with MDMA, which also appears to help autistic people – those locked in the box of their brain – enter into dialogue with the neurotypical world. Ayahuasca and psilocybin both have proven to be very effective at treating addictions, as these psychedelics allow substance abus- ers to powerfully experience just what their behaviour is doing to them and those within their circle. There is more than a little irony in the fact that psychedelics, considered evil and dangerous drugs by government agencies, can help addicts relinquish highly addictive chemicals such as opium-based concoctions like heroin and fentanyl, the very bogeymen at the centre of our ill-conceived 'War on Drugs'.

Our next golden era of psychopharmacology, I predict, will be with psychedelics, drugs not discovered but rediscovered, drugs so pure and powerful that they crack the thin veneer we call reality and show us a show the likes of which we do not forget. Psychedelics may be more potent in treating many psychiatric disorders than anything we have right now, and in some strange way they reunite us with the father of psychoanalysis, Sigmund Freud, who believed that awareness was the vehicle by which we could be cured of our ills. At once brand-new and ancient, psyche- delics allow us a radical awareness of our place and purpose in the universe; they actually seem to set us straight, these tie-dye drugs of long-gone hippiedom.

Thus it may be that we need to get high in order to finally act right. I hope, however, that we do not go so far as to forget the men and women who found the first cures, even if they have turned out to be radically less than perfect. The drugs presented in this book all have their flaws, for sure. But they all, in one manner or another, have helped numerous people to live a life, and that's no small thing. Even if the price has been steep, and the side effects sometimes severe, nevertheless the first golden era gave people back their minds and their days, long hours of light and water, serenity in the gaps where there used to be screeches, with the possibilities pure and seemingly endless, at least for a little while.

Acknowledgements

Thanks go to my editor at Little, Brown, Ben George, for seeing me the whole way through, for pulling this book up by its bootstraps and, to mix my metaphors here, hand-planing its many rough edges, doing the long, hard work of an editor with a vision and a belief, so much so that I feel the product comes not from me but from a joint effort, although any mistakes, soft spots, brown spots or rust ridges are mine and mine alone.

I could not have even conceived of this book were it not for my extraordinary agent, Dorian Karchmar, who heard, one day, five years ago, the delicate thrum of an idea and from that thrum pulled out a whole soft skein that came to be called 'the proposal'. I have written eight other books and seven of them were born on the backs of proposals, but no one has ever guided me from the first stray glitters of an unformed notion to a whole exposition of ideas and structure, and done it so patiently and insistently, so calmly and forcefully – for this I am deeply indebted.

Anna Jaffe read early drafts of this book and gave me the confidence to go on when I felt I could not. Alberta Nassi provided similar support. My children, while involved in no explicit way, nevertheless gave me motivation, because they were living proof that I am capable of producing at least two beautiful beings, and thus my manuscript stood a slim chance. A book, of course, is not a human, but still, if it is any good, it has a heart, and legs too; a book should skip and beat and, if it's really doing its job, it should exert some force upon your heart, the reader's heart, and thus I have, as well, to thank you, the reader, for putting these pages in your palm, or on your tablet, or wherever they may be. It is a great honour to be held in such a fashion. I hope I can return the favour.

Notes

1. Chlorpromazine

Sea change in policy regarding mental health treatment: Steven J. Taylor, 'Caught in the Continuum: A Critical Analysis of the Principle of the Least Restrictive Environment', *Research and Practice for Persons with Severe Disabilities* 29 (2004): 218–30.

History of treatments preceding chlorpromazine: Elliot Valenstein, *Great and Desperate Cures* (New York: Free Press, 1988), 15–20.

Manfred Sakel coma therapy: David Healy, *The Creation of Psychopharmacology* (Cambridge, MA: Harvard University Press, 2004), 52–53.

Depth of hypoglycaemic comas: Heinz Lehmann and Thomas Ban, 'The History of the Psychopharmacology of Schizophrenia', *Canadian Journal of Psychiatry* 42 (1997): 152.

Meduna experiments: Ibid.

Lucio Bini's use of electroconvulsive therapy: Norman S. Endler, 'The Origins of Electroconvulsive Therapy (ECT)', *Convulsive Therapy* 4, no. 1 (January 1988): 5–23.

Lehmann's use of fever in treatment: Maureen Muldoon, 'From Psychiatrist-Researcher to Psychiatrist and Researcher: Heinz Lehmann', *Journal of Ethics in Mental Health* 6 (2011): 222.

Moniz, the invention of psychosurgery: Healy, *The Creation of Psychopharmacology*, 40–41. See also Mical Raz, *The Lobotomy Letters: The Making of American Psychosurgery* (Rochester, NY: University of Rochester Press, 2013), 5–7.

The doctor-turned-pilot and the virtuoso violinist: Jack El-Hai, *The Lobotomist: A Maverick Medical Genius and His Tragic Quest to Rid the World of Mental Illness* (New York: Wiley, 2005), 196, 277.

Use of an ice pick in the first lobotomy: Jenell Johnson, *American Lobotomy: A Rhetorical History* (Ann Arbor: University of Michigan Press, 2014), 24.

Chemical make-up of chlorpromazine: Healy, *The Creation of Psychopharmacology*, 80–81.

Methylene blue protects against Alzheimer's: H. Atamna and R. Kumar, 'Protective Role of Methylene Blue in Alzheimer's Disease via Mitochondria and Cytochrome C Oxidase', *Journal of Alzheimer's Disease* 20, no. 2 (2010): 439–52.

Methylene blue staining nerve cells of frogs: Healy, *The Creation of Psychopharmacology*, 44.

Treating neuralgia with methylene blue: Ibid.

Pietro Bodoni treating manic patients with methylene blue: Ibid.

Methylene blue transformed into chlorpromazine: Ibid., 39.

'no drug company would market an old drug even if it worked': Ibid., 45.

'competing therapies or interest groups': Ibid., 44–45.

Phenothiazine nucleus having antihistamine effects: Judith Swazey, *Chlorpromazine in Psychiatry: A Study of Therapeutic Innovation* (Cambridge, MA: MIT Press, 1974), 58.

Promethazine synthesised in 1947: Ibid., 77.

Promethazine precursor to chlorpromazine: Ibid., 78.

The sinking of the *Sirocco*: Henri Laborit, *L'esprit du grenier* (Paris: Grasset, 1992), 103–53.

Laborit's use of promethazine: Fernando Alemanno and Ferdinando Auricchio, 'Sedation in Regional Anesthesia', in *Anesthesia of the Upper Limb: A State of the Art Guide,* eds. Fernando Alemanno, Mario Bosco and Aldo Barbati (New York: Springer, 2014), 233.

Artificial hibernation and Laborit's use of promethazine: Swazey, *Chlorpromazine in Psychiatry*, 62.

'euphoric quietude': Laborit in *La Presse Médicale* (1950), cited ibid., 79.

'tense and anxious Mediterranean type': Ibid.

Description of surgical shock: Ibid., 62.

Courvoisier and Charpentier test discoveries: Healy, *The Creation of Psychopharmacology*, 82.

'a completely different molecule': Ibid., 81.

Pierre Koetschet on the usefulness of chlorpromazine: Swazey, *Chlorpromazine in Psychiatry*, 96.

'The idea of an antipsychotic': Healy, *The Creation of Psychopharmacology*, 84.

Laborit's 'lytic cocktail': Ibid., 79.

Chlorpromazine included in soldiers' battlefield kits: Ibid., 82.

'possible use of the product in psychiatry': Swazey, *Chlorpromazine in Psychiatry*, 106.

Quarti's account of chlorpromazine's effects: Ibid., 117–18.

Treatment of Jacques Lh.: Ibid., 119–20.

Jean Delay's reputation: David Healy, *The Psychopharmacologists*, vol. 1 (Boca Raton, FL: CRC Press, 4 September 1998), 2.

Patients given rectal enemas: Jean Thuillier, *Ten Years That Changed The Face of Mental Illness* (Boca Raton, FL: CRC Press, September 1999), 5.

Woman getting second-degree burns in the bath at Sainte Anne's: Ibid.

Sigwald and Bouttier: Swazey, *Chlorpromazine in Psychiatry*, 126.

Madame Gob: D. G. Cunningham Owens, *A Guide to the Extrapyramidal Side Effects of Antipsychotic Drugs* (New York: Cambridge University Press, 1999), 7.

Hamon's results: Ibid., 112.

Delay and Deniker first learned of chlorpromazine: Owens, *A Guide to the Extrapyramidal Side Effects of Antipsychotic Drugs*, 7.

The case of Phillippe Burg: Healy, *The Creation of Psychopharmacology*, 91.

Responses to chlorpromazine of catatonic patients versus paranoid patients: Elliot Valenstein, *Blaming the Brain: The Truth about Drugs and Mental Health* (New York: Free Press, 1988), 25.

The barber's reaction to chlorpromazine treatment: Healy, *The Creation of Psychopharmacology*, 91.

The barber shaves the psychiatrist: Ibid., 93.

Account of the juggler's reaction to chlorpromazine treatment: Ibid., 91.

Jean Thuillier to the fish dealer: David Healy, *The Psychopharmacologists*, vol. 3, 3rd ed. (Boca Raton, FL: CRC Press, 2000), 551.

Glaziers' work reduced: David Healy, *The Antidepressant Era* (Cambridge, MA: Harvard University Press, 1997), 63.

Laborit suggests Largactil as name: Swazey, *Chlorpromazine in Psychiatry*, 141.

Smith, Kline & French's marketing: Valenstein, *Blaming the Brain*, 141.

Smith, Kline & French's response to Rhône-Poulenc's inquiry: Ibid., 160.

Difficult to get chlorpromazine into North American treatment programmes: Swazey, *Chlorpromazine in Psychiatry*, 196.

Henry Brill on resistance to chlorpromazine: Ibid.

'No one in his right mind was working with drugs': Ibid., 196–97.

Patients would have taken the two years of restored life: Healy, *The Creation of Psychopharmacology*, 97.

'One of them would even rip radiators right off the wall': R. Walter Heinrichs, *In Search of Madness* (New York: Oxford University Press, 2001), 151.

A clean somatic approach: Swazey, *Chlorpromazine in Psychiatry*, 217.

'That was perhaps the most spectacular demonstration': Ibid., 201.

'Lest everything be evaluated in terms of decibels': Ibid.

Mortgaging his house to buy shares of chlorpromazine: Healy, *The Creation of Psychopharmacology*, 98.

Within a year chlorpromazine had been prescribed: Sarah Linsley Starks and Joel T. Braslow, 'The Making of Contemporary American Psychiatry, Part 1: Patients, Treatments, and Therapeutic Rationales Before and After World War II', *History of Psychology* 8, no. 2 (May 2005): 181.

The patient populations in asylums: Swazey, *Chlorpromazine in Psychiatry*, 222.

Ayd's patient dismissed as 'hysterical': Healy, *The Creation of Psychopharmacology*, 110.

Parkinson's seen as repressed anger: Ibid., 112–13.

Naming and history of the double-bind theory: Gregory Bateson, Don D. Jackson, Jay Haley and John Weakland, 'Toward a Theory of Schizophrenia', *Systems Research and Behavioral Science* 1, no. 4 (1956): 251–64.

Acetylcholine given to schizophrenic patients: Edward Shorter, *A History of Psychiatry* (New York: Wiley, 1988), 247.

Chemical versus electrical signalling: Elliot Valenstein, *The War of the Soups and the Sparks* (New York: Columbia University Press, 2005), 3.

An alkaloid from the Rauwolfia plant: Healy, *The Creation of Psychopharmacology*, 102.

Bowman invented a machine called the spectrophotofluorometer: Victoria A. Harden, Ph.D., and Claude Lenfant, M.D., 'The AMINCO-Bowman Spectrophotofluorometer', Stetten Museum Office of NIH History, Web.

Brodie used the new machine: Healy, *The Creation of Psychopharmacology*, 106.

Rabbits became lethargic, apathetic: Scott Stossel, *My Age of Anxiety* (New York: Knopf, 2013), 174.

Arvid Carlsson discovering that dopamine: Vikram K. Yeragani, 'Arvid Carlsson, and the Story of Dopamine', *Indian Journal of Psychiatry* 52 (2010): 87–88.

The 'dopamine hypothesis of schizophrenia': Ralf Brisch et al., 'The Role of Dopamine in Schizophrenia from a Neurobiological and Evolutionary Perspective: Old Fashioned, but Still in Vogue', *Front Psychiatry* 5 (2014): 47.

Schizophrenics experiencing obstetrical trauma at birth: J. R. Geddes et al., 'Schizophrenia and Complications of Pregnancy and Labor: An Individual Patient Data Meta-Analysis', *Schizophrenia Bulletin* 25, no. 3 (1999): 413–23.

Schizophrenia caused by an error: Edward Shorter, *A History of Psychiatry, From the Era of the Asylum to the Age of Prozac* (New York: Wiley, 1988), 270.

Neurons were jumbled: Ibid., 268.

PET and fMRI technology: Ibid., 269.

In 2011, atypical antipsychotics were prescribed: Richard A. Friedman. 'A Call for Caution on Antipsychotic Drugs', *New York Times*, 24 September 2012.

'their psyches manipulated by therapists': Healy, *The Creation of Psychopharmacology*, 148.

The drug has been relegated: E. Estrada, 'Clinical Uses of Chlorpromazine in Veterinary Medicine', *Journal of the American Veterinary Medical Association* 128 (1956): 292–94.

'When it comes to antipsychotics': Personal interview with Alexander Vuckovic, 19 February 2015.

Hiroshi Utena pushed out of his office: Jon Agar, *Science in the 20th Century and Beyond* (Malden, MA: Polity Press, 2012), 243.

Students in France storming Sainte-Anne's asylum: Ibid.

The ransacking of Jean Delay's office: Healy, *The Creation of Psychopharmacology*, 176–77.

Spiders under the influence of hallucinogens: Ronald K. Siegel, *Intoxication: Life in the Pursuit of Artificial Paradise* (New York: Park Street Press, 1989), 73.

2. Lithium

Lithium found in space: Michael Pidwirny, *Understanding Physical Geography* (Kelowna, BC: Our Planet Earth Publishing, 2015), 3.

The element atomises on contact with air: Jaime Lowe, 'I Don't Believe in God, but I Believe in Lithium', *New York Times*, 25 June 2015.

Bonifácio de Andrada e Silva: Per Enghag, *Encyclopedia of the Elements: Technical Data—History—Processing—Applications* (New York: Wiley, 2004), 291.

Lithium found on Utö: F. Neil Johnson, *The History of Lithium Therapy* (New York: Macmillan, 1984), 3.

How lithium came to be called lithion: Ibid.

Lithium's ability to alkalise excessively acidic urine: Ibid., 8.

Doctors believing that excess uric acid: David Healy, *Mania: A Short History of Bipolar Disorder* (Baltimore: Johns Hopkins University Press, 1984), 90.

Lithium levels in tap water: N. Sugawara, 'Lithium in Tap Water and Suicide Mortality in Japan', *International Journal of Environmental Research and Public Health* 10 (2013): 6044–48.

Japanese research on tap water: Hirochika Ohgami et al., 'Lithium Levels in Drinking Water and Risk of Suicide', *British Journal of Psychiatry* (2009): 464–65.

'I was born in 1917': Johnson, *The History of Lithium Therapy*, 18.

Discovery and development of lithium's medicinal uses: Ibid., 5–22.

On the popularisation of lithium spas: Ibid., 18–19.

'For a person to obtain a therapeutic dose': Elliot Valenstein, *Blaming the Brain: The Truth about Drugs and Mental Health* (New York: Free Press, 1988), 41.

Lange first to use lithium prophylactically: Edward Shorter, 'The History of Lithium Therapy', *Bipolar Disorders* (2009): 4–9.

John Aulde's treatment: Johnson, *The History of Lithium Therapy,* 12.

Cocoanut Grove fire: Kathiann M. Kowalski, *Attack of the Superbugs: The Crisis of Drug-Resistant Diseases* (New York: Enslow Publishing, 2005). See also Stuart B. Levy, *The Antibiotic Paradox: How the Misuse of Antibiotics Destroys Their Curative Powers* (Cambridge, MA: Da Capo Press, 2002), 1–4.

By the 1940s you couldn't get your hands on a lithium tablet: Johnson, *The History of Lithium Therapy,* 31. See also Healy, *Mania,* 96.

Cade held as a prisoner of war in the Changi camp: Johnson, *The History of Lithium Therapy,* 32–34. See also Greg de Moore and Ann Westmore, *Finding Sanity: John Cade, Lithium, and the Taming of Bipolar Disorder* (Melbourne: Allen & Unwin, 2017). See also Jack F. Cade, 'John Frederick Joseph Cade: Family Memories on the Occasion of the Fiftieth Anniversary of His Discovery of the Use of Lithium in Mania', *Australian and New Zealand Journal of Psychiatry* 33, no. 5 (1999): 615–18. For conditions at the camp, see Roland Perry, *The Changi Brownlow* (Sydney: Hachette Australia, 2012).

How and when Cade developed his ideas: Healy, *Mania,* 100; Johnson, *The History of Lithium Therapy,* 32–34.

'mourning the wasted years': John Cade, quoted in Johnson, *The History of Lithium Therapy,* 34.

Cade's powers of observation: David Healy, *The Psychopharmacologists,* vol. 2 (Boca Raton, FL: CRC Press, 1998), 262.

'Because I did not know': Johnson, *The History of Lithium Therapy,* 35.

Cade storing urine samples in family refrigerator: Ibid., 36.

Urine 'from the manic patients': Valenstein, *Blaming the Brain,* 44.

'all that had been demonstrated so far': Samuel Gershon et al., eds., *Lithium: Its Role in Psychiatric Research and Treatment* (New York: Springer, 1973), 9.

Cade injected large doses: Johnson, *The History of Lithium Therapy,* 36.

'the animals, although fully conscious': Ibid., 36.

Cade trying lithium on himself: Jack F. Cade, *Australian and New Zealand Journal of Psychiatry,* 33, no. 5 (1999): 615–18.

Cade believed that 'spontaneous remission is far less likely to occur': John F. Cade, 'Lithium Salts in the Treatment of Psychotic Excitement', *Bulletin of the World Health Organization* 78, no. 4 (2000): 518–20.

'How to proceed?': Johnson, *The History of Lithium Therapy,* 108.

'Our kitchen refrigerator': Ibid., 37.

In total Cade treated nineteen patients: Philip B. Mitchell, 'On the 50th Anniversary of John Cade's Discovery of the Anti-Manic Effect of Lithium', *Australian and New Zealand Journal of Psychiatry* 33, no. 5 (1999): 624.

'in a state of typical manic excitement': Cade, 'Lithium Salts in the Treatment of Psychotic Excitement', 518–20.

'enjoyed preeminent nuisance value': Valenstein, *Blaming the Brain*, 44.

Cade's 'expectant imagination': Ibid., 46.

'he found normal surroundings and liberty of movement strange at first': Healy, *Mania*, 102.

'I readmitted him to the hospital': Johnson, *The History of Lithium Therapy*, 39.

'very first scientific evidence': Barry Blackwell, *Bits and Pieces of a Psychiatrist's Life* (Bloomington, IN: Xlibris, 2012), 218.

'E.A., a male, aged forty-six years': Cade, 'Lithium Salts in the Treatment of Psychotic Excitement', 518–20.

Patients lithium did and did not help: Johnson, *The History of Lithium Therapy*, 38.

Cade's hypothesis on the effects of lithium deficiency: Cade, 'Lithium Salts in the Treatment of Psychotic Excitement', 518–20.

Young found that lithium salts: Johnson, *The History of Lithium Therapy*, 59.

W. B. was 'back to his old form again': Cade, 'Lithium Salts in the Treatment of Psychotic Excitement', 518–20.

Cade reported that W. B.'s skin: Johnson, *The History of Lithium Therapy*, 40.

The paper stirred little interest: Healy, *Mania*, 105.

Young 'found a supply of effervescent lithium': Johnson, *The History of Lithium Therapy*, 58–59.

Schou recalled how his father: Healy, *The Psychopharmacologists*, vol. 2, 259.

Schou clearly remembered: Ibid.

Mogens Schou on Cade's paper: Ibid., 263.

Schou's study was the first: Ibid.

Schou publishes findings consistent with Cade's: Shorter, 'The History of Lithium Therapy'. See also Johnson, *The History of Lithium Therapy*, 68.

Danish researchers learning to use the flame spectrophotometer: Johnson, *The History of Lithium Therapy*, 61.

Two reports of thirty-five patients: Ibid., 69.

A common substrate for mania and depression: Ibid., 70.

Baastrup on patients who chose to continue lithium: Ibid., 71. See also Healy, *Mania*, 113.

Baastrup's findings: Healy, *Mania*, 114.

Geoffrey P. Hartigan gives lithium to twenty of his patients: Ibid.

Five of the seven recovered: Johnson, *The History of Lithium Therapy*, 72.

Wife reporting that her husband: G. P. Hartigan, 'Experience of Treatment with Lithium Salts', cited ibid., 187.

'has kept very well since': Ibid.

In 1961 Schou wrote to Hartigan: Ibid.; Johnson, *The History of Lithium Therapy*, 75.

'From the age of twenty he suffered': Ibid.

Dangers of lithium-based salt substitutes: Ibid., 49.

Most asylums had huge canisters of lithium left over: Ibid.

On Shepherd and Blackwell's criticisms of Schou: Healy, *Mania*, 115–19.

It was an impression: Healy, *The Psychopharmacologists*, vol. 2, 267.

He 'clearly felt that when I showed gratification': Ibid.

Blackwell and Shepherd's criticisms of Schou and Baastrup: Johnson, *The History of Lithium Therapy*, 80.

'How ... could I put him': Ibid., 87.

'He was a genial man': Healy, *The Psychopharmacologists*, vol. 2, 249–50.

'Critical debate is what science thrives on': Ibid., 268.

Blackwell countered that Schou's entire professional life: Johnson, *The History of Lithium Therapy*, 85.

Schou's study design and trial: Ibid., 88.

'They saw a killing here': Healy, *The Psychopharmacologists*, vol. 2, 250.

Clinicians in the United States began applying to the FDA: Johnson, *The History of Lithium Therapy*, 102.

Lithium approved in the United States: Ibid.

'therapeutic effects of complicated compounds': Johnson, *The History of Lithium Therapy*, 67.

'But it has never really excited neuroscientists': Personal interview with Alexander Vuckovic, McLean Hospital, Belmont, MA, 21 May 2015.

'as good a symbol of the vacuity': Healy *Mania*, 168.

Valproate semisodium an effective treatment for mania: Daniel Goleman, '2 Drugs Get a New Use: Soothing Mania', *New York Times*, 13 July 1994.

Numerous anticonvulsants were repurposed: Healy, *Mania*, 168.

The term 'mood stabiliser': Ibid., 174.

Gabapentin grossed $1.3 billion: Ibid.

'I've found it to be as effective': Personal interview with Alexander Vuckovic, McLean Hospital, Belmont, MA, 21 May 2015.

3. Early Antidepressants

Evidence that depression is genetic: Maria Neves-Pereira, Emanuela Mundo, Pierandrea Muglia, Nicole King, Fabio Macciardi and James L. Kennedy, 'The Brain Derived Neurotrophic Factor Gene Confers Susceptibility to Bipolar Disorder: Evidence from a Family Based Association Study', *American Journal of Human Genetics* 71, no. 3 (September 2002): 651.

Broadhurst's first impressions of the Geigy office: Alan D. Broadhurst, 'The Discovery of Imipramine from a Personal Viewpoint', in *The Rise of Psychopharmacology and the Story of CINP*, eds. T. A. Ban, D. Healy and E. Shorter (Budapest: Animula Press, 1998), 69.

'nothing intrinsically special': David Healy, *The Creation of Psychopharmacology* (Cambridge, MA: Harvard University Press, 2002), 37.

'making life did not require': Ibid.

Broadhurst and the executives at Geigy aware of developments: Broadhurst, 'The Discovery of Imipramine from a Personal Viewpoint', 69.

Desire of Broadhurst to avoid creating a 'me too' drug: Ibid.

'the spotlight fell on iminodibenzyl': Ibid., 71.

Geigy's organic chemists created derivatives of the substance: Peter Kramer, *Ordinarily Well: The Case for Antidepressants* (New York: Farrar, Straus and Giroux, 2016), 5.

Eventually the team narrowed in on G22150, the least toxic and most sedative: Ibid., 72.

Kuhn agreed to test G22150 on patients at Münsterlingen: Broadhurst, 'The Discovery of Imipramine from a Personal Viewpoint', 69.

Kuhn believed that the best way to test a drug was not through clinical trials: Holger Steinberg and Hubertus Himmerich, 'Roland Kuhn—100th Birthday of an Innovator of Clinical Psychopharmacology', *Psychopharmacology Bulletin* 45, no. 1 (2012): 48–50.

Geigy abandoned G22150: David Healy, *The Psychopharmacologists*, vol. 2 (Boca Raton, FL: CRC Press, 1998), 72.

Their scientists soon identified a new focus, G22355: Broadhurst, 'The Discovery of Imipramine from a Personal Viewpoint', 69.

'The road to Münsterlingen was already well trodden' and the trial of G22355: Ibid., 72–73.

The word 'antidepressant' was not in existence: David Healy, *The Creation of Psychopharmacology* (Cambridge, MA: Harvard University Press, 2002), 52.

'we wondered if the apparent mood elevation': Ibid., 73.

'I well remember the look of suspicious disbelief on his face': Broadhurst, 'The Discovery of Imipramine from a Personal Viewpoint', 74.

Kuhn's new clinical trial, entirely uncontrolled: Ibid.

Kuhn's approach to patients: Kramer, *Ordinarily Well*, 30.

The first patient to show a change was Paula J. F.: David Healy, *The Antidepressant Era* (Cambridge, MA: Harvard University Press, 1997), 52.

'It was clear that G22355': Broadhurst, 'The Discovery of Imipramine from a Personal Viewpoint', 74.

'the last person [he] would have expected': Ibid., 75.

'I remember how amazed Abraham was': Ibid.

Kuhn's claims and reputation: Ibid., 50.

Kuhn's style of psychotherapy: Healy, *The Antidepressant Era*, 49.

Those suffering from vital depression: Steinberg and Himmerich, 'Roland Kuhn—100th Birthday of an Innovator of Clinical Psychopharmacology'.

Lehmann managed to get his hands on some samples: Healy, *The Antidepressant Era*, 57.

The drug would be most useful: Ibid., 52.

World Health Organization series of studies: Ibid., 59.

Böhringer was made aware of Geigy's work on G22355: Kramer, *Ordinarily Well*, 8.

G22355 becoming imipramine; Kline, Kuhn and MAOIs: Healy, *The Antidepressant Era*, 54–69.

Reserpine also an effective antipsychotic: A. A. Baumeister, M. F. Hawkins and S. M. Uzelac, 'The Myth of Reserpine-Induced Depression: Role in the Historical Development of the Monoamine Hypothesis', *Journal of the History of the Neurosciences* 12, no. 2 (2003): 207–20.

Kline abandoned reserpine: David Healy, *Let Them Eat Prozac* (New York: NYU Press, 2004), 1–40. See also Chaitra T. Ramachandraih et al., 'Antidepressants: From MAOIs to SSRIs and More', *Indian Journal of Psychiatry* 53, no. 2 (2011): 180–82.

Reserpine did become an indispensable research tool: Healy, *The Antidepressant Era*, 64.

Rabbits pretreated with either imipramine: Ibid., 66.

Pretreated rabbits' synapses: C. Lebrand et al., 'Transient Uptake and Storage of Serotonin in Developing Thalamic Neurons', *Neuron* 17, no. 5 (1996): 823–35.

Two-thirds showed marked improvement: Healy, *The Antidepressant Era*, 64.

Kline alerted company executives to his findings: Ibid., 67.

Kline reported his study results to the *New York Times*: Ibid.

Within the first year 400,000 people: Rebecca Kreston, 'The Psychic Energizer! The Serendipitous Discovery of the First Antidepressant', *Discover Magazine*, 27 January 2016, Web.

Kline preferred the term 'psychic energiser': M. Rapley, J. Moncrieff and J. Dillon, eds., *De-Medicalizing Misery: Psychiatry, Psychology and the Human Condition* (New York: Palgrave Macmillan, 2011), 179.

Reserpine has been shown in other studies: Ramachandraih et al., 'Antidepressants: From MAOIs to SSRIs and More', 180.

Rats treated with reserpine became *more* active: Alan A. Boulton, Glen B. Baker, William G. Dewhurst and Merton Sandler, eds., *Neurobiology of the Trace Amines: Analytical, Physiological, Pharmacological, Behavioral, and Clinical Aspects* (New York: Springer Science & Business Media, 12 March 2013), 221.

Differing levels of serotonin in depressed people: Elliot Valenstein, *Blaming the Brain: The Truth about Drugs and Mental Health* (New York: Free Press, 2002), 104.

Side effects of the tricyclics and the MAOIs: Healy, *The Antidepressant Era*, 116–17.

Account of David Foster Wallace's struggle: D. T. Max, *Every Love Story Is a Ghost Story: A Life of David Foster Wallace* (New York: Viking, 2012), 297–301. See also D. T. Max, 'The Unfinished', *The New Yorker,* 9 March 2009; David Lipsky, 'The Lost Years and Last Days of David Foster Wallace', *Rolling Stone,* 30 October 2008; and Los Angeles County coroner's report, 13 September 2008.

Pharmacist writes to Blackwell: Barry Blackwell, 'Adumbration: A History Lesson', *International Network for the History of Neuropsychopharmacology* (2014): 201.

Blackwell and a colleague ingesting cheese: Ibid., 208.

Patients on MAOIs having bad reactions to cheese: Barry Blackwell, *Bits and Pieces of a Psychiatrist's Life* (Bloomington, IN: Xlibris, 2012), 156.

Blackwell claimed that there were forty deaths: Barry Blackwell, 'Adumbration'.

A prominent study in Britain: Healy, *The Antidepressant Era,* 119.

Debates about the safety of the medication: Robert Whitaker, *Anatomy of an Epidemic: Magic Bullets, Psychiatric Drugs, and the Astonishing Rise of Mental Illness in America* (New York: Crown, 2010), 54.

4. SSRIs

The monoamine hypothesis of depression: P. L. Delgado, 'Depression: The Case for a Monoamine Deficiency', *Journal of Clinical Psychiatry* 61, no. 6 (2000): 7–11.

Theory predominated until Arvid Carlsson further refined it: David Healy, *The Antidepressant Era* (Cambridge, MA: Harvard University Press, 1997), 165–66.

Zimelidine made some people ill: National Center for Biotechnology Information, PubChem Compound Database, CID=5365247, https://pubchem.ncbi.nlm.nih.gov/compound/5365247.

Serotonin is omnipresent in the body: Elizabeth DePoy and Stephen

French Gilson, *Human Behavior Theory and Applications: A Critical Thinking Approach* (New York: Sage Publications, 2012), 107.

Eli Lilly considering fluoxetine as a possible weight-loss drug: David Healy, *Let Them Eat Prozac: The Unhealthy Relationship between the Pharmaceutical Industry and Depression* (New York: NYU Press, 2004), 31.

'more human suffering has resulted from depression': Nathan S. Kline, M.D., 'The Practical Management of Depression', *JAMA* 190, no. 8 (1964): 732–40.

Serotonin is one of the oldest neurotransmitters: Efrain C. Azmitia, 'Serotonin and Brain: Evolution, Neuroplasticity, and Homeostasis', *International Review of Neurobiology* 77 (2006): 31–56.

Annual sales reached $350 million: Joseph Glenmullen, *Prozac Backlash: Overcoming the Dangers of Prozac, Zoloft, Paxil, and Other Antidepressants with Safe, Effective Alternatives* (New York: Simon and Schuster, 2001), 15.

Americans receiving disability payments: Robert Whitaker, *Anatomy of an Epidemic* (New York: Crown, 2010), 6–7.

Incidences of depression have increased a thousandfold: Healy, *Let Them Eat Prozac*, 31.

Infant animals secrete the stress hormone cortisol: Xiaoli Feng et al., 'Maternal Separation Produces Lasting Changes in Cortisol and Behavior in Rhesus Monkeys', *Proceedings of the National Academy of Sciences of the United States of America* 108, no. 34 (2011): 14312–17.

'I have forfeited my estate to the king': Andrew Solomon, *The Noonday Demon: An Atlas of Depression* (New York: Scribner, 2001), 386.

'The secret of life's greatest mystery': *Happy* [film], dir. Roko Belic (Wadi Rum Productions, 2011).

Bolo grew despondent after the birth of her daughter: Personal interview with Ann Bolo, 7 July 2014.

'the psychiatrist as psychotherapist is an endangered species': Daniel J. Carlat, *Unhinged: The Trouble with Psychiatry—A Doctor's Revelations about a Profession in Crisis* (New York: Free Press, 2010), 4–5.

'Doing psychotherapy doesn't pay well enough': Ibid., 5.

Even in Eli Lilly's published research: Irving Kirsch, 'Antidepressants and the Placebo Effect', *Zeitschrift für Psychologie* 222, no. 3 (2014): 128–34.

Pharmaceutical companies need only come up with two studies: Glenmullen, *Prozac Backlash*, 287.

The six major antidepressants beat the placebo less than half the time: Gary Greenberg, 'Is It Prozac? Or Placebo?', *Mother Jones*, November–December 2003.

antidepressants outperform placebos, but only minimally: Ibid.

Difference in performance between antidepressants and placebos 'trivial' and 'clinically meaningless': Irving Kirsch, quoted ibid.

The FDA approved fluoxetine after just six to eight weeks of clinical trials: Thomas Insel, 'Antidepressants: A Complicated Picture', National Institute of Mental Health blog, 6 December 2011. See also Andrea Rossi, Alessandra Barraco and Pietro Donda, 'Fluoxetine: A Review on Evidence Based Medicine', *Annals of General Hospital Psychiatry* 3, no. 2 (12 February 2004); Nili Buchman and Rael D. Strous, 'Side Effects of Long-Term Treatment with Fluoxetine', *Clinical Neuropharmacology* 25, no. 1 (January 2002): 55–57.

Few studies on the long-term side effects of serotonin boosters: Glenmullen, *Prozac Backlash,* 10.

'I think the industry is concerned about the possibility': Donald Klein, quoted ibid., 105.

Bolo was told that taking a serotonin booster: Personal interview with Ann Bolo, 25 January 2015.

Psychiatric disorders are not tied to a chemical imbalance: Irving Kirsch, Ph.D., *The Emperor's New Drugs* (New York: Basic Books, 2010), 5–6.

Lilly package insert for fluoxetine: Prozac package insert, Eli Lilly and Co., Indianapolis, 2017.

60 to 75 per cent of people experience sexual dysfunction: James M. Ferguson, 'SSRI Antidepressant Medications: Adverse Effects and Tolerability', *Journal of Clinical Psychiatry* 3, no. 1 (February 2001): 22.

As serotonin rises, dopamine decreases: Glenmullen, *Prozac Backlash,* 122.

Fluoxetine caused facial and bodily spasms: Ibid.

Dexfenfluramine damaged the serotonin neurons: Ibid., 95.

Hoehn-Saric reported on a 23-year-old man with obsessive-compulsive disorder: Ibid., 102.

Fluoxetine makes it difficult to maintain an erection: Lauren Slater, 'How Do You Cure a Sex Addict?', *New York Times,* 19 November 2000. See also Drogo K. Montague et al., 'Pharmacologic Management of Premature Ejaculation', American Urological Association, *Journal of Urology* 172, no. 1 (July 2004): 290–94.

Surprisingly conventional existences: Ibid.

Dependency on a drug causing vulnerability: Alvaro Alonso et al., 'Use of Antidepressants and the Risk of Parkinson's Disease: A Prospective Study', *Journal of Neurology, Neurosurgery, and Psychiatry* 80, no. 6 (2009): 671–74.

Statistics on American women: Laura A. Pratt, Ph.D., Debra J. Brody, M.P.H., and Qiuping Gu, Ph.D., 'Antidepressant Use in Persons Aged 12 and Over: United States, 2005–2008', National Center for Health Statistics Brief 76, October 2011.

antidepressants can be responsible for 'emotional blunting': H. E. Fisher and J. A. Thomson Jr, 'Lust, Romance, Attachment: Do the Sexual Side Effects of Serotonin-Enhancing Antidepressants Jeopardize Romantic Love,

Marriage, and Fertility?', *Evolutionary Cognitive Neuroscience*, eds. S. Platek, J. Keenan and T. Shackelford (Cambridge, MA: MIT Press, 2006), 245.

'serotonin-enhancing antidepressants can jeopardize one's ability to fall in love': Ibid., 245–65.

Women will be more orgasmic: B. Fink, N. Neave, J. T. Manning and K. Grammer, 'Facial Symmetry and Judgments of Attractiveness, Health and Personality', *Personality and Individual Differences* (2001): 491–99.

Oxytocin is tightly tied: Michael D. Breed and Janice Moore, *Animal Behavior* (Cambridge, MA: Academic Press, 2015), 3–4. See also Milt Freudenheim, 'The Drug Makers Are Listening to Prozac', *New York Times*, 12 January 1994.

Over a billion dollars in sales of Prozac in 1993: Peter Breggin and Ginger Ross Breggin, *Talking Back to Prozac: What Doctors Won't Tell You about Prozac and the Newer Antidepressants* [e-book] (Open Road Media, 1 April 2014).

'intense, violent suicidal preoccupation': M. Teicher, M.D., Ph.D., C. Glod, R.N., M.S.C.S, and J. Cole, M.D., 'Emergence of Intense Suicidal Preoccupation during Fluoxetine Treatment', *American Journal of Psychiatry* 147, no. 2 (February 1990): 207–10.

'Death would be a welcome result': Ibid.

She banged her head repeatedly against the floor: Ibid.

The drug agitated them: Glenmullen, *Prozac Backlash*, 146.

Wesbecker on fluoxetine: Ibid., 137.

Account of Wesbecker massacre: Mark Ames, *Going Postal: Rage, Murder, and Rebellion from Reagan's Workplaces to Clinton's Columbine and Beyond* (New York: Soft Skull Press, 2005), 7–8.

'like a zombie, an automaton': Glenmullen, *Prozac Backlash*, 181.

Account of the Wesbecker trial: Ibid., 170–74. See also Richard DeGrandpre, *The Cult of Pharmacology: How America Became the World's Most Troubled Drug Culture* (Durham, NC: Duke University Press, 2006), 35–38.

'My profession now practises': Jeffery Lieberman, *Shrinks: The Untold Story of Psychiatry* (New York: Little, Brown, 2015), 310.

Scientists have searched for evidence: Kirsch, *The Emperor's New Drugs*, 4–5.

Happy subjects do not necessarily: Whitaker, *Anatomy of an Epidemic*, 72–73.

'Several weeks later': Ibid., 81.

The likelihood of relapse: Ibid., 158, 169.

Rats' neurons were 'swollen' and 'twisted like corkscrews': Ibid., 170. See also S. K. Kalia et al., 'Injury and Strain-Dependent Dopaminergic Neuronal Degeneration in the Substantia Nigra of Mice after Axotomy or MPTP', *Brain Research* 994, no. 2 (2003): 243–52.

Helen Mayberg reported in 2013: Helen Mayberg et al., 'Toward a

Neuroimaging Treatment Selection Biomarker for Major Depressive Disorder', *JAMA Psychiatry* 70, no. 8 (2013): 821–29. See also Richard Friedman, M.D., 'To Treat Depression, Drugs or Therapy?', *New York Times,* 8 January 2015.

Long-term exposure to cortisol: Christopher Bergland, 'Cortisol: Why the "Stress Hormone" Is Public Enemy No. 1', *Psychology Today,* 22 January 2013.

Depressed 'patients showed significantly more decline': T. Frodl, M.D., et al., 'Depression-Related Variation in Brain Morphology Over 3 Years', *Archives of General Psychiatry* 65, no. 10 (2008): 1156–65.

Possibility that antidepressants are neurotrophic: M. Sairanen, G. Lucas, P. Ernfors, M. Castrén and E. Castrén, 'Brain-Derived Neurotrophic Factor and Antidepressant Drugs Have Different but Coordinated Effects on Neuronal Turnover, Proliferation, and Survival in the Adult Dentate Gyrus', *Journal of Neuroscience* 25, no. 5 (2005): 1089–94.

Elizabeth Loftus on inducing false memories: E. F. Loftus and J. E. Pickrell, 'The Formation of False Memories', *Psychiatric Annals* 25 (1995): 720–25.

Diazepam another instigator of diagnostic drift: Erik MacLaren, Ph.D., and Amanda Lautieri, eds., Sober Media Group, 'Valium History and Statistics', DrugAbuse.com, 21 December 2016.

Time **magazine's report on patient Susan:** Anastasia Toufexis, 'The Personality Pill', *Time,* 24 June 2001.

Psychiatrists prescribe fluoxetine: Ashley Pettus, 'Psychiatry by Prescription', *Harvard Magazine,* July–August 2006.

'Dial-A-Prozac': Glenmullen, *Prozac Backlash.*

Distinction between the solid science involved: Edward Shorter, *A History of Psychiatry: From the Era of the Asylum to the Age of Prozac* (New York: Wiley, 1998), 324.

Pharmacological hedonism: Carlat, *Unhinged,* 104–5.

Serotonin boosters cause subjects to become peppier: Simon Sobo, 'Psychotherapy Perspectives in Medication Management', *Psychiatric Times,* 1 April 1999.

Fluoxetine reduces frequency of ultrasonic cries in baby rats: Ibid.

Ann Bolo on going off of fluoxetine: Personal interview with Ann Bolo, 18 December 2016.

'A profession undergoing intellectual rejuvenation': Lieberman, *Shrinks,* 234.

'hard to think of a single truly novel psychotropic drug': Richard A. Friedman, 'A Dry Pipeline for Psychiatric Drugs', *New York Times,* 19 August 2013.

Sufferers complaining of a light head: Solomon, *The Noonday Demon,* 288.

Cauliflower as a cure for depression: Ibid.

Patients of Rufus of Ephesus: Ibid., 305.

Sexual stimulation of genitals as treatment: Ibid., 291.

Depression was seen as a sin: S. S. Asch, 'Depression and Demonic Possession: The Analyst as an Exorcist', *Hillside Journal of Clinical Psychiatry* 7, no. 2 (1985): 149.

Rufus's 'sacred remedy': Solomon, *The Noonday Demon*, 290.

5. Placebos

'Placebos are extraordinary drugs': Robert Buckman and Kark Sabbagh, *Magic or Medicine? An Investigation of Healing and Healers* (Toronto: Key Porter, 1993), 246.

'febrile, gasping for air, completely bedridden': B. Klopfer, 'Psychological Variables in Human Cancer', *Journal of Projective Techniques* 21, no. 4 (December 1957): 331.

X-rays showing that the tumours had shrunk: Ibid.

Mr Wright's tumours reappeared: Ibid., 333.

Ancient medicine consisted almost entirely of placebos: Arthur K. Shapiro and Elaine Shapiro, 'The Placebo: Is it Much Ado about Nothing?', *The Placebo Effect: An Interdisciplinary Exploration,* ed. Anne Harrington (Cambridge, MA: Harvard University Press, 1997), 12–36.

Theriac was an especially popular placebo: Ibid., 13.

In the 1970s endorphins were discovered: J. Hughes, T. W. Smith, H. W. Kosterlitz, L. A. Fothergill, B A. Morgan and H. R. Morris, 'Identification of Two Related Pentapeptides from the Brain with Potent Opiate Agonist Activity', *Nature* 258 (December 1975): 577–80.

Most patients were given a placebo: Daniel Moerman, *Meaning, Medicine and the 'Placebo Effect'* (New York: Cambridge University Press, 2002), 103–4, 125.

How placebos might work, colour correlation: Ibid., 104.

Sumatriptan versus placebo: Ibid., 52.

People with Alzheimer's: Robert Trivers, *The Folly of Fools: The Logic of Deceit and Self-Deception in Human Life* (New York: Basic Books, 2011), 73.

Diazepam affects a person: Steven Poole, *Rethink: The Surprising History of New Ideas* (New York: Scribner, 2016), 214. See also Beth Israel Deaconess Medical Center, 'Knowingly Taking Placebo Pills Eases Pain, Study Finds', *ScienceDaily,* 14 October 2016.

No definitive profile of a placebo person: Moerman, *Meaning, Medicine and the 'Placebo Effect',* 33–34.

Outcome of sham surgeries: Ibid., 59.

67 per cent reported subjective improvement: Ibid., 33–34.

Patient estimates that he is 95 per cent better: Ibid. For statistics on later treatment, see also Daniel Moerman, 'Explanatory Mechanisms for Placebo Effects: Cultural Influences and the Meaning Response', in *Science of the Placebo: Toward an Interdisciplinary Research Agenda,* eds. Harry Guess, Linda Engel, Arthur Kleinman and John Kusek (London: The BMJ, 2002), 86.

'Electrical machines have great appeal': Alan G. Johnson, 'Surgery as Placebo', *The Lancet,* 22 October 1994, quoted in Moerman, *Meaning, Medicine and the 'Placebo Effect',* 64.

The belief in the surgery sparks an increase of dopamine production: Jo Marchant, 'Parkinson's Patients Trained to Respond to Placebos', *Nature,* 10 February 2016.

Making medications so strong they trump placebo: Gary Greenberg, 'Is it Prozac? Or Placebo?', *Mother Jones,* November–December 2003; see also Irving Kirsch, *The Emperor's New Drugs: Exploding The Antidepressant Myth* (New York: Basic Books, 2010), 78.

Psychotherapeutic treatment in the United States: Moerman, *Meaning, Medicine and the 'Placebo Effect',* 89.

People respond similarly to all types of psychotherapy: Ibid., 90.

those who receive psychotherapy: Ibid., 90–92, 96–97.

Pennebaker's experiment with college students: Moerman, *Meaning, Medicine and the 'Placebo Effect',* 96–97.

Use of 'causal words' improves health: Jessica Wapner, 'He Counts Your Words (Even Those Pronouns)', *New York Times,* 13 October 2008.

Correlation of the effect between experience of therapist and outcome is 0.01: Moerman, *Meaning, Medicine and the 'Placebo Effect',* 92.

Study involving skilled therapists and kindly non-therapists: Ibid., 93.

'healing effects of a benign human relationship': Hans H. Strupp and Suzanne W. Hadley, 'Specific vs. Nonspecific Factors in Psychotherapy: A Controlled Study of Outcome', *Archives of General Psychiatry* 36 no. 10 (1979): 1135.

Account of overdose on placebo antidepressants: Joseph Stromberg, 'What Is the Nocebo Effect?', Smithsonian.com, 23 July 2012. See also R. R. Reeves, M. E. Ladner, R. H. Hart and R. S. Burke, 'Nocebo Effects with Antidepressant Clinical Drug Trial Placebos', *General Hospital Psychiatry* 29, no. 3 (2007): 275–77.

Voodoo death accounts: Walter Bradford Cannon, '"VOODOO" Death', *American Journal of Public Health* 92, no. 10 (2002): 1593.

Researchers believe that nocebos precipitate: W. Häuser, E. Hansen and P. Enck, 'Nocebo Phenomena in Medicine: Their Relevance in Everyday Clinical Practice', *Deutsches Ärzteblatt International* 109 no. 26 (2012): 459–65.

When a newspaper releases a story about a suicide: Daniel Goleman, 'Pattern of Death: Copycat Suicides among Youths', *New York Times,* 18 March 1987. See also Madelyn Gould, Patrick Jamieson and Daniel Romer,

'Media Contagion and Suicide among the Young', *American Behavioral Scientist* 46, no. 9 (1 May 2003): 1269–84.

When an accident is reported: Harrington, *The Placebo Effect,* 65.

Account of Frau Troffea and the 'dancing plague' of Strasbourg: Jennifer Viegas, '"Dancing Plague" and Other Odd Afflictions Explained', *Discovery News,* 1 August 2008; and F. Sirois, 'Perspectives on Epidemic Hysteria', in *Mass Psychogenic Illness: A Social Psychological Analysis.* eds. M. J. Colligan, J. W. Pennebaker and L. R. Murphy (Abingdon-on-Thames: Routledge, 1982), 217–36.

The more care you lavish on a person: Ted J. Kaptchuk, John M. Kelley, Lisa A. Conboy, Roger B. Davis, Catherine E. Kerr, Eric E. Jacobson et al., 'Components of Placebo Effect: Randomised Controlled Trial in Patients with Irritable Bowel Syndrome', *BMJ* 336 (2008): 999. See also Elaine Schattner, 'The Placebo Debate: Is It Unethical to Prescribe Them to Patients?', *The Atlantic,* 19 December 2011.

6. Psilocybin (Magic Mushrooms)

Carol Vincent found a strange swelling: Personal interview with Carol Vincent, 14 April 2016.

He believes meditation 'opened up a spiritual window': David Jay Brown and Louise Reitman, 'An Interview with Roland Griffiths, Ph.D.', https://www.maps.org/news-letters/v20n1/v20n1-22to25.pdf. See also Olga Khazan, 'The Life-Changing Magic of Mushrooms', *The Atlantic,* 1 December 2016, Web.

His landmark study of the drug: Roland Griffiths et al., 'Psilocybin Can Occasion Mystical-Type Experiences Having Substantial and Sustained Personal Meaning and Spiritual Significance', *Psychopharmacology* 187 no. 3 (27 May 2006): 284–92.

Huxley's written request to inject him: Laura Huxley, *This Timeless Moment* (San Francisco: Mercury House, 1991), 320.

Kast's statistical analysis: Stanislav Grof, *The Ultimate Journey: Consciousness and the Mystery of Death* (Santa Cruz, CA: MAPS, 2006), 204–6.

Kast went on to study 128 cancer patients: Ibid., 205.

Kast's study with eighty people: Ibid.

Wasson hated mushrooms: R. Gordon Wasson, 'Seeking the Magic Mushroom', *Life,* 10 June 1957. See also Valentina Pavlova Wasson and R. Gordon Wasson, *Mushrooms, Russia, and History,* vol. 1 (New York: Pantheon, 1957), 22.

Wasson had heard stories: Wasson, 'Seeking the Magic Mushroom'.

'they cried out in rapture over the firmness': Ibid.

'I am a cloud person, a dew-on-the-grass person': Ibid.

The mushrooms were sacred to them: Ibid.

'everything took on a Mexican character': Michael Pollan, 'The Trip Treatment', *The New Yorker,* 9 February 2015.

Timothy Leary learning about the magic mushrooms: Jim Parker, 'Intelligent People Keep Growing and Changing: The DSN Interview with Dr. Timothy Leary', *Drug Survival News,* part 1 (September–October 1981): 12–19.

Grof's description of 'psychedelic therapy': Grof, *The Ultimate Journey,* 207.

'all our patients transcended the realm of postnatal biography': Ibid.

'fear of their own physiological demise diminished': Ibid., 209–10.

'I was taken to a fresh windswept world': Ibid., 213–14.

Untimely death of Walter Pahnke: Ibid., 196–97, 215.

Method and process of Grof's psychedelic sessions: Ibid., 215–28.

Case study of Matthew: Stanislav Grof and Joan Halifax, *The Human Encounter with Death* (New York: Dutton, 1977), 66–68.

On Matthew's psychedelic session: Grof, *The Ultimate Journey,* 239–41.

Case study of Jesse: Grof and Halifax, *The Human Encounter with Death,* 80–81.

On Jesse's psychedelic session: Grof, *The Ultimate Journey,* 253.

'The perspective of another incarnation': Ibid.

'I don't really have altogether a definitive answer': Personal interview with Charles Grob, 3 February 2012.

'On psychedelics you have an experience': Personal interview with John Halpern, 8 February 2012.

Pahnke's Good Friday experiment: Thomas B. Roberts and Robert N. Jesse, 'Recollections of the Good Friday Experiment: An Interview with Huston Smith', *Journal of Transpersonal Psychology* 29, no. 2 (1997): 99–103.

Eight said they had a mystical experience: Pollan, 'The Trip Treatment'.

Psilocybin high shared many aspects: Ibid.

Doblin finding methodological flaws: Ibid.

Patient thinking he was meant to announce the next Messiah: Rick Doblin, 'Pahnke's "Good Friday Experiment": A Long-Term Follow-Up and Methodological Critique', *Journal of Transpersonal Psychology* 23, no. 1 (1991): 1–25.

Critiques of 'chemical mysticism': Grof, *The Ultimate Journey,* 222.

The counterargument, 'chemical mysticism': Ibid.

Psychedelic plants at the root of all religions: Richard J. Miller, 'Religion as a Product of Psychotropic Drug Use', *The Atlantic,* 27 December 2013.

Leary's prison experiment: Ralph Metzner, Ph.D. 'Reflections on the Concord Prison Experiment and the Follow-Up Study', *Journal of Psychoactive Drugs* 30, no. 4 (1998): 427–28. See also Timothy Leary, Ralph

Metzner, Madison Presnell, Gunther Weil, Ralph Schwitzgebel and Sarah Kinne, 'A New Behavior Change Program Using Psilocybin', *Psychotherapy* 2, no. 2 (July 1965): 61–72.

Ayahuasca experiment in Brazil: Simon Romero, 'In Brazil, Some Inmates Get Therapy with Hallucinogenic Tea', *New York Times,* 28 March 2015.

Importance of set and setting: J. Huston Smith, *The Huston Smith Reader* (Berkeley: University of California Press, 26 March 2012), 165.

'It feels a little bit like Rip Van Winkle': Personal interview with Charles Grob, 18 March 2012.

'It is enormously exciting': Ibid.

Psilocybin as 'existential medicine': Ibid.

Grob envisioning treatment centres: Ibid.

'Why confine this to just the dying?': Personal interview with Rick Doblin, 3 March 2012.

Griffiths's 2006 psilocybin study: Griffiths et al., 'Psilocybin Can Occasion Mystical-Type Experiences', 268.

Fourteen-month follow-up: Ibid.

Griffiths's study and personality domains: Ibid.

'The core feature of the mystical experience': Brown and Reitman, 'An Interview with Roland Griffiths, Ph.D.'

Importance of priming the patient: Personal interview with Charles Grob, 18 March 2012.

Nutt et al. MRI study: David Nutt et al., 'Neural Correlates of the Psychedelic State as Determined by fMRI Studies with Psilocybin', *PNAS* 109, no. 6 (7 February 2012): 2138–43.

All patients displayed marked improvement, and five had had a complete remission: Zoe Cormier, 'Magic-Mushroom Drug Lifts Depression in First Human Trial', *Nature,* 17 May 2016.

Additional studies done at New York University: Pollan, 'The Trip Treatment'.

Charles Grob's findings from his psilocybin study: Charles S. Grob, 'Commentary on Harbor-UCLA Psilocybin Study', *MAPS Bulletin* 20, no. 1 (2010): 28–29.

'an intuition that consciousness is alive': Brown and Reitman. 'An Interview with Roland Griffiths, Ph.D.'

Griffiths exploring the role of psilocybin: Roland Griffiths et al., 'Pilot Study of the 5-HT$_{2A}$R Agonist Psilocybin in the Treatment of Tobacco Addiction', *Journal of Psychopharmacology* 28, no. 11 (11 September 2014): 983–92. See also Lauren Nelson, 'Hallucinogen in "Magic Mushrooms" Helps Longtime Smokers Quit in Hopkins Trial', John Hopkins University, *The Hub,* 11 September 2014, Web.

William's experience in Griffiths's study: Personal interview with Roland Griffiths, 10 October 2015.

'the ultimate existential medicine': Personal interview with Charles Grob, 18 March 2012.

Rick Doblin's mission to legalise psychedelics: Personal interview with Rick Doblin, 8 April 2017.

Doblin's opinion regarding how psilocybin may prove useful: Ibid.

Carol Vincent listening to black spirituals: Personal interview with Carol Vincent, 3 March 2016.

7. MDMA (Ecstasy)

Thomas and Kelly Shuge's marital problems: Personal interview with Thomas and Kelly Shuge, 8 November 2014.

On the history and development of MDMA: Roland W. Freudenmann, Florian Öxler and Sabine Bernschneider-Reif, 'The Origin of MDMA (Ecstasy) Revisited: The True Story Reconstructed from the Original Documents'. *Addiction* 101, no. 9 (September 2006): 1241–45. See also Alexander T. Shulgin, 'History of MDMA', in *Ecstasy: The Clinical, Pharmacological and Neurotoxicological Effects of the Drug MDMA,* ed. S. J. Peroutka (Boston: Kluwer, 1990), 1–20, esp. 4–6; also Alexander T. Shulgin, 'The Background and Chemistry of MDMA', *Journal of Psychoactive Drugs* 18, no. 4 (1986): 291–304, esp. 291, 297.

Shulgin feeling 'absolutely clean': Alexander Shulgin and Ann Shulgin, *PiHKAL: A Chemical Love Story* (Berkeley, CA: Transform Press, 1991), entry 109.

Therapists using MDMA in their practice: Myron J. Stolaroff, *The Secret Chief Revealed* (Santa Cruz, CA: MAPS, 2005).

Effectiveness of MDMA in couples counselling: Matthew J. Baggott et al., 'Intimate Insight: MDMA Changes How People Talk about Significant Others', *Journal of Psychopharmacology* 29, no. 6 (28 April 2015): 669–77.

Doblin's critique of Leary: Personal interview with Rick Doblin, 11 October 2015.

Percentage of Americans who have used psychedelics: Jeremy Travis, 'Rise in Hallucinogen Use', *NIJ Research in Brief,* October 1997.

Doblin discussing social stigma of psychedelics: Personal interview with Rick Doblin, 24 August 2016.

Charles Grob and Alicia Danforth on MDMA for autistic adults with social anxiety: Alicia Danforth et al., 'MDMA-Assisted Therapy: A New Treatment Model for Social Anxiety in Autistic Adults', *Progress in Neuro-Psychopharmacology and Biological Psychiatry* 64 (4 January 2016): 242.

91 per cent of respondents report an increase in feelings of connectedness: Ibid.

LSD experiments with autistic children in 1960s: Ibid., 242–43.

LSD was also given to mute catatonic schizophrenics: Ibid.

The need for 'good medical research' into MDMA: Personal interview with John Halpern, 8 May 2015.

The need for high-quality research: Personal interview with John Halpern, 13 November 2015.

Mithoefer's MDMA study for post-traumatic stress disorder: Michael C. Mithoefer, Mark T. Wagner, Ann T. Mithoefer, Lisa Jerome, Scott F. Martin, Berra Yazar-Klosinski, Yvonne Michel, Timothy D. Brewerton and Rick Doblin, 'Durability of Improvement in Posttraumatic Stress Disorder Symptoms and Absence of Harmful Effects or Drug Dependency after 3,4-Methylenedioxymethamphetamine-Assisted Psychotherapy: A Prospective Long-Term Follow-Up Study', *Journal of Psychopharmacology* 27, no. 1 (20 November 2012), Web.

Second phase of Mithoefer's study: Michael C. Mithoefer et al., 'The Safety and Efficacy of {+/-}3,4-Methylenedioxymethamphetamine-Assisted Psychotherapy in Subjects with Chronic, Treatment-Resistant Posttraumatic Stress Disorder: The First Randomized Controlled Pilot Study', *Journal of Psychopharmacology* 25, no. 4 (2011): 452.

MDMA allowing patients to reframe trauma: M. B. Young, R. Andero, K. J. Ressler and L. L. Howell, '3,4-Methylenedioxymethamphetamine Facilitates Fear Extinction Learning', *Translational Psychiatry* 5, e634 (2015): 138.

MDMA helped Kelly Shuge: Personal interviews with Thomas Shuge and Kelly Shuge, 3 January 2015 and 15 April 2016.

Oxytocin increasing when on MDMA: G. J. Dumont, F. C. Sweep, R. van der Steen, R. Hermsen, A. R. Donders, D. J. Touw, J. M. van Gerven, J. K. Buitelaar and R. J. I. Verkes, 'Increased Oxytocin Concentrations and Prosocial Feelings in Humans after Ecstasy (3,4-Methylenedioxymethamphetamine Administration', *Social Neuroscience* 4(4) (2009): 359–66.

Brain is 'flooded' with oxytocin when on MDMA: Personal interview with Rick Doblin, 11 May 2016.

Prairie voles and oxytocin: Thomas R. Insel and Terrence J. Hulihan, 'A Gender-Specific Mechanism for Pair Bonding: Oxytocin and Partner Preference Formation in Monogamous Voles', *Behavioral Neuroscience* 109, no. 4 (August 1995): 782–89.

MDMA made in Boston and Texas: Torsten Passie and Udo Benzenhöfer, 'The History of MDMA as an Underground Drug in the United States, 1960–1979', *Journal of Psychoactive Drugs* 48, no. 2 (2016): 67–75. See also Bruce Eisner, *Ecstasy: The MDMA Story* (Berkeley, CA: Ronin Publishing, 1989) 6, 14–15.

Senator in Texas grows concerned about MDMA: AP, 'U.S. Will Ban 'Ecstasy,' a Hallucinogenic Drug', *New York Times,* 1 June 1985. See also Jerome Beck and Marsha Rosenbaum, *Pursuit of Ecstasy: The MDMA Experience* (Albany, NY: SUNY Press, 1994), 18–20.

MDMA caused neurotoxicity in rats: G. A. Ricaurte et al., '(±)3,4-Methylenedioxymethamphetamine ("Ecstasy")-Induced Serotonin

Neurotoxicity: Studies in Animals', *Neuropsychobiology* 42 (2000): 5–10.

'We saw it coming': Personal interview with Rick Doblin, 14 October 2013.

Doblin challenges Ricaurte's study: Ibid.

Doblin wins lawsuit: Ibid.

'For me the work has to be not about what we've achieved': Personal interview with Rick Doblin, 5 November 2013.

Doblin fighting the Drug Enforcement Administration (DEA): Ibid.

Ricaurte claiming primates are dying from MDMA: G. A. Ricaurte, J. Yuan, G. Hatzidimitriou, B. J. Cord and U. D. McCann, 'Severe Dopaminergic Neurotoxicity in Primates after a Common Recreational Dose Regimen of MDMA ("Ecstasy")', *Science* 297, no. 5590 (27 September 2002).

'They shut us right down': Personal interview with Rick Doblin, 5 November 2013.

'We've seen thousands of people safely use MDMA': Personal interview with Julie Holland, 6 November 2013.

'MDMA is just not a significant cause of psychiatric crisis': Ibid.

Ricaurte's retraction: George A. Ricaurte et al., 'Letters: Retraction', *Science* 301, no. 5639 (12 September 2003): 1479. See also Leo John, 'RTI Denies It Made Mistake That Torpedoed Results of a $1.3M Study', *Triangle Business Journal,* 10 November 2003, Web.

'The Ricaurte study has definitely added to the stigma': Personal interview with Rick Doblin, 10 March 2016.

Efficacy of MDMA in treating post-traumatic stress disorder: Mithoefer et al., 'The Safety and Efficacy of {+/-}3,4-Methylenedioxymethamphetamine-Assisted Psychotherapy'.

MDMA has many applications beyond the treatment of post-traumatic stress disorder: Personal interview with Rick Doblin, 12 October 2013.

MDMA stored at Purdue University: Ibid.

Doblin against using MDMA for couples counselling: Ibid.

Marriage is not a disease: Ibid.

'My life's goal is to see the psychedelics made into prescription drugs': Ibid.

8. PKMzeta/Zip (Memory Drugs)

Population doubling: Jennifer M. Ortman and Victoria A. Velkoff, 'An Aging Nation: The Older Population in the United States', United States Census Bureau, May 2014.

Recalling events reactivates fear circuitry: Alain Brunet, Ph.D., Joaquin Poundja, B.Sc., Jacques Tremblay, M.D., Éric Bui, M.D., Émilie Thomas, B.Sc., Scott P. Orr, Ph.D., Abdelmadjid Azzoug, B.Sc., Philippe Birmes, M.D., Ph.D., and Roger K. Pitman, M.D., 'Trauma Reactivation under the Influence of Propranolol Decreases Posttraumatic Stress Symptoms and Disorder: 3 Open-Label Trials', *Journal of Clinical Psychopharmacology* 31, no. 4 (August 2011): 547–50.

Propranolol inhibits adrenaline: A. Brunet et al., 'Effect of Post-Retrieval Propranolol on Psychophysiologic Responding during Subsequent Script-Driven Traumatic Imagery in Post-Traumatic Stress Disorder', *Journal of Psychiatric Research* 42, no. 6 (2008): 503–6.

Beta blocker works to dilute traumatic memories: Ibid.

Todd Sacktor studying protein kinase C: Personal interview with Todd Sacktor, 12 February 2014.

Sacktor influenced by father: Ibid.

Loftus discovering suggestibility in recall: E. F. Loftus and J. E. Pickrell, 'The Formation of False Memories', *Psychiatric Annals* 25 (1995): 720–25.

Phelps and Hirst, flashbulb memories: William Hirst, Elizabeth A. Phelps et al., 'Long-Term Memory for the Terrorist Attack of September 11: Flashbulb Memories, Event Memories, and the Factors That Influence Their Retention', *Journal of Experimental Psychology General* 138, no. 2 (2009): 161–76. See also William Hirst, Elizabeth A. Phelps, Robert Meksin, Chandan J. Vaidya, Marcia K. Johnson, Karen J. Mitchell, Randy L. Buckner, Andrew E. Budson, John D. E. Gabrieli, Cindy Lustig, Mara Mather, Kevin N. Ochsner, Daniel Schacter, Jon S. Simons, Keith B. Lyle, Alexandru F. Cuc, Andreas Olsson, 'A Ten-Year Follow-Up of a Study of Memory for the Attack of September 11, 2001: Flashbulb Memories and Memories for Flashbulb Events', *Journal of Experimental Psychology* 144, no. 3 (9 March 2015): 604–23.

Act of repeating a narrative somehow contaminates it: E. Loftus, 'Our Changeable Memories: Legal and Practical Implications', *Nature Reviews Neuroscience* 4 (March 2003): 231–34.

Shift in mental weight alters the network of neurons: Tony W. Buchanan, 'Retrieval of Emotional Memories', *Psychological Bulletin* 133, no. 5 (2007): 761–79. See also Jonah Lehrer, 'The Forgetting Pill Erases Painful Memories Forever', *Wired,* 17 February 2012.

PKMzeta always present in the brain: Personal interview with Todd Sacktor, 30 May 2015.

Jerry Yin did a similar experiment with fruit flies: Lewis D. Solomon, *The Quest for Human Longevity* (Livingston, NJ: Transaction Publishers, 2006), 130.

PKMzeta and addictions: Personal interview with Todd Sacktor, 12 February 2014.

Sacktor's comparison of PKMzeta to a sheepdog: Michael Humphrey, 'Todd Sacktor's Search for the Memory Enzyme', *Forbes,* 25 May 2011.

The mice had no memory attenuation: Lenora J. Volk, Julia L. Bachman, Richard Johnson, Yilin Yu and Richard L. Huganir, 'PKM-ζ Is Not Required for Hippocampal Synaptic Plasticity, Learning and Memory', *Nature* 493 (January 2013): 420–23.

Memory's back-up system: Ibid.

'It turns out that when PKMzeta is genetically eliminated': Todd Sacktor, email correspondence, 31 May 2015.

He says he hated school and was always the fat, shy, smart kid: Personal interview with Todd Sacktor, 30 May 2015.

ZIP undoing memories in rodents' brains: Ewen Callaway, 'Long-Term Memory Gets Wiped', *Nature,* August 2007, Web.

ZIP not damaging the rodents' brains: Todd Charlton Sacktor, 'Memory Maintenance by PKMζ—An Evolutionary Perspective', *Molecular Brain,* 18 September 2012.

Chronic pain linked to memory: D. S. Choi, D. Y. Choi, R. A. Whittington and S. S. Nedeljković, 'Sudden Amnesia Resulting in Pain Relief: The Relationship between Memory and Pain', *Pain* 132, nos. 1–2 (November 2007): 206–10.

'ZIP might be injected to try to "reset' the synapses in that region': Interview with Todd Sacktor, 'Erasing Your Memories', *New York Times,* 13 April 2009.

'I am somewhat hesitant': Elie Wiesel, 'Never Forget', op-ed, *New York Daily News,* 10 April 2009.

'imagining the future depends': Daniel L. Schacter et al., 'Remembering the Past to Imagine the Future: The Prospective Brain', *Nature Reviews Neuroscience* 8 (September 2007): 657.

Reader comments in response to Sacktor interview: Sacktor, 'Erasing Your Memories'.

By 2050 more than 16 million Americans will have Alzheimer's: Paola Scommegna, 'Dementia Cases Expected to Triple by 2050 as World Population Ages', Population Reference Bureau, November 2012, Web.

If the molecule is available to the brain in larger amounts: Personal interview with Todd Sacktor, 30 May 2015.

'we don't have another treatment for [Alzheimer's]': Gwenn Smith, 'A Stimulating Finding in Mild Alzheimer's', *Hopkins Medicine Magazine,* Spring–Summer 2012.

DBS for memory disorders discovered via obese man: C. Hamani, et al., 'Memory Enhancement Induced by Hypothalamic/Fornix Deep Brain Stimulation', *Annals of Neurology* 63. no. 1 (2008): 119–23. See also Carl Erik Fisher, 'Psychiatrists Embrace Deep-Brain Stimulation: Brain-Stimulation Procedures for Psychiatric Disorders Are on the Rise. Should We Be Concerned?', *Scientific American Mind,* 1 January 2014, Web.

Electrodes implanted in patients with Alzheimer's: Andres M. Lozano et al., 'A Phase II Study of Fornix Deep Brain Stimulation in Mild Alzheimer's Disease', *Journal of Alzheimer's Disease* 54, no. 2 (2016): 777–87.

9. Deep Brain Stimulation

Mario Della Grotta case: Series of personal interviews with Mario Della Grotta, June 2003–September 2004.

Pierre Paul Broca confirms theory of localisation in 1861: Maria Konnikova, 'The Man Who Couldn't Speak and How He Revolutionized Psychology', *Scientific American,* 8 February 2013.

Moniz looking for suitable lobotomy patients: Dominik Gross, Ph.D., M.D., D.D.S., and Gereon Schäfer, Ph.D., 'Egas Moniz (1874–1955) and the "Invention" of Modern Psychosurgery: A Historical and Ethical Reanalysis under Special Consideration of Portuguese Original Sources', *Journal of Neurosurgery* 30, no. 2 (February 2011): E8.

By the late 1950s, more than twenty thousand patients: Fiona Govan, 'Lobotomy: A History of the Controversial Procedure', *Telegraph,* August 2011, Web.

Heath implanted electrodes in human beings: James Hamblin, 'Deep Brain Stimulation for the Soul', *The Atlantic,* 25 June 2013.

Feelings of rage, fear, pleasure vary by electrode placement: Lauren Slater, 'Who Holds the Clicker?', *Mother Jones,* November 2005.

Heath's treatment of a homosexual man: Robert Heath, 'Pleasure and Brain Activity in Man: Deep and Surface Electroencephalograms during Orgasm', *Journal of Nervous and Mental Disease* 154, no. 1 (1972): 6–9. See also John Horgan, 'What Are Science's Ugliest Experiments?', *Scientific American* blog, 14 May 2012.

People had believed that thoughts and emotions: Michael S. Sweeney, *Brain: The Complete Mind* (Washington, DC: National Geographic, 2009).

Account of Delgado provoking an implanted bull: John A. Osmundsen, '"Matador" with a Radio Stops Wired Bull: Modified Behavior in Animals the Subject of Brain Study', *New York Times,* 17 May 1965.

Louis Jolyon West, the Vacaville Prison and the CIA: Harry V. Martin and David Caul, 'Mind Control', thirteen-part series, *Napa Sentinel,* 13 August–22 November 1991. See also Samuel Chavkin, *The Mind Stealers: Psychosurgery and Mind Control* (Boston: Houghton Mifflin, 1978), 13–15, 60–63, 96–109.

Implants were resurrected in 1987: A. L. Benabid, P. Pollak, A. Louveau, S. Henry and J. de Rougemont, 'Combined (Thalamotomy and Stimulation) Stereotactic Surgery of the VIM Thalamic Nucleus for Bilateral Parkinson Disease', *Applied Neurophysiology* 50, nos. 1–6 (1987): 344–46.

150,000 patients worldwide implanted for movement disorders: Helen Mayberg, email correspondence, 13 June 2017.

'It's how a lot of medicine happens': Personal interview with Jeff Arle, 21 January 2005.

'We want more than anything to find that sweet spot, and go there': Personal interview with Helen Mayberg, 5 January 2005.

'If you can get relief without invasive surgery': Personal interview with Harold Sackheim, 7 February 2005.

'We have searched and searched for the Holy Grail': Personal interview with William Burke, 17 June 2003.

Remission rates of 31 per cent after fourteen weeks: Thomas Insel, 'Antidepressants: A Complicated Picture', National Institute of Mental Health blog, 2011.

Of the 65 per cent who are helped: Personal interview with John Halpern, 19 August 2016.

Between 10 and 20 per cent of patients never improve: Ibid.

Surgeons choose the brain targets: Personal interview with Ben Greenberg, 13 March 2005.

'We chose the anterior limb': Personal interview with Don Malone, 14 March 2005.

Greenberg and colleagues see a minimum of 25 per cent: David Orenstein, 'Deep Brain Stimulation Helps Severe OCD, but Pioneer Advises Caution, Compassion', AAAS presentation, *News from Brown*, Brown University, 16 February 2011, Web.

'In the real world, the group of patients': Ibid.

Activity in Area 25 decreased: Helen Mayberg et al., 'Deep Brain Stimulation for Treatment-Resistant Depression', *Neuron* 45, no. 5 (March 2005): 651–60.

'Acute effects' felt by Mayberg's patients: Ibid.

Results of follow-up studies: Ibid.

Mayberg's study in Area 25: Sylvia Wrobel, 'Flipping the Switch', *Emory Medicine*, Spring 2015.

Deep brain stimulation in Dutch patient: Carl Erik Fisher, 'Psychiatrists Embrace Deep-Brain Stimulation', *Scientific American Mind*, 2 January 2014.

More than five hundred people around the world: Personal interview with Helen Mayberg, 21 May 2017.

'There are people falling off the boat': Danielle Egan, 'Adverse Effects: The Perils of Deep Brain Stimulation for Depression', *Mad in America: Science, Psychiatry and Social Justice*, 24 September 2015, Web.

Americans spend billions of dollars a year: Paul E. Holtzheimer III, M.D., and Helen S. Mayberg, M.D., 'Deep Brain Stimulation for Treatment-Resistant Depression', *American Journal of Psychiatry* 167, no. 12 (December 2010): 1437–44.

Sales reps sell medication: Patti Neighmond, 'That Prescription Might Not Have Been Tested for Your Ailment', *NPR Morning Edition: Your Health*, 12 May 2014, Web.

Freeman's assembly-line lobotomies: Elliot Valenstein, *Great and Desperate Cures: The Rise and Decline of Psychosurgery and Other Radical Treatments for Mental Illness* (New York: Basic Books, 1986), 268.

'Psychosurgery cured me': H. A. Dannecker, 'Psychosurgery Cured Me', *Coronet,* October 1942, quoted in Mary De Young, *Madness: An American History of Mental Illness and Its Treatment* (Jefferson, NC: McFarland & Company, 1949), 225–26.

Psychosurgery patients lost what Moniz called their 'vital spark': Jenell Johnson, 'A Dark History: Memories of Lobotomy in the New Era of Psychosurgery', *Medicine Studies* 1, no. 4 (2009): 367–78.

'We don't want to repeat the mistakes of the past': Personal interview with Ben Greenberg, 3 March 2005.

'With DBS the thing has a certain immediacy to it': Personal interview with Steven Rasmussen, 4 March 2005.

'That's one of the dangers': Personal interview with Ben Greenberg, 3 March 2005.

'We don't want hypomania': Personal interview with Don Malone, 4 March 2005.

Cosgrove's answer: 'The doctor': G. Rees Cosgrove, M.D., 'Session 6: Neuroscience, Brain, and Behavior V: Deep Brain Stimulation' [transcript], the President's Council on Bioethics, 25 June 2004.

'We don't even know what the optimal stimulation parameters are': Ibid.

'It's easy for any good neurosurgeon to do this now': Ibid.

Cosgrove described a patient: Slater, 'Who Holds the Clicker'.

Patient for the first implantable cardiac pacemaker: Denton A. Cooley, M.D., 'In Memoriam: Tribute to Åke Senning, Pioneering Cardiovascular Surgeon', *Texas Heart Institute Journal* 27, no. 3 (2000): 234–35.

Epilogue

Drugs that dampen dopamine: H. Steeds, R. L. Carhart-Harris and J. M. Stone, 'Drug Models of Schizophrenia', *Therapeutic Advances in Psychopharmacology* 5, no. 1 (2015): 43–58.

No correlation between high dopamine: Robert Whitaker, *Anatomy of an Epidemic: Magic Bullets, Psychiatric Drugs, and the Astonishing Rise of Mental Illness in America* (New York: Crown, 2010), 75.

Some depressed people have a lot of serotonin: Ibid., 71.

Penfield's various demonstrations of brain specificity: Rahul Kumar and Vikram K. Yeragani, 'Penfield—A Great Explorer of Psyche-soma-neuroscience', *Indian Journal of Psychiatry* 53, no. 3 (2011): 277. See also Wilder Penfield and Edwin Boldrey, 'Somatic Motor and Sensory Representation in the Cerebral Cortex of Man as Studied by Electrical

Stimulation', *Brain* 60, no. 4 (1937): 389–443; Wilder Penfield and Lyle Gage, 'Cerebral Localization of Epileptic Manifestations', *Archives of Neurological Psychiatry* 30, no. 4 (1933): 709–27.

Carlat questions why psychiatrists should go to medical school: Daniel Carlat, *Unhinged: The Trouble with Psychiatry—A Doctor's Revelations about a Profession in Crisis* (New York: Free Press, 2010), 63.

Proponents of the monoamine hypothesis: P. L. Delgado, 'Depression: The Case for a Monoamine Deficiency', *Journal of Clinical Psychiatry* 61, supplement 6 (2000): 7–11.

'the amount of good, solid science': Theodore Millon, quoted in Alix Spiegel, 'The Dictionary of Disorder', *The New Yorker*, 3 January 2005.

Rosenhan's experiment: David L. Rosenhan, 'On Being Sane in Insane Places', *Science* 179 (1973): 250–58.

'If melancholia wasn't the Holy Grail': Gary Greenberg, 'Does Psychiatry Need Science?', *The New Yorker*, 23 April 2013.

***DSM-V* rejects the use of the DST:** Ibid.

'the main obstacle was exactly what you would think was melancholia's strength': Ibid.

No novel drugs have come through the pipeline: Richard A. Friedman, 'A Dry Pipeline for Psychiatric Drugs', *New York Times*, 19 August 2013.

That medicine turned out, despite the huge hype: Don H. Hockenbury and Sandra E. Hockenbury, *Discovering Psychology* (New York: Macmillan, 2010), 612.

Many autistic patients have experienced: Alicia Danforth et al., 'MDMA-Assisted Therapy: A New Treatment Model for Social Anxiety in Autistic Adults', *Progress in Neuro-Psychopharmacology and Biological Psychiatry* 64 (4 January 2016): 237–49.

Danforth would also like to see MDMA utilised: Alicia Danforth, 'Findings from a Collective Case Study on the MDMA/Ecstasy Experiences of Adults on the Autism Spectrum', [transcript] lecture at Psychedelic Science 2013, April 2013.

Some theorise that the drug is neurotrophic: J. C. Ibla, H. Hayashi, D. Bajic and S. G. Soriano, 'Prolonged Exposure to Ketamine Increases Brain Derived Neurotrophic Factor Levels in Developing Rat Brains', *Current Drug Safety* 4, no. 1 (2009): 11–16.

One study shows that: Nancy DiazGranados, M.D., M.S., et al., 'Rapid Resolution of Suicidal Ideation after a Single Infusion of an NMDA Antagonist in Patients with Treatment-Resistant Major Depressive Disorder', *Journal of Clinical Psychiatry* 71, no. 12 (2010): 1605–11.

300 million people worldwide suffer from depression: World Health Organization, http://www.who.int/mediacentre/factsheets/fs369/en/; Rachel Martin, 'Working through Depression: Many Stay on the Job, Despite Mental Illness', *NPR Mental Health*, 2015, Web.

Ayahuasca and psilocybin both have proven to be very effective: Gerald Thomas et al., 'Ayahuasca-Assisted Therapy for Addiction: Results from a Preliminary Observational Study in Canada', *Current Drug Abuse Reviews* 6, no. 1 (2013): 30–42. See also Lauren Nelson, 'Hallucinogen in "Magic Mushrooms" Helps Longtime Smokers Quit in Hopkins Trial', John Hopkins University, *The Hub,* 11 September 2014, Web.

Select Bibliography

Adam, David. 'Truth about Ecstasy's Unlikely Trip from Lab to Dance Floor'. *The Guardian,* 18 August 2006. www.theguardian.com/uk/2006/aug/18/topstories3.drugsandalcohol.

Agar, Jon. *Science in the 20th Century and Beyond.* Malden, MA: Polity Press, 2012.

Alexander, Bruce. *The Globalization of Addiction.* New York: Oxford University Press, 2010.

———. *Peaceful Measures: Canada's Way Out of the 'War on Drugs'.* Toronto: University of Toronto Press, 1990.

Alonso, Alvaro, et al. 'Use of Antidepressants and the Risk of Parkinson's Disease: A Prospective Study'. *Journal of Neurology, Neurosurgery, and Psychiatry* 80, no. 6 (2009): 671–74.

American Psychiatric Association. *Diagnostic and Statistical Manual of Mental Disorders.* 5th ed. (*DSM-V*). Arlington, VA: American Psychiatric Association Press, 2013.

Ames, Mark. *Going Postal: Rage, Murder, and Rebellion from Reagan's Workplaces to Clinton's Columbine and Beyond.* New York: Soft Skull Press, 2005.

Andrews, Evan. 'What Was the Dancing Plague of 1518?'. History.com, 14 September 2015. www.history.com/news/ask/what-was-the-dancing-plague-of-1518.

Angell, Marcia. *The Truth about the Drug Companies: How They Deceive Us and What to Do about It.* New York: Random House, 2004.

Austin, Paul. *A Quick Guide to Microdosing Psychedelics: Everything You Want to Know about This Cutting-Edge Method of Psychedelic Use.* [Kindle edn] Seattle: Amazon Digital Services, 2016.

Ayd, Frank J. and Barry Blackwell (eds). *Discoveries in Biological Psychiatry.* Baltimore Ayd Medical Communications, 1984.

Azmitia, Efrain C. 'Serotonin and Brain: Evolution, Neuroplasticity, and Homeostasis'. *International Review of Neurobiology* 77 (2006): 31–56.

Baggott, Matthew J., et al. 'Intimate Insight: MDMA Changes How People Talk about Significant Others'. *Journal of Psychopharmacology* 29, no. 6 (28 April 2015): 669–77.

Bateson, Gregory, Don D. Jackson, Jay Haley and John Weakland. 'Toward a Theory of Schizophrenia'. *Systems Research and Behavioral Science* 1, no. 4 (1956): 251–64.

Baumeister, A. A., M. F. Hawkins and S. M. Uzelac. 'The Myth of Reserpine-Induced Depression: Role in the Historical Development of the Monoamine Hypothesis'. *Journal of the History of the Neurosciences* 12, no. 2 (2003): 207–20.

Baumeister, Alan. 'The Tulane Electrical Brain Stimulation Program: A Historical Case Study in Medical Ethics'. *Journal of the History of the Neurosciences* 9, no. 3 (2000): 262–78.

Beck, Jerome and Marsha Rosenbaum. *The Pursuit of Ecstasy: The MDMA Experience*. Albany, NY: SUNY Press, 1994.

Belic, Roko, dir. *Happy* [film]. Wadi Rum Productions, 2011.

Benedictus, Leo. 'End of the Affair'. *The Guardian,* 16 January 2004. ww.theguardian.com/society/2004/jan/16/drugsandalcohol.uk.

Bergland, Christopher. 'Cortisol: Why the "Stress Hormone" Is Public Enemy No. 1'. *Psychology Today*, 22 January 2013. https://www.psychology today.com/blog/the-athletes-way/201301/cortisol-why-the-stress -hormone-is-public-enemy-no-1.

Beth Israel Deaconess Medical Center. 'Knowingly Taking Placebo Pills Eases Pain, Study Finds'. *ScienceDaily*, 14 October 2016. www. sciencedaily.com/releases/2016/10/161014214919.htm.

Blackwell, Barry. 'Adumbration: A History Lesson'. *International Network for the History of Neuropsychopharmacology* (18 December 2014). inhn.org/controversies/barry-blackwell-adumbration-a-history-lesson.html.

———. *Bits and Pieces of a Psychiatrist's Life*. Bloomington, IN: Xlibris, 2012.

Boodman, Sandra G. 'Running Out of Wonder Drugs'. *Washington Post,* 16 March 1993.

Boulton, Alan A., Glen B. Baker, William G. Dewhurst and Merton Sandler, eds. *Neurobiology of the Trace Amines: Analytical,*

Physiological, Pharmacological, Behavioral, and Clinical Aspects. New York: Springer Science and Business Media, 12 March 2013.

Breed, Michael D. and Janice Moore. *Animal Behavior.* Cambridge, MA: Academic Press, 2015.

Breggin, Peter and Ginger Ross Breggin. *Talking Back to Prozac: What Doctors Won't Tell You about Prozac and the Newer Antidepressants.* [e-book] New York: Open Road Media, 1 April 2014.

Brisch, Ralf. 'The Role of Dopamine in Schizophrenia from a Neurobiological and Evolutionary Perspective: Old Fashioned, but Still in Vogue'. *Front Psychiatry* 5 (2014): 47.

Broadhurst, Alan D. 'The Discovery of Imipramine from a Personal Viewpoint'. In *The Rise of Psychopharmacology and the Story of CINP*, edited by T. A. Ban, D. Healy and E. Shorter, 69–73. Budapest: Animula Press, 1998.

Brown, David Jay and Louise Reitman. 'An Interview with Roland Griffiths, Ph.D'. *MAPS Bulletin* 20, no. 1 (Spring 2010): 22–25.

Brunet, A., et al. 'Effect of Post-Retrieval Propranolol on Psychophysiologic Responding during Subsequent Script-Driven Traumatic Imagery in Post-Traumatic Stress Disorder'. *Journal of Psychiatric Research* 42, no. 6 (2008): 503–6.

Brunet, Alain, Ph.D., Joaquin Poundja, B.Sc., Jacques Tremblay, M.D., Éric Bui, M.D., Émilie Thomas, B.Sc., Scott P. Orr, Ph.D., Abdelmadjid Azzoug, B.Sc., Philippe Birmes, M.D., Ph.D., and Roger K. Pitman, M.D. 'Trauma Reactivation under the Influence of Propranolol Decreases Posttraumatic Stress Symptoms and Disorder: 3 Open-Label Trials'. *Journal of Clinical Psychopharmacology* 31, no. 4 (2011): 547–50.

Buchanan, Tony W. 'Retrieval of Emotional Memories'. *Psychological Bulletin* 133, no. 5 (2007): 761–79.

Buchman, Nili and Rael D. Strous. 'Side Effects of Long-Term Treatment with Fluoxetine'. *Clinical Neuropharmacology* 25, no. 1 (January 2002): 55–57.

Cade, Jack F. 'John Frederick Joseph Cade: Family Memories on the Occasion of the 50th Anniversary of His Discovery of the Use of Lithium in Mania'. *Australian and New Zealand Journal of Psychiatry* 33, no. 5 (1999): 615–18.

Cade, John F. 'Lithium Salts in the Treatment of Psychotic Excitement'. *Bulletin of the World Health Organization* 78, no. 4 (2000): 518–20.

Callaway, Ewen. 'Long-Term Memory Gets Wiped'. *Nature,* 2007. www.nature.com/news/2007/070813/full/news070813-10.html.

Cannon, Walter Bradford. '"VOODOO" Death'. *American Journal of Public Health* 92, no. 10 (October 2002): 1593–96.

Carlat, Daniel. *Unhinged: The Trouble with Psychiatry—A Doctor's Revelations about a Profession in Crisis.* New York: Free Press, 2010.

Cooley, Denton A., M.D. 'In Memoriam: Tribute to Åke Senning, Pioneering Cardiovascular Surgeon'. *Texas Heart Institute Journal* 27, no. 3 (2000): 234–35.

Cormier, Zoe. 'Magic-Mushroom Drug Lifts Depression in First Human Trial'. *Nature,* 17 May 2016. https://www.nature.com/news/magic-mushroom-drug-lifts-depression-in-first-human-trial-1.19919.

Cosgrove, G. Rees, M.D. 'Session 6: Neuroscience, Brain, and Behavior V: Deep Brain Stimulation'. The President's Council on Bioethics, 25 June 2004.

Danforth, Alicia. 'Findings from a Collective Case Study on the MDMA/Ecstasy Experiences of Adults on the Autism Spectrum'. [Transcript] lecture at Psychedelic Science 2013, April 2013.

Dannecker, H. A. 'Psychosurgery Cured Me'. *Coronet,* October 1942, quoted in Mary De Young, *Madness: an American History of Mental Illness and Its Treatment.* Jefferson, NC: McFarland & Company, 1949. 225–26.

Danquah, M. N-A. *Willow Weep for Me.* New York: W. W. Norton, 1988.

De Young, Mary. *Madness: An American History of Mental Illness and Its Treatment.* Jefferson, NC: McFarland & Company, 1949.

Delgado, P. L. 'Depression: The Case for a Monoamine Deficiency'. *Journal of Clinical Psychiatry* 61, no. 6 (2000): 7–11.

DePoy, Elizabeth and Stephen French Gilson. *Human Behavior Theory and Applications: A Critical Thinking Approach.* New York: Sage Publications, 2012.

'Depression'. National Alliance on Mental Illness, undated. www.nami.org/learn-more/mental-health-conditions/depression.

'Depression'. World Health Organization Media Centre Fact Sheet, February 2017. www.who.int/mediacentre/factsheets/fs369/en/.

DiazGranados, Nancy, M.D., M.S., et al. 'Rapid Resolution of Suicidal Ideation after a Single Infusion of an NMDA Antagonist in Patients with Treatment-Resistant Major Depressive Disorder'. *Journal of Clinical Psychiatry* 71, no. 12 (2010): 1605–11.

Doblin, Rick. 'Pahnke's "Good Friday Experiment": A Long-Term Follow-Up and Methodological Critique'. *Journal of Transpersonal Psychology* 23, no. 1 (1991): 1–25.

Dumont, G. J., F. C. Sweep, R. van der Steen, R. Hermsen, A. R. Donders, D. J. Touw, J. M. van Gerven, J. K. Buitelaar and R. J. I. Verkes. 'Increased Oxytocin Concentrations and Prosocial Feelings in Humans after Ecstasy (3,4-Methylenedioxymethamphetamine) Administration'. *Social Neuroscience* 4(4) (2009): 359–66.

Egan, Danielle. 'Adverse Effects: The Perils of Deep Brain Stimulation for Depression'. *Mad in America: Science, Psychiatry and Social Justice,* 24 September 2015. https://www.madinamerica.com/2015/09/adverse-effects-perils-deep-brain-stimulation-depression.

Ehrenberg, Alain. *Weariness of the Self: Diagnosing the History of Depression in the Contemporary Age.* Montreal: McGill–Queen's University Press, 2010.

Eisner, Bruce. *Ecstasy: The MDMA Story.* Berkeley, CA: Ronin, 1989.

El-Hai, Jack. *The Lobotomist.* New York: Wiley, 2007.

Enghag, Per. *Encyclopedia of the Elements: Technical Data–History–Processing–Applications.* New York: Wiley, 2004.

Estrada, E. 'Clinical Uses of Chlorpromazine in Veterinary Medicine'. *Journal of the American Veterinary Medical Association* 128, no. 6 (1956): 292–94.

Evans, Dylan. *Placebo, Mind over Matter in Modern Medicine.* New York: Oxford University Press, 2004.

Fadiman, James. *The Psychedelic Explorer's Guide: Safe, Therapeutic, and Sacred Journeys.* New York: Park Street Press, 2011.

'Fascists in White Coats: The CIA's Dr. Louis Jolyon West and the UCLA Neuropsychiatric Institute'. *Constantine Report.* www.constantinereport.com/dr-louis-jolyon-west-the-ucla-neuropsychiatric-institute-and-fascists-in-white-coats.

Feng, Xiaoli, et al. 'Maternal Separation Produces Lasting Changes in Cortisol and Behavior in Rhesus Monkeys'. *Proceedings of the National Academy of Sciences of the United States of America* 108, no. 34 (2011): 14312–17.

Fink, B., N. Neave, J. T. Manning and K. Grammer. 'Facial Symmetry and Judgments of Attractiveness, Health and Personality'. *Personality and Individual Differences* 41, no. 3 (2006): 491–99.

Fisher, Carl Erik. 'Psychiatrists Embrace Deep-Brain Stimulation: Brain-Stimulation Procedures for Psychiatric Disorders Are on the Rise. Should We Be Concerned?', *Scientific American Mind,* 2014. https://www.scientificamerican.com/article/psychiatrists-embrace-deep-brain-stimulation.

Fisher, H. E. and J. A. Thomson Jr. 'Lust, Romance, Attachment: Do the Sexual Side Effects of Serotonin-Enhancing Antidepressants Jeopardize Romantic Love, Marriage, and Fertility?', *Evolutionary Cognitive Neuroscience,* edited by S. Platek, J. Keenan and T. Shackelford. Cambridge, MA: MIT Press, 2006.

Fisher, Helen. *Anatomy of Love: A Natural History of Mating, Marriage, and Why We Stray.* New York: Ballantine, 1994.

Fisher, Helen and J. Andrew Thomson Jr. 'Prozac and Sexual Desire'. *New York Review of Books,* 20 March 2008.

Freudenheim, Milt. 'The Drug Makers Are Listening to Prozac'. *New York Times,* 12 January 1994.

Freudenmann, Roland W., Florian Öxler and Sabine Bernschneider-Reif. 'The Origin of MDMA (Ecstasy) Revisited: The True Story Reconstructed from the Original Documents'. *Addiction* 101, no. 9 (September 2006): 1241–45.

Friedman, Richard A. 'A Call for Caution in the Use of Antipsychotic Drugs'. *New York Times,* 24 September 2012.

———. 'A Dry Pipeline for Psychiatric Drugs'. *New York Times,* 19 August 2013.

———, M.D. 'To Treat Depression, Drugs or Therapy?' *New York Times,* 8 January 2015.

Frodl, T., M.D., et al. 'Depression-Related Variation in Brain Morphology over 3 Years'. *Archives of General Psychiatry* 65, no. 10 (2008): 1156–65.

Fukada, Christine, M.Sc., Jillian Clare Kohler, Ph.D., Heather Boon, Ph.D., Zubin Austin, Ph.D., and Murray Krahn, M.D., M.Sc., FRCPC. 'Prescribing Gabapentin Off Label: Perspectives from Psychiatry, Pain and Neurology Specialists'. *Canadian Pharmacists Journal* 145, no. 6 (November 2012): 280–84, E1.

Gardner, John. 'A History of Deep Brain Stimulation: Technological Innovation and the Role of Clinical Assessment Tools'. *Social Studies of Science* 43, no. 5 (October 2013): 707–28.

Gershon, Samuel, et al., eds. *Lithium: Its Role in Psychiatric Research and Treatment.* New York: Springer, 1973.

Glenmullen, Joseph. *Prozac Backlash: Overcoming the Dangers of Prozac, Zoloft, Paxil, and Other Antidepressants with Safe, Effective Alternatives.* New York: Simon & Schuster, 2001.

Goleman, Daniel. '2 Drugs Get a New Use: Soothing Mania'. *New York Times,* 13 July 1994.

———. 'Pattern of Death: Copycat Suicides among Youths'. *New York Times,* 18 March 1987.

Gould, Madelyn, Patrick Jamieson and Daniel Romer. 'Media Contagion and Suicide among the Young'. *American Behavioral Scientist* 46, no. 9 (May 2003): 1269–84.

Govan, Fiona. 'Lobotomy: A History of the Controversial Procedure'. *Telegraph,* August 2011. www.telegraph.co.uk/news/world news/southamerica/argentina/8679929/lobotomy-a-history-of-the-controversial-procedure.html.

Greenberg, Ben, Loes Gabriels, D. A. Malone Jr and Bart Nuttin, et al. 'Deep Brain Stimulation of the Ventral Internal Capsule/ Ventral Striatum for Obsessive-Compulsive Disorder: Worldwide Experience'. *Molecular Psychiatry* 15, no. 1 (2010): 64–79.

Greenberg, Gary. *The Book of Woe: The DSM and the Unmaking of Psychiatry.* New York: Blue Rider Press, 2013.

———. 'Does Psychiatry Need Science?' *The New Yorker,* 23 April 2013.

———. 'Is It Prozac? Or Placebo?' *Mother Jones,* November–December 2003.

Griffiths, Roland, et al. 'Pilot Study of the $5\text{-}HT_{2A}R$ Agonist Psilocybin in the Treatment of Tobacco Addiction'. *Journal of Psychopharmacology* 28, no. 11 (September 2014): 983–92.

———. 'Psilocybin Can Occasion Mystical-Type Experiences Having Substantial and Sustained Personal Meaning and Spiritual Significance'. *Psychopharmacology* 187, no. 3 (2006): 268–83, discussion 284–92.

Grob, Charles S. 'Commentary on Harbor-UCLA Psilocybin Study'. *MAPS Bulletin* 20, no. 1 (2010): 28–29.

Grof, Stanislav. *Realms of the Human Unconscious: Observations from LSD Research.* London: Souvenir Press, 1996.

———. *The Ultimate Journey: Consciousness and the Mystery of Death.* Santa Cruz, CA: MAPS, 2006.

Grof, Stanislav and Joan Halifax. *The Human Encounter with Death*. New York: Dutton, 1977.

Grof, Stanislav and Albert Hofmann. *LSD Psychotherapy: The Healing Potential of Psychedelic Medicine*. Santa Cruz, CA: MAPS, 2008.

Gross, Dominik, Ph.D., M.D., D.D.S. and Gereon Schäfer, Ph.D. 'Egas Moniz (1874–1955) and the "Invention" of Modern Psychosurgery: A Historical and Ethical Reanalysis under Special Consideration of Portuguese Original Sources'. *Journal of Neurosurgery* 30, no. 2 (February 2011): E8.

Halem, Dann. 'Altered Statesman: Ecstasy Pioneer Alexander Shulgin Defends His Work; Making Mind-Bending Drugs Right Here in Contra Costa'. *Time Out*, 2002. www.mdma.net/alexander-shulgin/index.html.

Hamani, C., et al. 'Memory Enhancement Induced by Hypothalamic/Fornix Deep Brain Stimulation'. *Annals of Neurology* 63, no. 1 (2008): 119–23.

Hamblin, James. 'Deep Brain Stimulation for the Soul'. *The Atlantic*, 25 June 2013.

Hammock, Elizabeth A. D. 'Developmental Perspectives on Oxytocin and Vasopressin'. *Neuropsychopharmacology Reviews* 40, no. 1 (2015): 24–42.

Harden, Victoria A., Ph.D., and Claude Lenfant, M.D. 'The AMINCO-Bowman Spectrophotofluorometer'. Stetten Museum Office of NIH History. history.nih.gov/exhibits/bowman.

Harrington, Anne. *The Placebo Effect: An Interdisciplinary Exploration*. Cambridge, MA: Harvard University Press, 1999.

Harris, Ian. *Surgery, the Ultimate Placebo: A Surgeon Cuts through the Evidence*. Kensington: University of New South Wales Press, 2016.

Häuser, W., E. Hansen and P. Enck. 'Nocebo Phenomena in Medicine: Their Relevance in Everyday Clinical Practice'. *Deutsches Ärzteblatt International* 109, no. 26 (2012): 459–65.

Healy, David. *The Antidepressant Era*. Cambridge, MA: Harvard University Press, 1997.

———. *The Creation of Psychopharmacology*. Cambridge, MA: Harvard University Press, 2002.

———. *Let Them Eat Prozac: The Unhealthy Relationship between the Pharmaceutical Industry and Depression*. New York: New York University Press, 2004.

———. *Mania: A Short History of Bipolar Disorder*. Baltimore: Johns Hopkins University Press, 2008.

———. *Pharmageddon*. Berkeley, CA: University of California Press, 2012.

———. *Psychiatric Drugs Explained*. London: Churchill Livingstone, 2016.

———. *The Psychopharmacologists*. Vol. 1. Boca Raton, FL: CRC Press, 1998.

———. *The Psychopharmacologists*. Vol. 2. Boca Raton, FL: CRC Press, 1998.

———. *The Psychopharmacologists*. Vol. 3. 3rd ed. Boca Raton, FL: CRC Press, 2000.

Heath, Robert G., M.D., D.M.Sci. 'Pleasure and Brain Activity in Man: Deep and Surface Electroencephalograms during Orgasm'. *Journal of Nervous and Mental Disease* 154, no. 1 (January 1972): 3–18.

Heinrichs, R. Walter. *In Search of Madness: Schizophrenia and Neuroscience*. New York: Oxford University Press, 2001.

Higgins, Agnes, Michael Nash and Aileen M. Lynch. 'Antidepressant-Associated Sexual Dysfunction: Impact, Effects, and Treatment'. *Drug, Healthcare, and Patient Safety* 2 (2010): 141–50.

Hirst, William, et al. 'Long-Term Memory for the Terrorist Attack of September 11: Flashbulb Memories, Event Memories, and the Factors That Influence Their Retention'. *Journal of Experimental Psychology: General* 138, no. 2 (2009): 161–76. https://www.ncbi.nlm.nih.gov/pubmed/19397377.

Hockenbury, Don H. and Sandra E. Hockenbury. *Discovering Psychology*. New York: Macmillan, 2010.

Hoffman, Albert. *LSD, My Problem Child: Reflections on Sacred Drugs, Mysticism, and Science*. Santa Cruz, CA: MAPS, 2009.

Holtzheimer, Paul E. III, M.D., and Helen S. Mayberg, M.D. 'Deep Brain Stimulation for Treatment-Resistant Depression'. *American Journal of Psychiatry* 167, no. 12 (2010): 1437–44.

Hooper, Judith and Dick Teresi. *The Three Pound Universe*. New York: Tarcher, 1991.

Horgan, John. 'What Are Science's Ugliest Experiments?' *Scientific American* blog, 2014. https://blogs.scientificamerican.com/cross-check/what-are-sciences-ugliest-experiments.

Hughes, J., T. W. Smith, H. W. Kosterlitz, L. A. Fothergill, B. A. Morgan and H. R. Morris. 'Identification of Two Related Pentapeptides from the Brain with Potent Opiate Agonist Activity'. *Nature* 258 (1975): 577–80.

Humphrey, Michael. 'Todd Sacktor's Search for the Memory Enzyme'. *Forbes*, 25 May 2011.

Hunt, Morton. *The Story of Psychology*. New York: Doubleday, 1994.

Huxley, Laura. *This Timeless Moment: A Personal View of Aldous Huxley*. San Francisco: Mercury House, 1991.

Ibla, J. C., H. Hayashi, D. Bajic and S. G. Soriano. 'Prolonged Exposure to Ketamine Increases Brain Derived Neurotrophic Factor Levels in Developing Rat Brains'. *Current Drug Safety* 4, no. 1 (2009): 11–16.

Insel, Thomas. 'Antidepressants: A Complicated Picture'. National Institute of Mental Health blog, 6 December 2011. https://www.nimh.nih.gov/about/directors/thomas-insel/blog/2011/antidepressants-a-complicated-picture.shtml.

Insel, Thomas R. and Terrence J. Hulihan. 'A Gender-Specific Mechanism for Pair Bonding: Oxytocin and Partner Preference Formation in Monogamous Voles'. *Behavioral Neuroscience* 109, no. 4 (1995): 782–89.

Ironside, Wallace. 'Cade, John Frederick Joseph (1912–1980)', in *Australian Dictionary of Biography*. Vol. 13. Carlton, Vic: Melbourne University Press, 1993.

Jackson, Sarah. 'Alim-Louis Benabid and Mahlon DeLong Win the 2014 Lasker–DeBakey Clinical Medical Research Award'. *Journal of Clinical Investigation* 124, no. 10 (2014): 4143–47.

John, Leo. 'RTI Denies It Made Mistake That Torpedoed Results of a $1.3M Study'. *Triangle Business Journal,* 10 November 2003. https://www.bizjournals.com/triangle/stories/2003/11/10/story4.html.

Johnson, F. Neil. *The History of Lithium Therapy*. New York: Macmillan, 1984.

Johnson, Jenell. *American Lobotomy: A Rhetorical History*. Ann Arbor: University of Michigan Press, 2014.

Kalia, S. K., et al. 'Injury and Strain-Dependent Dopaminergic Neuronal Degeneration in the Substantia Nigra of Mice after Axotomy or MPTP'. *Brain Research* 994 (2003): 243–52.

Kaptchuk, Ted J., John M. Kelley, Lisa A. Conboy, Roger B. Davis, Catherine E. Kerr, Eric E. Jacobson, et al. 'Components of Placebo Effect: Randomised Controlled Trial in Patients with Irritable Bowel Syndrome'. *BMJ* 336 (2008): 999.

Keene, Michael T. *Mad House: The Hidden History of Insane Asylums in 19th-Century New York*. Fredericksburg, VA: Willow Manor Publishing, 2013.

Khazan, Olga. 'The Life Changing Magic of Mushrooms'. *The Atlantic*, 1 December 2016. https://www.theatlantic.com/heath/archive/2016/12/the-life-changing-magic-of-mushrooms/509246.

Kirsch, Irving. *The Emperor's New Drugs: Exploding the Antidepressant Myth*. New York: Basic Books, 2010.

Kleinman, Arthur, M.D. *The Illness Narratives: Suffering, Healing, and The Human Condition*. New York: Basic Books, 1998.

Kline, Nathan S., M.D. 'The Practical Management of Depression'. *JAMA* 190, no. 8 (1964): 732–40.

Klopfer, B. 'Psychological Variables in Human Cancer'. *Journal of Projective Techniques* 21, no. 4 (December 1957): 331–40.

Knight, Jonathan. 'Agony for Researchers as Mix-Up Forces Retraction of Ecstasy Study'. *Nature*, 11 September 2003. www.nature.com/articles/425109a.

Konnikova, Maria. 'The Man Who Couldn't Speak and How He Revolutionized Psychology'. *Scientific American*, 8 February 2013.

Kramer, Peter. *Listening to Prozac*. New York: Penguin, 1997.

———. *Ordinarily Well: The Case for Antidepressants*. New York: Farrar, Straus and Giroux, 2016.

Kreston, Rebecca. 'The Psychic Energizer! The Serendipitous Discovery of the First Antidepressant'. *Discover Magazine*, 27 January 2016. blogs.discovermagazine.com/bodyhorrors/2016/01/27/2081/#.Wi7UIVI-71.

Kumar, Rahul and Vikram K. Yeragani. 'Penfield—A Great Explorer of Psyche-soma-neuroscience'. *Indian Journal of Psychiatry* 53, no. 3 (2011): 276–78.

Laborit, Henri. *L'esprit du grenier*. Paris: Grasset, 1992.

Lambert, Craig. 'The Downsides of Prozac'. *Harvard Magazine*, May–June 2000.

Leary, Timothy. *The Psychedelic Experience: A Manual Based on the Tibetan Book of the Dead*. New York: Citadel, 2000.

Leary, Timothy, Ralph Metzner, Madison Presnell, Gunther Weil, Ralph Schwitzgebel and Sarah Kinne. 'A New Behavior Change Program Using Psilocybin'. *Psychotherapy* 2, no. 2 (July 1965): 61–72.

Lehmann, Heinz and Thomas Ban. 'The History of the Psychopharmacology of Schizophrenia'. *Canadian Journal of Psychiatry* 42, no. 2 (1997): 152–62.

Lehrer, Jonah. 'The Forgetting Pill Erases Painful Memories Forever'. *Wired*, 17 February 2012.

Lieberman, Jeffrey. *Shrinks: The Untold Story of Psychiatry*. New York: Little, Brown, 2015.

Loftus, E. 'Our Changeable Memories: Legal and Practical Implications'. *Nature Reviews Neuroscience* 4 (2003): 231–34.

Loftus, E. F. and J. E. Pickrell. 'The Formation of False Memories'. *Psychiatric Annals* 25 (1995): 720–25.

Loftus, Elizabeth F. *Memory: Surprising New Insights into How We Remember and Why We Forget*. Boston: Addison-Wesley, 1980.

Lowe, Jaime. 'I Don't Believe in God, but I Believe in Lithium'. *New York Times,* 25 June 2015.

Lozano, Andres M., et al. 'A Phase II Study of Fornix Deep Brain Stimulation in Mild Alzheimer's Disease'. *Journal of Alzheimer's Disease* 54, no. 2 (2016): 777–87.

MacLaren, Erik, Ph.D., and Amanda Lautieri, eds. 'Valium History and Statistics'. Sober Media Group, DrugAbuse.com, 21 December 2016. https://drugabuse.com/library/valium-history-and-statistics.

Magni, Laura R., Marianna Purgato, Chiara Gastaldon, Davide Papola, Toshi A. Furukawa, Andrea Cipriani and Corrado Barbui. 'Fluoxetine versus Other Types of Pharmacotherapy for Depression'. Cochrane Common Mental Disorders Group, 17 July 2013. www.cochrane.org/CD004815/DEPRESSN_fluoxetine-compared-with-other-antidepressants-for-depression-in-adults.

Marchant, Jo. 'Parkinson's Patients Trained to Respond to Placebos'. *Nature,* 10 February 2016.

Martin, Rachel. 'Working through Depression: Many Stay on the Job, Despite Mental Illness'. *NPR Mental Health,* 2015. www.npr.org/2015/04/12/398811515/working-through-depression-many-stay-on-the-job-despite-mental-illness.

Max, D. T. *Every Love Story Is a Ghost Story*. New York: Viking, 2012.

Mayberg, Helen S., et al. 'Deep Brain Stimulation for Treatment-Resistant Depression'. *Neuron* 45, no. 5 (March 2005): 651–60.

———. 'Toward a Neuroimaging Treatment Selection Biomarker for

Major Depressive Disorder'. *JAMA Psychiatry* 70, no. 8 (2013): 821–29.

Meade, Stephanie. 'The West's Strange Relationship to Babies and Sleep'. *InCultureParent*, 6 August 2011. www.incultureparent. com/2011/08/the-wests-strange-relationship-to-babies-and-sleep.

Merkin, Daphne. *This Close to Happy*. New York: Farrar, Straus and Giroux, 2017.

Metzner, Ralph, Ph.D. 'Reflections on the Concord Prison Experiment and the Follow-Up Study'. *Journal of Psychoactive Drugs* 30, no. 4 (1998): 427–28.

Meyer, Jerrold S. and Linda F. Quenzer. *Psychopharmacology: Drugs, the Brain, and Behavior.* 2nd ed. Sunderland, MA: Sinauer Associates, 2013.

Miller, Richard J. 'Religion as a Product of Psychotropic Drug Use'. *The Atlantic,* 27 December 2013.

Mitchell, Philip B. 'On the 50th Anniversary of John Cade's Discovery of the Anti-Manic Effect of Lithium'. *Australian and New Zealand Journal of Psychiatry* 33, no. 5 (1999): 623–28.

Mithoefer, M., et al. 'The Safety and Efficacy of {+/-}3,4-Methylenedioxymethamphetamine-Assisted Psychotherapy in Subjects with Chronic, Treatment-Resistant Posttraumatic Stress Disorder: The First Randomized Controlled Pilot Study'. *Journal of Psychopharmacology* 25, no. 4 (2011): 439–52.

Mithoefer, Michael C., Mark T. Wagner, Ann T. Mithoefer, Lisa Jerome, Scott F. Martin, Berra Yazar-Klosinski, Yvonne Michel, Timothy D. Brewerton and Rick Doblin. 'Durability of Improvement in Posttraumatic Stress Disorder Symptoms and Absence of Harmful Effects or Drug Dependency after 3,4-Methylenedioxymethamphetamine-Assisted Psychotherapy: A Prospective Long-Term Follow-Up Study'. *Journal of Psychopharmacology,* 27, no. 1, 20 November 2012.

Moerman, Daniel. 'Explanatory Mechanisms for Placebo Effects: Cultural Influences and the Meaning Response'. In *Science of the Placebo: Toward an Interdisciplinary Research Agenda,* edited by Harry Guess, Linda Engel, Arthur Kleinman and John Kusek, 77–107. London: The BMJ, 2002.

———. *Meaning, Medicine, and the Placebo Effect.* New York: Cambridge University Press, 2002.

Muldoon, Maureen. 'From Psychiatrist-Researcher to Psychiatrist and Researcher: Heinz Lehmann'. *Journal of Ethics in Mental Health* 6 (2011): 222.

Nasar, Sylvia. *A Beautiful Mind.* New York: Simon & Schuster, 2011.

Neighmond, Patti. 'That Prescription Might Not Have Been Tested for Your Ailment'. *NPR Morning Edition: Your Health,* 12 May 2014. www.npr.org/sections/health-shots/2014/05/12/307747891/that-prescription-might-not-have-been-tested-for-your-ailment.

Nelson, Lauren. 'Hallucinogen in "Magic Mushrooms" Helps Longtime Smokers Quit in Hopkins Trial'. Johns Hopkins University, *The Hub,* 11 September 2014. https://hub.jhu.edu/2014/09/11/magic-mushrooms-smoking.

Neves-Pereira, Maria, Emanuela Mundo, Pierandrea Muglia, Nicole King, Fabio Macciardi and James L. Kennedy. 'The Brain Derived Neurotrophic Factor Gene Confers Susceptibility to Bipolar Disorder: Evidence from a Family Based Association Study'. *American Journal of Human Genetics* 71, no. 3 (September 2002): 651–5.

Nutt, David. *Drugs without the Hot Air: Minimising the Harms of Legal and Illegal Drugs.* Cambridge: UIT Cambridge, 2012.

Nutt, David, et al. 'Neural Correlates of the Psychedelic State as Determined by fMRI Studies with Psilocybin'. *PNAS* 109, no. 6 (7 February 2012): 2138–43.

Ohgami, Hirochika, et al. 'Lithium Levels in Drinking Water and Risk of Suicide'. *British Journal of Psychiatry* 194, no. 5 (2009): 464–65.

Orenstein, David. 'Deep Brain Stimulation Helps Severe OCD, but Pioneer Advises Caution, Compassion'. AAAS presentation, Brown University, *News from Brown,* 16 February 2011. https://news.brown.edu/articles/2011/02/dbs.

Ortman, Jennifer M. and Victoria A. Velkoff. 'An Aging Nation: The Older Population in the United States'. United States Census Bureau, 2014.

Owens, D. G. Cunningham. *A Guide to the Extrapyramidal Side Effects of Antipsychotic Drugs.* New York: Cambridge University Press, 1999.

Park, Denise C., et al. 'The Impact of Sustained Engagement on Cognitive Function in Older Adults: The Synapse Project'. *Psychological Science* 25, no. 1 (January 2014): 103–12.

Parker, Jim. 'Intelligent People Keep Growing and Changing: The DSN

Interview with Dr. Timothy Leary'. *Drug Survival News* Part 1 (September–October 1981): 12–19.

Passie, Torsten and Udo Benzenhöfer. 'The History of MDMA as an Underground Drug in the United States, 1960–1979'. *Journal of Psychoactive Drugs* 48, no. 2 (2016): 67–75.

Peroutka, S. J., ed. *Ecstasy: The Clinical, Pharmacological and Neurotoxicological Effects of the Drug MDMA*. Boston: Kluwer, 1990.

Pettus, Ashley. 'Psychiatry by Prescription'. *Harvard Magazine*, July–August 2006.

Pidwirny, Michael. *Understanding Physical Geography*. Kelowna, BC: Our Planet Earth Publishing, 2015.

Pollan, Michael. 'The Trip Treatment'. *The New Yorker*, 9 February 2015.

Poole, Steven. *Rethink: The Surprising History of New Ideas*. New York: Scribner, 2003.

Porter, Roy. *Madness: A Brief History*. New York: Oxford University Press, 2003.

Pratt, Laura A., Ph.D., Debra J. Brody, M.P.H., and Qiuping Gu, Ph.D. 'Antidepressant Use in Persons Aged 12 and Over: United States, 2005–2008'. National Center for Health Statistics Brief 76, October 2011.

'Profiles in Cardiology, Åke Senning'. *Clinical Cardiology* 32, no. 8 (2009): 66–67.

Ramachandraih, Chaitra T., Narayana Subramanyam, Karl Jurgen Bar, Glen Baker and Vikram K. Yeragani. 'Antidepressants: From MAOIs to SSRIs and More'. *Indian Journal of Psychiatry* 53, no. 2 (2011): 180–82.

Rasmussen, Nicolas. *On Speed: The Many Lives of Amphetamine*. New York: NYU Press, 2009.

Raz, Mical. *The Lobotomy Letters: The Making of American Psychosurgery*. Rochester, NY: University of Rochester Press, 2013.

Ricaurte, G. A., et al. '(+/-)3,4-Methylenedioxymethamphetamine ("Ecstasy")-Induced Serotonin Neurotoxicity: Studies in Animals'. *Neuropsychobiology* 42 (2000): 5–10.

Ricaurte, G. A., J. Yuan, G. Hatzidimitriou, B. J. Cord and U. D. McCann. 'Severe Dopaminergic Neurotoxicity in Primates after a Common Recreational Dose Regimen of MDMA ("Ecstasy")'. *Science* 297, no. 5590 (27 September 2002).

Ricaurte, George A. 'Letters: Retraction'. *Science* 301, no. 5639 (12 September 2003): 1479.

Riedlinger, Thomas J., *Sacred Mushroom Seeker: Tributes to R. Gordon Wasson*. New York: Park Street Press, 1997.

Roberts, Thomas B. and Robert N. Jesse. 'Recollections of the Good Friday Experiment: An Interview with Huston Smith'. *Journal of Transpersonal Psychology* 29, no. 2 (1997): 99–103.

Roccatagliata, Giuseppe. *A History of Ancient Psychiatry*. New York: Praeger, 1986.

Romero, Simon. 'In Brazil, Some Inmates Get Therapy with Hallucinogenic Tea'. *New York Times,* 28 March 2015.

Rossi, Andrea, Alessandra Barraco and Pietro Donda. 'Fluoxetine: A Review on Evidence Based Medicine'. *Annals of General Hospital Psychiatry* 3, no. 2 (12 February 2004).

Sacktor, Todd. 'Erasing Your Memories'. *New York Times,* Consults blog, 13 April 2009. https://consults.blogs.nytimes.com/2009/04/13/memory-erasing.

Sacktor, Todd Charlton. 'Memory Maintenance by PKMζ – An Evolutionary Perspective'. *Molecular Brain,* 18 September 2012.

Sairanen, M., G. Lucas, P. Ernfors, M. Castrén and E. Castrén. 'Brain-Derived Neurotrophic Factor and Antidepressant Drugs Have Different but Coordinated Effects on Neuronal Turnover, Proliferation, and Survival in the Adult Dentate Gyrus'. *Journal of Neuroscience* 25, no. 5 (2005): 1089–94.

Saks, Elyn R. *The Center Cannot Hold: My Journey through Madness*. New York: Hachette, 2008.

Schacter, Daniel L. *Searching for Memory: The Brain, the Mind, and the Past*. New York: Basic Books, 2008.

Schacter, Daniel L., et al. 'Remembering the Past to Imagine the Future: The Prospective Brain'. *Nature Reviews Neuroscience* 8 (2007): 657–61.

Schattner, Elaine. 'The Placebo Debate: Is It Unethical to Prescribe Them to Patients?' *The Atlantic,* 19 December 2011.

Scommegna, Paola. 'Dementia Cases Expected to Triple by 2050 as World Population Ages'. Population Reference Bureau, November 2012. www.prb.org/Publications/Articles/2012/global-dementia.aspx.

Scull, Andrew. *Madhouse*. New Haven, CT: Yale University Press, 2007.

Seminowicz, D.A., H. S. Mayberg, A. R. McIntosh, K. Goldapple, S. Kennedy, Z. Segal and S. Rafi-Tari. 'Limbic-Frontal Circuitry in Major Depression: A Path Modeling Metanalysis'. *Neuroimage* 22, no. 1 (May 2004): 409–18.

Shapiro, Arthur K. and Elaine Shapiro. 'The Placebo: Is It Much Ado about Nothing?', *The Placebo Effect: An Interdisciplinary Exploration*, edited by Anne Harrington, 12–36. Cambridge, MA: Harvard University Press, 1997.

Shorter, Edward. *A History of Psychiatry: From the Era of the Asylum to the Age of Prozac*. New York: Wiley, 1998.

Shulgin, Alexander. *Pihkal: A Chemical Love Story*. Berkeley, CA: Transform Press, 1991.

Shulgin, Alexander T. 'The Background and Chemistry of MDMA'. *Journal of Psychoactive Drugs* 18, no. 4 (1986): 291–304.

———. 'History of MDMA'. In *Ecstasy: The Clinical, Pharmacological, and Neurotoxicological Effects of the Drug MDMA,* edited by S. J. Peroutka, 1–20. Boston: Kluwer, 1990.

Siegel, Ronald K. *Intoxication: Life in the Pursuit of Artificial Paradise*. New York: Park Street Press, 1989.

Sirois, F. 'Perspectives on Epidemic Hysteria'. In *Mass Psychogenic Illness: A Social Psychological Analysis,* edited by M. J. Colligan, J. W. Pennebaker, and L. R. Murphy, 217–22. Abingdon-on-Thames: Routledge, 1982.

Slater, Lauren. 'How Do You Cure a Sex Addict?', *New York Times*, 19 November 2000.

———. 'Who Holds the Clicker?' *Mother Jones,* November 2005.

Smith, Gwenn. 'A Stimulating Finding in Mild Alzheimer's'. *Hopkins Medicine Magazine,* Spring–Summer 2012.

Smith, J. Huston. *The Huston Smith Reader*. Berkeley: University of California Press, 26 March 2012.

Sobo, Simon. 'Psychotherapy Perspectives in Medication Management'. *Psychiatric Times,* 1 April 1999.

Solomon, Andrew. *The Noonday Demon*. New York: Scribner, 2001.

Solomon, Lewis D. *The Quest for Human Longevity*. Livingston, NJ: Transaction Publishers, 2006.

Spiegel, Alix. 'The Dictionary of Disorder'. *The New Yorker,* 3 January 2005.

Stahl, Stephen. *Prescriber's Guide: Stahl's Essential Psychopharmacology*. New York: Cambridge University Press, 2017.

Starks, Sarah Linsley and Joel T. Braslow. 'The Making of Contemporary American Psychiatry, Part 1: Patients, Treatments, and Therapeutic Rationales Before and After World War II'. *History of Psychology* 8, no. 2 (May 2005): 176–93.

Steeds, H., R. L. Carhart-Harris and J. M. Stone. 'Drug Models of Schizophrenia'. *Therapeutic Advances in Psychopharmacology* 5, no. 1 (2015): 43–58.

Steinberg, Holger and Hubertus Himmerich. 'Roland Kuhn—100th Birthday of an Innovator of Clinical Psychopharmacology'. *Psychopharmacology Bulletin* 45, no. 1 (2012): 48–50.

Stolaroff, Myron J. *The Secret Chief Revealed*. Santa Cruz, CA: MAPS, 2005.

Stossel, Scott. *My Age of Anxiety: Fear, Hope, Dread, and the Search for Peace of Mind*. New York: Knopf, 2013.

Stromberg, Joseph. 'What Is the Nocebo Effect? For Some Patients, the Mere Suggestion of Side Effects Is Enough to Bring on Negative Symptoms'. *Smithsonian*, 23 July 2012. https://www.smithsonianmag.com/science-nature-what-is-the-nocebo-effect-5451823.

Sugawara, N., et al. 'Lithium in Tap Water and Suicide Mortality in Japan'. *International Journal of Environmental Research and Public Health* 10, no. 11 (2013): 6044–48.

Swazey, Judith. *Chlorpromazine in Psychiatry: A Study of Therapeutic Innovation*. Cambridge, MA: MIT Press, 1974.

Sweeney, Michael S. *Brain, the Complete Mind*. Washington, DC: National Geographic, 2009.

Talbot, Margaret. 'The Placebo Prescription'. *New York Times Magazine*, 3 January 2000. www.nytimes.com/2000/01/09/magazine/the-placebo-prescription.html.

Tan, Siang Yong and Angela Yip. 'António Egas Moniz (1874–1955): Lobotomy Pioneer and Nobel Laureate'. *Singapore Medical Journal* 55, no. 4 (April 2014): 175–76.

Tansey, E. M. and D. A. Christie, eds. 'Drugs in Psychiatric Practice'. *Wellcome Witnesses to Twentieth Century Medicine* 2 (September 1998).

Taylor, Steven J. 'Caught in the Continuum: A Critical Analysis of the Principle of the Least Restrictive Environment'. *Research and Practice for Persons with Severe Disabilities* 29, no. 4 (2004): 218–30.

Teicher, M., M.D., Ph.D., C. Glod, R.N., M.S.C.S., and J. Cole, M.D. 'Emergence of Intense Suicidal Preoccupation during Fluoxetine Treatment'. *American Journal of Psychiatry* 147, no. 2 (February 1990): 207–10.

Thomas, Gerald, et al. 'Ayahuasca-Assisted Therapy for Addiction: Results from a Preliminary Observational Study in Canada'. *Current Drug Abuse Reviews* 6, no. 1 (2013): 30–42.

Toufexis, Anastasia. 'The Personality Pill'. *Time,* 24 June 2001.

Travis, Jeremy. 'Rise in Hallucinogen Use'. *NIJ Research in Brief,* October 1997. www.abtassociates.com/reports/hallucinogen.pdf.

Trivers, Robert. *The Folly of Fools: The Logic of Deceit and Self-Deception in Human Life.* New York: Basic Books, 2011.

'U.S. Will Ban "Ecstasy", a Hallucinogenic Drug'. *New York Times,* 1 June 1985.

Valenstein, Elliot. *Blaming the Brain: The Truth about Drugs and Mental Health.* New York: Free Press, 2002.

———. *Brain Control: A Critical Examination of Brain Stimulation and Psychosurgery.* New York: Wiley-Interscience, 1973.

———. *Great and Desperate Cures: The Rise and Decline of Psychosurgery and Other Radical Treatments for Mental Illness.* New York: Basic Books, 1986.

———. *The Psychosurgery Debate: Scientific, Legal, and Ethical Perspectives.* San Francisco, CA: W. H. Freeman, 1980.

———. *The War of the Soups and the Sparks: The Discovery of Neurotransmitters and the Dispute over How Nerves Communicate.* New York: Columbia University Press, 2005.

Viegas, Jennifer. '"Dancing Plague" and Other Odd Afflictions Explained'. *Discovery News,* 1 August 2008.

Volk, Lenora J., Julia L. Bachman, Richard Johnson, Yilin Yu and Richard L. Huganir. 'PKM-ζ Is Not Required for Hippocampal Synaptic Plasticity, Learning and Memory'. *Nature* 493 (2013): 420–23.

Wapner, Jessica. 'He Counts Your Words (Even Those Pronouns)'. *New York Times,* 13 October 2008.

Wasson, R. Gordon. 'Seeking the Magic Mushroom'. *Life,* 10 June 1957.

Wasson, Valentina Pavlova and R. Gordon Wasson. *Mushrooms, Russia, and History.* Vol. 1. New York: Pantheon, 1957.

Watkins, John. *Hearing Voices: A Common Human Experience*. Melbourne: Michelle Anderson Publishing, 2008.

Whitaker, Robert. *Anatomy of an Epidemic: Magic Bullets, Psychiatric Drugs, and the Astonishing Rise of Mental Illness in America*. New York: Crown, 2010.

———. *Mad in America*. New York: Basic Books, 2010.

Wiesel, Elie. 'Never Forget: Holocaust Survivor, Nobel Peace Prize Winner Warns Against Drugs That Erase Memory'. *New York Daily News*, 10 April 2009.

Wrobel, Sylvia. 'Flipping the Switch'. *Emory Medicine*, Spring 2015.

Yeragani, Vikram K. et al. 'Arvid Carlsson, and the Story of Dopamine'. *Indian Journal of Psychiatry* 52, no. 1 (2010): 87–88.

Young, M. B., R. Andero, K. J. Ressler and L. L. Howell. '3,4-Methylenedioxymethamphetamine Facilitates Fear Extinction Learning'. *Translational Psychiatry* 5, e634 (2015): 138.

'Zimelidine'. PubChem Compound Database. CID=5365247, https://pubchem.ncbi.nlm.nih.gov/compound/5365247.

Index